The Active W(
and Fitne~~ ~andbook

The Active Woman's Health and Fitness Handbook

Nadya Swedan, M.D.

A PERIGEE BOOK

To Rob: Since our first triathlon together, your love and pride prevails. I love how you love to have fun, and this always involves sports. Through smooth rides or flat tires, breezy or hot training runs, powdery or icy ski trails, tennis highs or lows, and short or long par fives, you have always been by my side. Your patience, mechanical talents, athletic skills and insight, and desire for us to be equal on the playing field are invaluable. Cherishing the athlete in me, and in all women, makes you the most amazing man. You have made me a better doctor, friend, advisor, and athlete. I hope all women can find a life partner as supportive as you.
—NADYA

ℙ

A Perigee Book
Published by The Berkley Publishing Group
A division of Penguin Group (USA) Inc.
375 Hudson Street
New York, New York 10014

Copyright © 2003 by Nadya Swedan
Text design by Richard Oriolo
Cover design by Wendy Bass
Cover photos copyright © by Superstock

FIRST EDITION: July 2003

This book has been cataloged by the Library of Congress.

Printed in the United States of America

10   9   8   7   6   5   4   3   2   1

Contents

Acknowledgments

This book would not have been possible without the support of Lisa Ekus, my literary agent, who believes in who I am and what I have to say. Thank you to Beth Shepard for your initial and ongoing support and enthusiasm for me as a women's sports health representative. Also to my editor, Sheila Curry Oakes, athlete, mother, and dedicated supporter of writers. Thanks to Laura Shepard at Penguin also. All these women have faith in the strength, power, and wisdom of women.

Thank you to my supportive peers and staff at Manhattan Orthopedics and Sports Medicine for your understanding, ease of scheduling, and mostly, for keeping me on top of my field. I especially thank the doctors, particularly Mark Klion, the most amazing sports medicine surgeon (and five-time Ironman Triathlete) for sharing your infinite knowledge and wise judgment in patient care. This is what keeps athletes "in the game."

Special thanks to my dear friend and invaluable assistant, Jenifer Silverman, a natural athlete with the greatest enthusiasm for (easily) participating in new athletic activities. I am indebted to you for your patience, time, and willingness to be both photographer and model. Your grace in handling the events surrounding your hockey-game ankle fracture, surgery, and recovery is inspirational.

To Ellie Krieger, R.D., for your advice on nutrition; your professional and personal philosophies exemplify the best of health. Also, thank you for your confidence and faith in me as a helpful resource for your programs, for introducing me to Beth, and for sharing all your experience with the challenges of publicity. I can't wait to read your book!

Thank you to my illustrator, Igor Nazarenko; you have been so professional, and your talents and flexibility have made this book much clearer and more captivating. Special thanks to my photographer and dear friend, Mark Eggleston.

And finally, thank you to my family, friends, past coaches, therapists, patients, and peers, who have contributed to my experiences and knowledge. Thanks also to the many other women who have written fitness and sports-related books and articles. All of you make the health and fitness world more exciting, healthier, educated, fulfilling, and fun.

Introduction

Welcome to your sports and fitness health handbook—everything you need to know about staying strong, fit, and healthy. Whether you are a recreational, competitive, or weekend athlete; someone interested in becoming active in fitness; or do not consider yourself a true "athlete" but exercise or are contemplating exercise, you will find this book useful. It is a resource for all active girls and women.

This book is unique in that it addresses issues specific to girls and women, issues that are different from men and not known to every doctor, trainer, or coach. Using this handbook will advise and assist you in reaching your sports and fitness goal while preserving health and preventing injury. It provides the foundation for your optimum sports and fitness health plan.

This book covers all up-to-date comprehensive medical, muscular, skeletal, social, and psychological concerns related to active women. It provides a philosophy more comprehensive than "sports medicine," as it includes overall health with respect to unique issues of being female. This handbook can help you understand your health and training issues more completely and add to the information you receive from your doctor or health-care professional.

The challenges of being active in athletic and fitness activities can be stressful to your mind and body occasionally. Too much training or sports accidents can lead to pain patterns or injuries that require attention to prevent them from limiting your activity. *The Active Woman's Health and Fitness Handbook* shares with you practical wisdom to improve fitness performance and keep you healthy. It will help you determine what "fitness" advice from coaches, trainers, magazines, TV, and even doctors is healthy and what can be risky. You will also learn how to avoid any new injuries or health problems.

This book is organized to allow you to appreciate general issues but also understand the details as you need them. The first section, "The Inner System: Staying Fit Inside Your Body and Mind," helps you assess your overall health, including internal, mental, and nutritional issues as well as body image and bone health. The second section, "The Musculoskeletal System: Understanding and Improving Movement and Strength," defines the workings of your muscles, ligaments, and joints and describes how to keep them healthy and strong. It also explains pain and injuries and how to prevent and avoid them. Each chapter includes exercises streamlined to be most effective to improve strength and to prevent and recover from injuries. The third section, "The Fitness System: Maximizing Athletic and Workout Performance," incorporates all the components of health and fitness, providing strategies to be the best athlete you can be. It offers insight into potential and common problems and how to avoid and correct them.

In anticipation of the joys, challenges, and occasional setbacks of living an active lifestyle as a woman, this book is for you. Whether you are struggling with an injury or health issue, want to prevent them, or simply want to improve your health and fitness, you will find this an easy-to-read, reliable, and understandable source of support and information. Congratulations! By reading this book, you are taking a giant step toward a longer, healthier, and happier life.

PART I

The Inner System: Staying Fit Inside Your Body and Mind

CHAPTER ONE

Inner Body and Medical Management

You feel good, work out, and try to eat healthy. But are you as healthy as you can possibly be inside? Fitness is good for all your body systems, and as a regular exerciser, you are much less likely to have health problems. Still, do you have some habits that are not so healthy? Is there anything you need to be careful of? Are you at risk of certain diseases or injuries? These questions are important to consider, because the answers help define your overall fitness and health.

Because medicine becomes more complicated almost every day as new research is done and more information gained, it can be difficult to know what is best for your health. Knowing what to do and what to avoid will help you define what is healthy and help you make your fitness program as good as it can be. This will maximize not only your performance in fitness, but also your performance in life.

Your Doctor's Examination

Your internal organ systems are screened by your general doctor with a physical every or every other year if you are without risks. This includes the doctor's examination of your heart, lungs, abdomen, and skin; blood pressure and pulse measurements; blood tests to establish liver and kidney functions, blood cell count, iron levels, and cholesterol levels; and discussion of your lifestyle, disease risks, and health prevention techniques that are most effective. If you have any disease risk factors or take any regular medications, you might need to see your doctor more often than every year or two. As a woman, you should also see your gynecologist once a year for a Pap test and breast and pelvic examinations. Seeing your doctor regularly is an important step to preventing health problems.

You might be referred to a specialist after a routine screening exam. There are medical specialists, who train in internal medicine and then continue with a specialty in their area or expertise, and surgical specialists, who train in surgery and go on to surgical specialties. Because medicine and surgery are so complex, you might need to see more than one specialist for the best care. For muscle, bone, or joint problems, you will likely be referred to an orthopedist, physiatrist, or sports medicine specialist. The following tables list different areas of speciality.

Medical Specialties and Their Areas of Expertise

Cardiology	Heart and blood vessels
Dermatology	Skin
Gastroenterology	Stomach, intestines, colon
Gynecology	Women's reproductive systems
Hematology	Blood
Hepatology	Liver diseases
Neurology	Brain and nerves
Oncology	Cancer
Pediatrics	Children, adolescents
Physiatry	Muscles, nerves, bones; injury recovery
Pulmonology	Lungs and breathing

Rheumatology	Immune system, joints
Urology	Bladder, kidneys

Surgical Specialties and Their Areas of Expertise	
Cardiothoracic	Heart and lungs
Neurosurgery	Brain and spinal cord
Obstetric and gynecologic	Women's reproductive organs
Oncology	Cancer removal
Orthopedic	Bones/joints
Plastic	Skin

It is wise to proceed with any referrals and follow up with doctors or health-care providers as recommended. Return visits are extremely important to establish that treatment is working without undesirable side effects, measure any progression of the problem, and fine-tune methods to cure and prevent further disease processes. Many diseases can be prevented, at least from becoming life-threatening—they just need to be identified and treated early. Remember: Prevention is the best medicine.

Internal Systems

Heart and Lungs

Heart and lung disease is a concern to women as much as to men. Hopefully, you already know if you have any heart or lung trouble, as this can be established during your physical examination. Blood pressure and pulse measurements are very easy ways to rule out some serious heart and blood vessel diseases. Because heart and lung disease can be life-threatening, it is helpful to know the signs and symptoms. The heart pumps blood to and from the lungs and into the body to deliver oxygen and remove carbon dioxide. Because the heart and lungs are so closely connected and essential to life and movement, problems with either heart or lungs may cause similar symptoms.

Heart diseases can cause trouble with exertion, shortness of breath, swelling in your legs, chest pains, chest tightness, arm or shoulder pain or numbness, breathing trouble, lightheadedness, passing out, decreased energy, or decreased ability to exercise as efficiently. Symptoms more specific to the lungs include breathing difficulties, coughing, wheezing, tightness, chest pains, and blue lips or nails. Anxiety or feelings of doom are also recognized symptoms of possible heart or lung problems. These are all symptoms for which you should call your doctor immediately; if your doctor is unavailable, go to an emergency room.

Signs of Heart Problems

Chest pain*

Shortness of breath*

Burning in your chest

Easy fatigue

Leg swelling

Coughing

Feeling your heart miss a beat

Feeling your heart race

Passing out*

Feeling light-headed

Shoulder or arm pain or numbness*

Feelings of anxiety or doom*

Chest heaviness*

*Call your doctor as soon as possible if you have any of these symptoms or go to an emergency room.

Signs of Lung Problems

Wheezing

Shortness of breath

Coughing

Blue nails or lips

Easy fatique

Feeling unable to catch your breath

Chest pain

If you have heart or lung disease, it is recommended that you do not exercise alone. The people you work out with, your coach, trainer, or health club, should know how to contact a relative or friend in case of emergency. Even the safest of activities can have unpredictable risks with heart or breathing problems (such as light-headedness leading to dizziness and falls). If you have been diagnosed with a problem, follow the recommendations of your doctor, especially with regard to medications and follow-up visits. These return visits are an essential part of improving your symptoms and ensure that the treatment is working effectively for you.

The most commonly diagnosed heart abnormality in women is mitral valve prolapse. This is a condition where the mitral valve in the heart does not completely close. It causes a heart murmur and might make you feel an occasional heart flutter, but unless it is associated with another heart abnormality, it usually does not cause any problems or limitations to activity.

The most common lung problem among women is asthma. This can be life-threatening if not managed properly. There are many types of medications available to control asthma, and if you feel you have any shortness of breath, wheezing, or chest tightness, even if just once in a while, see your doctor as soon as possible for treatment options. Exercise-induced asthma is coughing, wheezing, or chest tightness related to exercise, especially in cold environments, extremely dry or humid conditions, polluted air, or during allergy seasons. (See "Breathing Problems" in chapter 13.) Exercise-induced asthma is often overlooked by physicians because the symptoms only occur during exercise, so be sure to emphasize this to your doctor.

Digestive System

Your digestive system, medically termed the gastrointestinal (GI) system, includes your esophagus, stomach, intestines, and colon, and gallbladder. These organs are in a delicate balance; disturbing that balance is a common source of frustration for many women as it leads to such unpleasant side effects as indigestion, heartburn, abdominal pain, nausea, gas, diarrhea, and constipation. The GI system is regulated by the same nerves that react to stress, so physical and emotional stress can negatively affect the GI tract.

Irritable bowel syndrome (IBS) is a condition occurring in women more than men and is characterized by cramping, gas, and diarrhea after eating certain foods or also due to stress (including pre-competition stress). Foods that can trigger an attack include fatty foods, milk products, leafy greens, and certain fruits. If irritable bowel syndrome is a daily problem, it can interfere with nutrition and electrolyte balance. In mild cases, limiting triggering foods to smaller portions, combining them with nonirritating foods, or eliminating them altogether can solve the problems. Stress management and relaxation techniques along with diet modification can also help control flare-ups. Because IBS can be so disturbing to life activities, especially sports, if you have these symptoms frequently, see a gastroenterologist, who might prescribe medication.

Vomiting and diarrhea due to viruses or bacteria can make you dehydrated, weak, dizzy, and light-headed. You should avoid intense exercise for at least 24 hours if you have been vomiting or have had repeated diarrhea, and especially if you have a fever. As much as you can, replenish your electrolytes with sports drinks, and try to eat bland foods to restore your strength. A recommended prescribed diet for gastrointestinal infection is the BRAT diet: bananas, rice, applesauce, and tea.

One of the most common causes of gastrointestinal problems is medications, especially pain medicines. Medications can disrupt the acid and bacterial balance in the stomach and intestines, leading to diarrhea or vomiting. Strong (narcotic) painkillers often cause nausea and vomiting; narcotics specifically can cause constipation. Anti-inflammatories, steroids, and antibiotic medications tend to cause stomach upset and occasional diarrhea.

Constipation is usually due to poor diet or not enough fluids; rarely is it a sign or cause of serious bowel problems. Iron and calcium supplements can lead to constipation. Constipation can be resolved with stool softeners or laxatives, although you should not make these a habit, as your body can develop a tolerance to them. Drinking warm fluids, especially caffeinated coffee or tea, can provide relief from constipation. (Cutting down on them can lead to constipation as your bowel readjusts to not having that trigger.) The most natural way to resolve and prevent constipation is to increase the amount of fiber and fluids in your diet.

Bladder and Kidneys

Some women, especially those who are sexually active, are prone to urinary tract infections (UTIs). These can be very irritating, as they cause pain, burning, and frequent urination. Urinary tract infections can be prevented by drinking plenty of water and urinating before and after sex; the uncomfortable symptoms can be avoided by drinking cranberry juice or eating cranberries or cranberry products. (Blueberries have also recently been found to provide similar relief.) Urinary tract infections can become serious if they are left untreated, as they can spread into the kidneys. See your doctor if you have pain or burning with urination or cloudy or foul-smelling urine lasting for more than a few days and especially if you have a fever. Thorough treatment of UTIs is with antibiotics.

Another problem among women that can occur after childbirth is stress incontinence, the condition where physical pressure, such as that caused by running and jumping, causes urine to leak out. This is usually due to loosening and stretching of the supporting muscles and ligaments around the bladder and urethra. Stress incontinence improves with Kegel exercises and can be managed by avoiding caffeine or other diuretic foods or products. Fluids can be limited before impact exercise, although this should not be done in hot weather. Wearing an absorbable pad is helpful; occasionally inserting a tampon into the vagina during exercise helps close flow of urine. There are also medications that sometimes help, and in severe cases, surgery can resolve the problem.

Kegel exercises are important for every woman to preserve urogenital health and are especially beneficial during and after pregnancy. These exercises strengthen the muscles that support your bladder and uterus, the same muscles you use to stop the flow of urine. To perform Kegel exercises, contract your internal pelvic muscles as if you are holding back urine. Do this 10–15 times, 5 times a day, increasing the time you hold each contraction to up to 10 seconds.

Managing Incontinence

Kegel exercises
Avoid caffeine or diuretics
Limit fluids before impact activities
Wear an absorbable pad
Try inserting a tampon
Medications
Surgery

Blood and Lymph

The fluid systems in your body circulate nutrients into your cells and eliminate waste products. Blood is made up of red cells, which carry oxygen;

white cells, which carry disease fighters; platelets, which allow clotting; and plasma, the fluid. Lymph is a fluid drainage system in addition to blood that is especially active in eliminating wastes produced by infection.

The most important function of blood is to transport oxygen, without which we cannot live. Oxygen is carried by the iron in the red cells of your blood. If there are not enough red cells, or not enough iron, this is called anemia. Anemia is more common in women, due to menstruation. Signs of anemia include feeling easily cold, tired, and out of breath. Anemia can occur in women who exercise a lot, as the body breaks down the iron and red cells during vigorous exercise. Anemia is diagnosed with a blood test. The best sources of iron are red meats; therefore, vegetarians are at greater risk of having anemia. Do not try to treat anemia by yourself by taking iron supplements; this is not the only answer for anemia, and the dose should be monitored. Consult your doctor if you think you might be anemic.

The lymphatic system does not usually cause problems unless you have an infection, cancer, or lymphedema. During an infection, lymph nodes become swollen and tender. In cases of cancer, they can become hard. If you notice bumps (lymph nodes) that you have not noticed before that are present for longer than one week, see your doctor for an evaluation. Lymphedema is a swelling of one arm or leg that can develop after surgery, such as in the arm after mastectomy, after injury, or for unknown reasons. Lymphedema should be managed daily with movement exercises to promote circulation. In more severe cases, compressive wraps are used to reduce uncomfortable swelling. Light weight training or exercises such as swimming are helpful, but heavy lifting should be avoided.

Brain and Nerves

Problems with the brain and nerves include weakness, numbness, headaches, vision or hearing problems, and seizures. These problems can be due to a pinched nerve, stroke, or lesion on the spinal cord, nerve, or brain. Neurological diseases such as multiple sclerosis, Parkinson's, meningitis, or viruses can cause other problems. If you have any of the above-mentioned symptoms, see a neurologist and limit exercise until you have been evaluated.

The most common neurological problem in active women is headaches. Because there are many causes and treatments, headaches that occur frequently or interfere with your daily or sports activities should be evaluated by a neurologist. (See chapter 13 for more on headaches.)

Hormones

Hormones are proteins that have special controlling and signaling functions in the body and maintain the body's delicate metabolic and functional balance. Important hormones include insulin, made by the pancreas; thyroxine and triiodothyronine, made by the thyroid; and estrogen and progesterone, made by the ovaries. Other important hormones are made in the pituitary gland, the hypothalamus, and the adrenal gland. Occasionally, they can be over- or underproduced.

Diabetes, a lack of insulin or resistance to insulin's effect in the body, is classified into two types. Type I, juvenile onset, "insulin dependent," diabetes, starts early in life and is managed with insulin. Type II, adult-onset, "insulin resistant," diabetes is a condition where your body does not respond to insulin and is managed sometimes with diet alone, but often with other medications. Signs you might have diabetes include increased urination, thirst, and hunger; sudden weight loss; fatigue; blurry vision; numbness; and frequent infections of the bladder, vagina, and skin. Diabetes does have genetic risk factors, although its exact causes are not known. Type II diabetes is associated with obesity and lack of exercise. Also, gestational diabetes (in pregnancy) is a strong risk factor for type II diabetes later in life.

Diabetes is a life-long condition, with sometimes life-threatening complications, although strict diet control, a consistent exercise regime, and monitoring of blood sugars can allow a life without the other complications that makes diabetes a life-threatening disease. Exercise plays a vital role in this process, as it helps lower and control blood sugar, increases blood flow, and reduces heart and other risk factors associated with diabetes.

Thyroid hormones control metabolism, temperature, heart rate, and other body systems including fertility and bone metabolism. Many women become hypothyroid, or have low thyroid levels. An overactive thyroid is called Graves' disease. These treatable conditions should be managed by an endocrinologist. Signs you might have thyroid problems include a change in appetite or weight, trouble with tolerating heat or cold, dry skin, brittle fingernails, or a swelling at the base of the neck.

Health Screening

You can screen yourself for possible medical problems by answering the following questions. Similar to the questions given at school physicals before clearing an athlete for participation in sports, the following list of questions is designed to identify disease or injury risks. A "yes" answer suggests that you discuss this with your primary care physician or health-care professional. You might also see a sports medicine doctor, especially if your problem is related to pain. If you have already seen a doctor in regards to the questions here, be sure you are following her recommendations as you continue your exercise or sports activity.

Do you have any pain that often limits your activity?	YES	NO
Do you have a pain that has come and gone for more than one week?	YES	NO
Do you have any muscle weakness that does not seem to get stronger?	YES	NO
Do you feel you tire out more easily than others?	YES	NO
Do you easily get short of breath?	YES	NO
Have you ever passed out during or after exercise?	YES	NO
Have you ever been told you have a heart murmur?	YES	NO
Do you ever feel chest pain?	YES	NO
Does your heart race or skip beats?	YES	NO
Has anyone in your family died from a heart condition before age 50?	YES	NO
Do you ever wheeze or have trouble catching your breath?	YES	NO
Do you cough a lot?	YES	NO
Do you get colds or sinus problems more than once every two months?	YES	NO
Have you recently had an illness lasting longer than one week?	YES	NO
Have you been in the hospital in the past year for an illness?	YES	NO
Have you ever had a sudden rash or hives?	YES	NO
Have you ever hit your head hard enough to pass out?	YES	NO

Do you ever feel light-headed or dizzy?	YES	NO
Do you suffer from daily or weekly headaches?	YES	NO
Have you ever had a seizure?	YES	NO
Have you ever lost your memory?	YES	NO
Do you have any loss of feeling anywhere?	YES	NO
Do you experience muscle cramps lasting more than five minutes?	YES	NO
Do you have trouble with diarrhea or constipation?	YES	NO
Have you ever had blood in your stool or urine?	YES	NO
Do you bruise easily?	YES	NO
Do you get cold easier than others and have trouble keeping warm?	YES	NO
Have you recently lost weight without trying?	YES	NO
Do you feel you have been urinating more than usual?	YES	NO
Do you have swelling of a joint or limb?	YES	NO
Have you had repeated sprains or fractures to the same area?	YES	NO
Have you had fractures that were not due to a fall or accident?	YES	NO
Have you ever had frostbite?	YES	NO
Have you ever passed out from heat or dehydration?	YES	NO

If you are diagnosed with a medical problem, you will probably still be allowed to exercise, but you might have some limitations or precautions. If you have any questions, make sure you ask your doctor specifically about the type of activity you are interested in, how often you will be doing it, at what level of competition, and for how long each exercise session will last. Some doctors are more knowledgeable than others with regard to exercise activity and risk factors; you might want to see a primary care sports medicine specialist (one who is a family practitioner, internist, or pediatrician). Some common medical problems and their associated limitations to exercise are outlined in the following chart.

Medical Problems and Their Risks with Exercise

PROBLEM	LIMITATIONS/RISKS
Bleeding problems	be careful with injuries and falls
Carditis (inflammation of the heart)	severe restrictions of exercise intensity
High blood pressure	avoid heavy weight lifting
Congenital heart disease	possibly limited per doctor
Irregular heartbeat	possibly limited per doctor
Mitral valve prolapse	usually no limits
Hear murmur	possibly limited per doctor
Diabetes	watch blood sugars if more than 30 minutes exercise
Diarrhea	watch fluid status and increase salt/potassium
Eating disorders	limited if severe and nutrition poor
Fever	do not exercise
HIV infection	no restrictions if currently healthy
Kidney disease	possibly limit contact sports
Liver disease	possibly limit contact sports
Cancer	possible limits after surgery or chemotherapy
Concussion	no contact sports if more than three in lifetime
Seizures	possibly limited, make sure medications taken
Obesity	avoid overheating and dehydration
Asthma	might need to modify environment, take medications
Bronchitis	possibly limit exertion
Sickle cell disease	avoid overheating/overcooling, dehydration
Skin diseases	if contagious, contact not allowed
Enlarged spleen (mononucleosis)	no contact sports

Lifestyle

There are also lifestyle risk factors that can lead to medical problems. These can be screened with the following questions. If you can answer any of these questions with a "yes," reconsider your behavior, as this might lead to serious problems. Behaviors can be hard to correct; if you need help, speak to your health-care provider, therapist, school counselor, social worker, or a family member or close friend you feel you can talk to and confide in.

Do you smoke?	YES	NO
Do you drink more than seven alcoholic drinks a week?	YES	NO
Have you ever used any street drugs?	YES	NO
Do you often forget to wear a seatbelt?	YES	NO
Do you forget to wear a helmet while biking or motorcycling?	YES	NO
Do you have trouble sleeping on more than two nights a week?	YES	NO
Do you feel stressed out with no relief in sight?	YES	NO
Do you throw up after eating?	YES	NO
Do you use laxatives on a regular basis because you "feel full"?	YES	NO
Do you take pills or teas to help you lose water weight?	YES	NO
Have you ever taken anything to help you lose weight?	YES	NO
Have you ever taken anything to help you gain muscle or strength?	YES	NO
Have you ever taken any drugs to keep you awake or alert?	YES	NO

Nutritional Health

Nutrition is an essential part of inner body health and athletic performance and, thus, is an important area of assessment and monitoring in athletic women. Health and performance problems can be due to poor nutrition, and poor nutrition can be due to poor health and performance. Athletic performance is one of the best indicators of nutrition. With the right nutrition, you perform at your best with low incidence of injury or illness. If you are feeling tired and run down, weak, irritable, or cramping, nutrition can be a factor. Weight is, of course, a good guide, as any quick change of weight can signal nutrition problems. It is always recommended to take a multivitamin daily to ensure nutrient balance. This along with a well-rounded diet of proteins, carbohydrates, and fats is essential. To quickly assess your nutritional habits, ask yourself the following questions:

Do you skip meals?	YES	NO
Do you always feel hungry?	YES	NO
Do you restrict yourself of certain foods?	YES	NO
Do you feel that you cannot quench your thirst?	YES	NO
Do you crave salty, sugary, or fatty foods often?	YES	NO
Do you take more than three vitamins or supplements a day?	YES	NO
Do you worry about your nutrition or weight on a daily basis?	YES	NO

If you have more than two "yes" answers, refer to chapter 3, "Nutritional Health," for more information, and make an appointment to see a doctor or nutritionist.

Exercise and Cancer

Cancer is very common; there is a one in eight chance any woman will get breast cancer at some time in her life. Other common types of cancer are colon, skin, cervical, ovarian, uterine, brain, bone, and lymphoma (cancer within the lymph nodes). We are fortunate to have various treatments and cures for many of these cancers, and researchers continue to search for more.

Cancer treatment is stressful on the body and can interfere with a regular exercise plan. It is important to try to maintain a flexible exercise schedule, because it is hard to predict how you will feel or how your body will react. Still, there are many people who stay physically active at moderate levels while being treated with chemotherapy or radiation. In fact, light to moderate exercise has been shown recently to improve survival, decrease uncomfortable side effects and fatigue, and improve appetite, mood, stamina, and energy. Exercise can be difficult at first, as the body can become weak after surgery or treatments. Returning to pre-treatment levels of activity might take anywhere from half the time since treatment started to twice the time.

During treatment with chemotherapy, in particular, there are a few precautions and some measures that indicate you should take a break from exercise until your body is responding better. These include avoiding exercise on days of treatment and mornings of blood tests and avoiding crowded exercise settings and pools where germs can easily spread. Blood levels of potassium and sodium must be close to normal (above 3 and 130, respectively) to prevent heart or muscle problems, and your blood count should include a platelet count more than 25,000 and a hemoglobin of more than 11 to prevent bleeding problems or poor oxygen supply to necessary organs.

Avoid Aerobic Exercise If You Have These Symptoms

Extreme fatigue

Confusion

Fever

Dizziness

Bleeding

Blurry vision

Irregular pulse or heartbeat

Light-headedness

Sudden swelling in an arm or leg

Nausea or vomiting

More than three episodes of diarrhea in the past 24 hours

Unable to eat more than 1,000 calories in the past 24 hours

Shortness of breath

Chest pain

Chemotherapy treatment in the past 24 hours

Platelets less than 25,000

Hemoglobin less than 11

Sodium less than 130

Potassium less than 3

On days you cannot exercise for one of the above reasons, consider gentle/beginning yoga with simple sitting or floor postures including breathing and relaxation components. Gentle pilates exercises or stretching classes are usually tolerated as well.

If you have had surgery, check with your surgeon to see when you can safely return to aerobic activity. For breast cancer patients who have had a lymph node resection or mastectomy, lifting on that side is usually not recommended for at least four weeks to prevent lymphedema (arm swelling). You should, however, begin moving the shoulder and arm through its full range within the first week after surgery and continue every day thereafter to prevent scar tissue from forming.

Both chemotherapy and radiation cancer treatments can lead to dry, irritated, and sun-sensitive skin. This can be managed and relieved by using sunscreen, covering up with clothing when possible, using ointments liberally to prevent chafing, and using generous amounts of moisturizer. A humidifier can help, as can drinking lots of fluids and eating fruits and vegetables. Exercise also improves skin conditions, as it increases blood flow to the skin.

Tips for Exercising While Recovering from Cancer

Start with gentle walking or cycling

Try light exercise three days a week with rest days in between

Alternate aerobic activity days with stretching and conditioning days

If you cannot tolerate 20 to 30 minutes, break the sessions into 10 minutes each

Start low, go slow, and increase gradually—no more than 10 percent a week

Do not get discouraged if you have a "tired" day—rest and try again tomorrow!

Make exercise enjoyable with good music, a good friend, or in front of a good TV show

---

Reproductive Health

There is an entire specialty of medicine devoted just to women—obstetrics and gynecology (OBGYN). Family practitioners also are trained in basic obstetric and gynecological care, although they do not do surgery. Seeing your gynecologist or family practitioner once a year to maintain reproductive health and screen for problems is highly recommended. For women without other health problems, OBGYNs sometimes function as their primary care doctors. However, your health care is more comprehensive if you also have an internist or primary care doctor.

As with all physicians, making an appointment is the best way to get answers to your health questions. This is why it is recommended that you see your OBGYN yearly and your primary health doctor at least once every two years. As a reminder, the following screening questions will help you determine whether you have any issues of possible concern. A "yes" answer to any of the following questions is a sign that you should see your gynecologist or family physician.

Do you have any foul-smelling discharge from your vagina?	YES	NO
Do you have any pain in the pelvis?	YES	NO
Do you have pain when you have sex?	YES	NO
Do you feel any breast lumps?	YES	NO
Do you have any drainage from your breasts?	YES	NO
Do you think you might be pregnant?	YES	NO
Have you missed your period more than twice in the past year?	YES	NO
Do you frequently miss your periods?	YES	NO
Do you have very heavy, painful periods?	YES	NO
Do you leak urine?	YES	NO

For women, preventive health measures include screening tests that rule out the most common types of cancers. Breast cancer, the greatest risk, is usually treatable if diagnosed early. Detection methods now may also include genetic screening, along with mammograms, recommended for women yearly after age 40 or 35 if you have risk factors. Breast self-exams should be done every month a few days after your period, once you have started having regular periods and for the rest of your life. Pap smears are done yearly after the age of 21 or if you are sexually active. After menopause, another screening test important for women is bone density testing; this should be done at least once to establish a baseline level of fracture risk.

If you are between the ages of 14 and 45, you should be getting your period every month unless you are pregnant or starting menopause. Stress,

FIGURE 1-1 **Breast Self-Exam: Breast self-exams should be done monthly, right after your period, when your breasts are not swollen. If you do not get your period, or are pregnant, check your breasts on the same day of each month in the following way:**

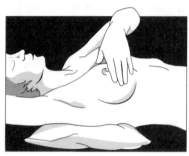

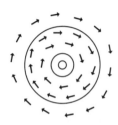

FIGURE 1-1A **Lying on your back with your right arm up or behind your head, pillow underneath your right upper back, left hand fingers flat, use your middle three fingers on your left hand to feel your breast for lumps or thickening.**

FIGURE 1-1B **Start in the center of your nipple and gently press in a circular pattern, making several concentric circles to cover the entire breast area along with the area under your right arm. Repeat with the left side.**

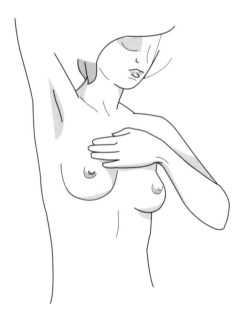

FIGURE 1-1C **Exam can also be done in the shower with arm elevated over head. Also, stand in front of a mirror and look at your breasts for any irregular pitting or bumps that you can see. Check with your doctor if you feel any lumps or thickening, or notice any irregular shape.**

*Illustrations reprinted with the permission of the American Cancer Society, Inc.

excessive exercise, and illness can cause a skipped period, but if this occurs more than two months in a row, speak with your doctor. Having your period means your hormones are balanced and your body is producing normal amounts of estrogen.

Premenstrual syndrome (PMS) is the occurrence of uncomfortable body changes a few days before your period. Treatment of PMS is based on preventing and relieving symptoms. Prevention strategies include a low-salt diet, low-sugar diet, proper sleep, and plenty of exercise. Calcium supplements, vitamin E, vitamin B_6, or magnesium in an extra dose the week before your period can help, and adequate amounts of calcium and vitamins should be taken throughout the month (see Chapter 3, "Nutritional Health").

Symptoms of PMS

Mood changes—	nervousness, moodiness, irritability, anger, anxiety, depression, edginess
Physical feelings—	sweet or salty cravings, hunger, headaches, feeling tired
Body changes—	bloating and water retention; weight gain; swollen, tender, and sore breasts
Depressive symptoms—	sleep problems, memory loss, confusion, fluctuating emotions, tears, suicidal thoughts

PMS with severe mood symptoms is medically classified and treated as premenstrual dysthymic disorder (PMDD). This is a mood disorder that disrupts work and other life activities related to the premenstrual part of the menstrual cycle. Medications have been approved for the treatment of PMDD and are typically taken for the last two weeks of the month of your cycle. If you are suffering from premenstrual symptoms that interfere with relationships, work, or athletic schedule, discuss possible treatment with your doctor.

Menopause

Every woman's body and mind respond differently to menopause. Occurring usually between the ages of 50 and 55, menopause has a bad reputation for causing unpleasant side effects such as hot flashes, moodiness, memory disturbance, and vaginal dryness. Menopause is not a disease, but rather simply a natural process that occurs as the amount of estrogen and progesterone in the body changes, sometimes causing strange sensations. For those who have trouble with the uncomfortable side effects of menopause, medications can be helpful. Until recently, the most commonly prescribed medication was hormone replacement therapy (HRT), usually a combination of estrogen and progesterone. Treatment with HRT is less frequently prescribed after the 2002 Women's Health Initiative study found HRT to slightly increase risk of breast cancer in some women if taken for more than five years. Instead, lower doses are prescribed for a few years, or medications used to treat mood disorders (including Zoloft, Paxil, and Prozac) are also effective. Natural treatments for symptoms of menopause can also be helpful and include soy and black cohosh.

After menopause, your risk of heart disease goes up slightly. Speak with your doctor if you have any other health risks of cardiovascular disease such as high blood pressure, high cholesterol, had a mother or daughter with heart disease, or have diabetes. It might be worth it for you to take a "statin" medication to prevent heart disease. Also, your risk of osteoporosis increases after menopause; this risk can be established with a bone density test (see chapter 5, "Bone Health and Osteoporosis").

There are no limitations to exercise before, during, or after menopause. In fact, exercise can help manage and lessen uncomfortable symptoms experienced before and during menopause. Exercise can also lower the risks of health problems that can occur after menopause: Cardiovascular (aerobic) exercise prevents cardiovascular disease, and weight-bearing exercise (walking, jogging, weight lifting) prevents osteoporosis. Skill sports involving balance challenges such as golf and tennis help maintain posture, motion, flexibility, and balance and prevent joint stiffness, weakness, and falls.

Ideally, all your body systems are as healthy as they can possibly be. Occasional setbacks or flare-ups of problems are part of life, but if they do not take you out of exercise for more than one week, they should be easy to recover from. When you experience serious illness or surgeries that require more than one week of rest, recovery can sometimes take longer than the illness. Anesthesia can also contribute to feeling tired and weak for anywhere from several days to several weeks. If you are weak or limited by illness, try basic yoga moves, light weight lifting exercises, or toning exercises or classes. Advance to walking a few times a week, then add cycling or swimming. Gradually, you should be able to return to your previous level of activity.

Do not hesitate to see a doctor if you have concerns about unusual symptoms or feel unhealthy. Make an appointment, as this is the best way to get correct and appropriate answers to your questions. The earlier a problem is diagnosed and treated, the earlier it will be resolved and the more likely it will be fully healed. If you do not feel comfortable speaking with your doctor, find another one.

Your exercise program should make you feel stronger and healthier. Your nutrition program should provide you with fuel for life and exercise. By taking care of yourself, you will need no (or fewer) medications and avoid illness and injury. Each day will feel great. Staying active will keep you looking and feeling young and healthy. Remember, your health is your greatest resource.

CHAPTER TWO

Stress and Sports Psychology Techniques

Stress has a very influential role on your entire body. How you respond to stress influences your personality, mood, hormones, stamina, appearance, weight, and overall health. Exercise challenges your body and mind and helps channel stress positively, improving your mental, emotional, and physical state. Because exercise helps you clear your mind, lift your mood, and improve your self-esteem, it is a major stress reducer.

All active girls and women face stress as they strive for goals. For those with goals for serious, competitive athletic achievement, and for women with multiple life responsibilities, stress-managing techniques are required daily. The athletic role model can be transferred to all challenging activities, as both the mind and body must work together. Athletes face mental challenges at each practice as they strive to achieve perfection and peak physical conditioning. As athletes, they are susceptible to pressures from athletic peers, coaches, and parents. Frustration can also occur if finding time for practice is a challenge.

Women usually function as the primary caregivers in their families. Stress can come from a time-limited schedule, excessive work, family demands, illness, injury, or poor sleep. The demands of others, including peers, bosses, and family members, can also contribute to stress. The pressures of performance, life schedule and activities, and responsibilities for those you love and care for can become overwhelming.

Still, for every challenge, there is opportunity to grow stronger. The ability to rise to a challenge, take control over stress, overcome any adversity, and finish successfully is the goal. Nurturing a clear, calm, productive, and healthy mind allows for happiness, enjoyment, success, and amazing athletic achievements.

Emotional Fitness

Just as you can train and condition your body, you can also train and condition your mind to think more clearly and feel less stress. Enlisting the help of other supportive people, or a therapist or counselor, can be very helpful. Therapists most commonly have degrees in social work or psychology. Sometimes, psychiatrists or educational counselors also specialize in sports counseling.

Sports and exercise therapists are specialists who are trained to identify, manage, and prevent the pressures and negative stressors in sports and athletics. These therapists recognize the role of stress and the pressures that active women at all levels of competition and achievement face with the realization that stress can become overwhelming enough to interfere with other aspects of life. They can provide training in the most effective way to gain the "mental edge" needed to excel. This is essential to peak performance among top athletes who cannot afford to mentally fall apart.

The mind can also be controlled by the effects of exercise. One of the most pleasing benefits of exercise is the release of chemicals called endorphins, which make you feel good. Your body responds to endorphins like a mood-enhancing drug; endorphins can even be addictive. Because of this, you can develop exercise dependence and addiction, in which your body and mind crave exercise. Addiction to exercise is only dangerous when female athletes overdo their training and sports to a point of poor health, which can also lead to injury. Meeting with a sports psychologist is recommended to help with feeling controlled or overwhelmed by expectations and performance obligations in sports and life.

Mood

A positive mood and positive emotions include happiness, pride, confidence, and high self-esteem. A positive, healthy emotional outlook is key to success in all aspects of life. Knowing that you are willingly working hard for your sport or task at hand puts you in charge of the training for the challenge. This makes it a positive experience for you, one for which you have control and accept eagerly. A negative mood and negative emotions include depression, poor self-esteem, self-criticism, anger, and bitterness. Negative emotions prevent success and drain the energy needed for your daily routine and activities.

Depression is the most common negative emotion in women. It is commonly treated with therapy and medications, but research has shown that regular exercise can be as effective as medications to treat depression. One example is the "runner's high," which can occur in all sports and is due to the release of hormones called endorphins. This feeling of euphoria, happiness, and bliss often occurs with intense sports activity. When you are happy, you feel less pain. When you smile, you can work harder. When you feel the pleasure and rush of endorphins, you can push yourself farther.

Self-Esteem

Self-esteem is having a feeling of self-importance and self-value. This is an essential quality to many aspects of life, particularly those related to success. Self-esteem allows you to feel more control over your situation, because you are able to speak up for and defend yourself if there is a problem. Standing up for yourself contributes to a sense of accomplishment with great satisfaction and overall happiness.

Self-esteem is vital to achieving goals, being independent, and allowing your life and sports goals to be as you want them to be. You are ruled by yourself, not by others, and this allows you to make wise decisions. You know right from wrong and will not be bullied. Self-esteem is important in situations of sexual discrimination and for preventing and defending yourself from dangerous attacks. Self-esteem allows you to stand up to anyone and not let them interfere with your success or take advantage of you.

Stress

Stress is caused by the mental and physical response you have to overwhelming demands. Demands can be both positive, such as a qualifying for the Olympics, or negative, such as an injury. The response can be positive and productive, such as eating healthier, or negative and destructive, such as not sleeping. There can often be a fine line between the productive and destructive effects of stress. This line is different for everyone, just as stress and the effects of stress are different for everyone. The mind interprets events to define them as stressful, and each woman is unique in her experiences and interpretations.

Productive Stress

In a positive sense, stress can make you alert, motivated, and productive. To this end, stress can be beneficial. It inspires you to meet the challenge of the task at hand. You push yourself and learn how to best handle the situation so it will be less stressful in the future. Some women "thrive" on stress, appreciating the motivation it provides.

Stress is common to women. Because women are capable of doing many things at once, they are more susceptible to the stresses of all the activities they take on. Women are social organizers, mediators, planners, mothers, wives, spouses, girlfriends, daughters, friends, athletes, teammates, managers, employees, cleaning ladies, cooks, partners, athletes, and therapists. Positive stress can lead to a full, very active life that keeps you young in spirit and in health. Athletic girls in organized sports have a full schedule as they go from school to athletic activity, and learn to balance school, fitness, friendships, and family. These girls grow into women who regularly exercise and who have the ability to manage their busy lives with multiple responsibilities, squeezing the most out of every day.

Some people need both physical and mental stress to be productive; some athletes need stress to stay at the top of their game. Their rewards are good health, personal satisfaction, and positive acknowledgment or compensation. Some athletes compete at high levels with the reward of enjoyment. Regardless, the stress must be worth it, otherwise the athlete will lose her edge, competitiveness, and desire.

Commonly Identified Positive Causes of Stress

Being involved in multiple activities

Qualifying for elite competition

Starting a new sport or job

Moving up a position or ranking

New relationship/marriage/living arrangement

Moving or going away to college

Joining a new team

A new contract or scholarship

Being responsible for others

Hormone fluctuations

Negative Stress

At high levels or for long periods of time, stress can be dangerous. Not only can it cause crying, anger, or inability to get work done, it can also cause physical illness or problems. Sometimes it can lead to negative coping behaviors, which lead to even more problems and a vicious cycle of never-ending stress. These negative coping behaviors include eating too little or too much, eating unhealthy foods, sleeping too much or too little, skipping work or practice, smoking, drinking, taking drugs, or taking too many prescribed medications. Even if you are not conscientiously engaging in negative coping behaviors, your body might be doing it for you. Signs of this are frequent colds, cold sores, canker sores, appetite and weight changes, heart disease, heart attacks, and even cancer. Too much stress can also lead to injuries or accidents, as it can cause you to be distracted from the task at hand.

Commonly Identified Negative Causes of Stress

Death of a loved one or friend

End of a relationship

A move, change of schools, or change of jobs

Money problems

Loss of position, standing, or ranking

Physical, sexual, or verbal abuse

Overwhelming pressure from coaches, peers, employers, or family

An accident or injury

Hormones

Hormonal fluctuations can be a source of stress in girls and women. This varies in intensity from one person to the next, but it is quite common. Premenstrual syndrome (PMS) can include feeling sad, hopeless, suicidal; tense, anxious, tearful, irritable, anger affecting others, disinterest in daily activities and relationships, trouble concentrating, fatigue, low energy; food cravings, bingeing, sleep disturbances, and feeling out of control. Physical symptoms include appetite changes, bloating, breast tenderness, headaches, and joint or muscle pain. In approximately 5 percent of women, the mood problems are so severe that the medical diagnosis is premenstrual dysthymic disorder (PMDD). This disorder is now treatable with antidepressants and mood-altering medications, either daily or just for the week before your period. PMDD has been discovered to be a cause of marriage, family, and social problems. Some athletes feel so disturbed by mood and physical changes around their period that they try not to compete during this time. While emotional changes may affect performance, there is no research suggesting impaired athletic performance at certain times of the cycle.

The more complicated life becomes, the more stressful it can be. As you try to juggle multiple activities, responsibilities, and roles, you might feel less in control of your life. Also, the more people involved in a situation, the less control you have (think of a big team versus a smaller one). It is important to know how to manage, control, and relieve negative stress so it does not cause negative effects in your life. It is important to know if you are under too much stress, because this can take a toll on many of your body systems as well as your sports performance.

Controlling Stress

The best way to manage any problem is to take control. First, you must evaluate the situation and determine how it can be changed. Often, being able to change your attitude toward the stressful situation is all you need to make it less stressful. Start by identifying your stress. If there is more than one type or cause of stress, make a chart for each one. Then identify your goals and desired positive results, both in the short term (one week) and long term (one year). Now make a list of positive and negative consequences and feelings associated with the stress, both short term (one week) and long term (one year). If the negatives total more than the positives, seriously think about changing whatever has caused the stress. If you have equal numbers of positives and negatives, just having the stress written down along with a goal and the positive end results will help you gain understanding and control. This worksheet can be used to help clarify all types of stressors, from an upcoming athletic event, to a school exam, to pregnancy!

Stress Worksheet

My stress is _____

Goal/positive results of stress this week _____

POSITIVE EFFECTS OF STRESS THIS WEEK	NEGATIVE EFFECTS OF STRESS THIS WEEK

Goal/positive results of stress this year _____

POSITIVE EFFECTS OF STRESS THIS YEAR	NEGATIVE EFFECTS OF STRESS THIS YEAR

If you prefer, keep a journal to chronicle your stress. This helps to assess your levels of anxiety surrounding the stress. You should note the level of anxiousness related to stress by rating it either high, medium, or low or on a scale of 1 to 10. You should also note any triggers of stress such as other people, situations, or time of day. Most important, note what relieved the anxious feeling you had. Try to note this every day, or even each time you have stress. Use the journal as a sounding board for you to discuss and understand your stress and how you respond to it.

In addition to using various techniques to understand and manage stress, controlling the amount is also important, as too much can be detrimental. Even too much positive stress can become negative (think of a nationally ranked high school athlete who has trouble with school). You can maintain healthy balance by scheduling time off from stressful competition, practice, work, or other pressures. Because stress can be so overwhelming that it is hard to identify, pay attention to emotional and physical symptoms that interfere with your other activities.

Signs You Are Under Too Much Stress

You are more irritable.

You are anxious.

You have nightmares about realistic life situations turning out poorly.

You feel exhausted.

You are very emotional.

You feel nervous.

You are having trouble sleeping.

Your friends and family irritate you.

You have lost friends.

You cannot possibly think about doing an enjoyable activity.

Your complexion is a problem.

You have either too much or too little appetite.

You stop getting your period, or get it less regularly.

To evaluate if your stress is worth the time and energy spent on the stressful activity, answer the following questions. If answers to the following questions are "no," "none," or "I don't know," you must consider changing your activity schedule to eliminate or decrease the stress to you.

What is my reward from all this?

Do I have significant personal satisfaction when the stress is resolved?

Do the stress factors go away when the stress is over?

Do I enjoy the stress?

Do I feel this stressful event as an exciting challenge?

If you are still having difficulty evaluating and controlling your stress, speaking with a therapist, or a mentor, parent, friend, co-worker, or coach can be very enlightening. Although it is possible to sort your problems out alone, having someone to help makes it much easier. The investment of a few hundred dollars in therapy is well worth the reduction in stress from the understanding and management skills you will learn. Health insurance often covers counseling sessions, making therapy easier to access.

If your stress analysis suggests you do not have enough positive end results or have too many negative effects, you need to consider changes. This might mean changing a relationship with friend or spouse, changing a job or team, changing a coach or trainer, staying away from negative people, or changing sports or activities. These changes can be difficult, but you will be more successful in situations that do not provide negative stress.

Stress Relief

One of the best stress relievers is regular exercises. Exercise is a natural stress reducer, increasing endorphins in the blood, relaxing your mind, and raising your heart rate. Simply taking a short walk outdoors, going up and down some steps, or doing jumping jacks in place can also help alleviate and manage stress.

Other less physical stress relievers that can work instantly include deep breathing, inhaling for a slow count of four and exhaling for the same slow count, reaching your arms overhead and breathing deep, and closing your eyes for five to ten minutes and imagining you are somewhere peaceful. Short meditations require practice but can be very effective, along with calming personal chants or "mantras." Because most people hold most of their stress in their neck and shoulders, a simple way to relieve stress is shoulder rolls—slowly rolling the shoulders forward 10 times and back 10 times. Follow this with 10 neck rolls alternating clockwise and counterclockwise.

If you are stressed before or during competition, try deep breathing, take a quick water break, shake your legs and arms out, and focus on the horizon for a minute. Open your mouth for a deep breath followed by a relaxing yawn. Recall all your positive imagery. Imagine your successful finish.

Relaxation Techniques

Count your breathing: Count to four on a slow inhale and four on a slow exhale.

Try to focus on each part of your body, relaxing first your toes, heels, ankles, and all the way up.

Think of a peaceful place and imagine all the sounds, smells, and sensations.

Do 10 shoulder rolls forwards, 10 backward, and follow with 10 alternating neck circles.

Stress-Reducing Techniques

Exercise

Stretching

Yoga

Meditation

Vacation

Calling a friend

Attacking your goal with enthusiasm and focus

Slowly indulging in one portion of a favorite food

Spending time with a loved one

Spending time with a pet

Taking a break

Making a schedule

Watching a funny TV show

Most beneficial is reminding yourself that this stress is temporary. Think briefly on an enjoyable moment ahead of or behind you. Think of the positive reasons why you are in this stressful place—you like the game, the pay, the feeling of accomplishment. Reflect on your stress chart or journal and your goals for renewed clarity, confidence, and sense of control.

Sleep

Sleep is necessary to allow the brain and body to recover from and absorb all the day's events, allowing you to think clearer and perform better in all aspects of life. Researchers have shown that the ideal amount of sleep in order to perform the best in both sports and mental tasks is between seven and eight hours nightly. This amount might vary a little from person to person but is overall an effective guideline. It is also evidenced that the better rested you are, the quicker and more efficiently you accomplish tasks, making that extra hour out of your day used to sleep worthwhile because you gain it back by being more efficient!

PERFORMANCE TIP **The most effective amount of sleep for athletic and mind function is seven to eight hours each night.**

Trouble Sleeping

Sleep and stress are very closely related. Stress can often deprive you of sleep by occupying both your mind and your scheduled time for sleep. Stress can also occasionally cause you to sleep too much, or oversleep due to fatigue. Trouble sleeping for a few nights or even a few weeks can be common at times of both positive and negative stress. If sleep is a problem for more than one week, however, or is interfering with daily functioning such as missed work or practice, you should see a doctor for effective ways to improve this. Chronic lack of sleep can result in both physical illness and emotional instability. In the short term, not sleeping impairs your reflexes, alertness, and brain, body, and nerve response. Sleep deprivation can be similar to being under the influence of alcohol or sedating drugs and can make driving and activities that require balance dangerous.

Caffeine is a major reason for disturbed sleep. If you are having trouble sleeping, avoid caffeine after noon because caffeine actually stays in the body for more than 12 hours (see "Caffeine" in chapter 14, "Exercise Fuel"). Certain medications, such as antibiotics, antidepressants, and steroids, can also interfere with sleep, especially when mixed with caffeine. Check with your doctor or pharmacist if your sleep problems are recent and you are taking a new medication.

Of course, children, a snoring spouse, or even a problem pet can interfere with your sleep. Try to manage this by arranging for help or changing sleeping arrangements on noisy nights of the week. Taking naps when your children do can also help replenish sleep. Although the ideal way to achieve rest is at night, naps can be effective for recharging the mind and body during the day. Some elite athletes swear by them.

Improving Sleep

There are many natural ways to improve your sleep, including relaxation techniques, natural herbs, or scents such as lavender and valerian, calming decaffeinated teas, warm milk, or even a small snack. A warm bath, warm sheets, or soothing music can also lull you to sleep.

There are a few things you should avoid: Do not use alcohol to induce sleep—alcohol interferes with the quality of sleep and your body can become dependent on it, requiring more and more over time to help you "relax." Also, do not make a habit of taking over-the-counter sleeping pills, as they can be addictive. These include melatonin, valerian, and diphenhydramine (the common ingredient in "PM" medicines and Benadryl). If you need to take a pill to help you sleep on a nightly basis for more than one week, let your doctor know. Prescription sleeping pills can be a better treatment, as newer pills to the market are less addictive. For sleep that does not improve after one month, seeking the help of a therapist or counselor is beneficial and recommended.

Tips to Improve Your Sleep

Avoid caffeine, especially after noon.

Do not work out within two hours of going to bed.

Do not eat a heavy meal two hours before going to bed.

Try lavender-scented sprays, candles, and lotions.

Use relaxation techniques to help yourself fall asleep.

Imagine yourself in a dreamlike place; begin a happy dream in your mind.

Think carefree thoughts, not about work.

Keep a notepad by your bed for thoughts that might be keeping you awake.

Turn off your telephone ringer so no one can call and wake you up.

If you are nervous about your alarm not going off, set a second one.

Turn off the TV before a show starts so you are not tempted to stay up to watch it.

Indulge in comfy pillows, sheets, a teddy bear, or a body pillow.

Keep stressful reminders or work-related items out of your bedroom.

If you are bothered by noise, purchase a "white noise" maker or turn on a fan.

Try a warm bath before bedtime.

Drink (decaffeinated) herbal tea or warm milk with vanilla and sugar before bed.

Finding Balance

We women have the opportunity to do anything. We can now play every sport, do every job, have children, cook, and make ourselves attractive.

But we also need to rise to the challenge of finding balance among all our activities and roles. If you can manage the potential stress from all these roles and challenges, you will not only shine but have a blast! Do not be afraid to ask for help or delegate responsibilities; this is key to successfully meeting all your challenges in life. By incorporating all the principles of health into your lifestyle, and keeping perspective of major versus minor stressors you should feel optimal mental health and happiness. By taking control, you will find balance.

Nutrition and the Mind

A healthy mind is also fueled by healthy food. People under stress can require more B vitamins, calcium, iron, and protein. Make sure you eat three meals a day, along with two small healthy snacks to keep blood sugars level. Avoid high-sugar foods, which will send blood sugars soaring and then plummeting, affecting your mood. Low blood sugar, resulting from a rebound after a high-sugar snack or meal can result in irritability and depression.

Your Coaches, Trainers, and Support Team

Successful athletic performance and success at all tasks is very closely related to the people you work with. You must have supportive coaches or trainers who assist you in positive ways, giving you constructive criticism and encouragement. They should be respectful of your training and emotional needs and have a coaching and personality style that suits you. Sometimes, having a coach or trainer of a certain sex motivates you more. You must carefully assess and monitor the effect of these people.

In younger athletes involved in school sports, there is often no choice of coaches. Still, there is usually an assistant who you might relate to better if you have a problem with the coach. Otherwise, having friends and fellow athletes as mentors can help. Supportive parents can also help with a difficult coach by allowing you to continue the sport in a nonschool setting with a coach you like better. This can do a lot for your performance. This is a very important point, as it is a shame when athletes lose their love of a sport due to coaching issues.

Likewise, parents can put too much pressure on children to perform. The parent who tries to "coach" a child rarely does it effectively, because there are too many emotions at stake. Also, this puts the child in a position of never getting a break from the sport—they are constantly reminded of the sport, bringing these pressures from the field to home. This is a difficult situation to resolve. If you are an athlete feeling this pressure, speak to a supportive coach, counselor, or teacher. Usually sports pressure involves only one parent; try to enlist the nonpressuring parent to help. Extreme pressure to perform in a sport reduces the enjoyment and ultimately negatively affects the athlete's performance. This can lead to a shortened athletic career.

Injury, Illness, and Stress

Keep in mind that stress can have detrimental effects on the body and is closely related to pain, injury, and illness. Stress weakens immunity, and physical stress weakens muscles and joints. It can cause immediate symptoms, including a runny nose, tears, a twitchy eye or face, sweating, trembling, and a greatly increased or decreased appetite. Some people get stomach and gastrointestinal symptoms, including diarrhea, cramps, and nausea. Vomiting, hives, and severe headaches are also quite common.

Body Responses to Stress

IMMEDIATE RESPONSE	LONG-TERM RESPONSE
Sweating	Illness
Twitching	Chronic fatigue
Crying	Fibromyalgia
Tremors	Asthma
Nausea	Neck and shoulder pain
Vomiting	Back pain
Itchiness	Trouble falling asleep
Headache	High blood pressure
Stomach cramps	New medical problem
Diarrhea	Ulcer
Irritability	Infertility
Trouble concentrating	Stroke

Injury or Illness Caused by Stress

There are various medical conditions, including allergies, neck and back pain, and even infertility, that have all been linked to stress. Stress can lower immunity, so you are less able to defend yourself from viruses or bacterial infections. This can lead to a cascade of poor health, as viruses have been known to trigger even more serious diseases such as diabetes, rheumatoid arthritis, and other autoimmune diseases that are often lifelong. There are some schools of thought that believe some cancer is also triggered by stress. High blood pressure, often connected with stress, can lead to heart disease and strokes.

Stress in other aspects of life can affect your fitness and training or lead to injury or negative consequences as well. For example, if you are overwhelmed or anxious, you might forget the proper equipment. Not only does this lead to poor performance, it can also cause injury. Stress on your schedule for time can lead you to work out at odd times of the day, perhaps running when it is dark out. Not only can you trip and fall, but also you are at the mercy of drivers who could hit you or criminals looking for a vulnerable woman.

There has been research on the links between poor stress management and higher injury rates. Not only can the body and immunity become weaker, but muscles are more tense, concentration is poor, and self-confidence is down. The distraction of stress on the mind interferes with focus and concentration, which can contribute to injuries. Also, pessimists and people more easily angry, aggressive, and depressed are more likely to injure themselves.

Mood Problems Secondary to Injury

Coping methods are very important during times of injury. A serious athlete who identifies herself with a certain sport can be devastated by an injury that takes her out of the game. She might fear losing her skills, strength, conditioning, and experience of a season. She might also fear losing her position. Additionally, she is unable to exercise as before due to the limitations of her injury. Even though she might now have a lot of time on her hands, she might feel great stress and turmoil.

There are many uncertainties related to injury. It is common to wonder if she will ever be able to play as well again. She might become anxious waiting for healing to take place and develop depression. She might also lose touch with her athletic friends and find new friends and interests. If these behaviors or feelings are affecting coping skills, feelings of self-worth, and identity problems, it is valuable to see a psychologist, counselor, social worker, or psychiatrist. The sooner she can start talking to someone, the sooner she will feel better and avoid negative mood problems.

Other problems related to injury are related to weight. An active athlete who cannot exercise due to injury might fear weight gain and start dieting.

This can be detrimental to healing because nutrition is crucial at times of injury. If the injury is to a leg, calories burned are actually higher than you think, as it takes more calories to hop on one leg, use crutches, or use your upper body to move around. Also, your body requires more calories to heal the injury. Therefore, although the injured athlete might have to cut back a little on caloric intake, there is really little risk of weight gain during this time.

For competitive athletes who are having trouble coping with injury, involving themselves in aggressive rehabilitation with a physical therapist and/or athletic trainer can be very helpful. Also, exercising the noninjured body parts can relieve stress. For some athletes going to practice and games can be helpful, although be aware that it might also be frustrating for the injured athlete to be a spectator rather than a participant.

Having a sports counselor or therapist is also very helpful for the injured athlete. She can help discuss and find ways to control the athlete's healing and rehabilitation process, focus on goals, and practice visualization and imagery of sports performance to keep the athlete mentally "in the game." The counselor or therapist can also help encourage mental imagery and have the athlete try other sports or activities during the healing process.

Strategies to Cope with the Stress of Illness or Injury

Have goals for therapy and rehabilitation.

Focus on the outcome.

Keep an active social schedule.

Read inspirational books about other athletes' injuries.

Work out regularly, incorporating rehabilitation strategies into your training.

Add stretching routines incorporating breathing and relaxation (such as yoga) into your training.

Practice visualization and imagery every day.

Optimum Athletic Performance

Recent research has focused on what makes an athlete most successful and ready for performance. It has been determined that mental attitude plays a large part in optimal performance; many would say it is the difference between an Olympian and a National Qualifier. There are many terms for the mental state that is optimum for athletic functioning: "The Zone" is the term most frequently used. The feelings experienced while in the Zone are closely linked to positive emotions felt before competition such as excitement, anxiety, and arousal. Negative emotions that have also been related to successful sports performance include anger, impatience, nervousness, and irritation. Emotions not associated with the Zone that poorly affect performance include depression, exhaustion, and sorrow.

Physical sensations can also be associated with being in the Zone. Examples of these are hunger, tightness, raciness, irritability, and anxiety. Again, these can vary for different athletes. It has been shown that by trying to remember the emotions felt before a successful athletic performance and repeating these emotions, the Zone is more likely to recur.

The Zone is also known as the "flow" in which all brain and body functions are fully concentrated on the task at hand. Knowing you are willingly facing the particular challenge and greeting it with excitement, will make you happy and allow your mind to work with your body fully to most successfully reach your goal.

Visualization and Imagery

Both visualization and imagery are terms used to describe a mental picture of success. When you visualize, you picture the event in your mind. You picture the last mile of the course, the cheering fans, the finish line. You picture yourself gaining speed and feeling that last "kick." You can also visualize tougher parts of a race and picture yourself running through the pain of exertion, feeling your body work despite its fatigue. Successful athletes often use visualization as part of their training.

In her book, *Peak Fitness for Women,* Paula Newby-Fraser, known as the greatest women's Ironman champion in history, describes "mental training" as an essential component of the last 14 days of training before an Ironman distance triathlon. She also emphasizes the need to focus on doing your best, both in visualization and in thoughts related to the race, rather than comparing yourself to others. This is the basis for a positive experience based on your own performance, not that of others. No matter what the other race participants are doing, you are focused on your strength, your success, and meeting your challenge.

Visualization and imagery are part of all successful athletes' preparation. It is important when you visualize to think these positive thoughts, focusing on yourself and not what others are doing. This is what establishes a feeling of success, self-satisfaction, and happiness.

Pre-Event Calm

Calm is a word to describe a peaceful, composed, serene feeling that allows focus, relaxation, and confidence. Although you might feel eager, energetic, and even anxious to compete in the sport, you are calm enough to make sure your equipment is as it should be, your position and technique is correct, and your mind focused. This is not only a very pleasant way to approach competition, it is also the most effective. If you are calm, your mind and body are in sync and each body movement is on track to help you meet your goal of best performance. This is especially important for success in skill sports such as golf, archery, or tennis.

Some athletes use distraction to keep them calm, focusing on the weather, the scenery, or a song in their head. Others talk, hold a good luck charm, or use deep breathing. If you are a competitive athlete and you put pressure on yourself to perform, you should develop techniques to become calm. Making last-minute race preparation details routine by practicing them can provide a calming ritual. You should also have a strategy for relaxation the night before your athletic event so you can sleep and rest well. A massage, warm bath, pedicure, or other pampering service can also help you feel nurtured and calm before a stressful competition.

Stay Positive

Athletic and fitness events were designed for one reason: fun! If you are not having fun, you might want to think about why. There are many other things in life that are not fun that you have to do; athletics are for enjoyment and improving self-worth and overall health. You must feel positively about the event you have trained so hard for and the workouts you do, or your performance will be disappointing. Having a positive attitude allows you to think more clearly, feel stronger, have less pain, and stay focused and calm. Repeating positive phrases to yourself about your strengths and athletic achievements is an essential part of this satisfaction.

Having a healthy, clear, calm, focused mind promotes your happiness, best performance, and overall health. It improves your confidence, self-esteem, and mental and physical strength. It allows you to rise to challenges that are not just physical as you learn the best coping mechanisms for stress. As a competitive athlete, this is essential to performance. As a regular exerciser, it is essential for life.

CHAPTER THREE

Nutritional Health

Nutritional health provides a foundation for optimum fitness, perfor-mance, and overall health. Excellent nutrition results in more energy, better athletic performance, and less risk of illness. Poor nutrition can cause poor performance, low energy, mental and physical stress, and greater inci-dence of injuries. A balanced diet is achieved by eating healthy foods, plenti-ful nutrients, and adequate calories. Reaching this balance can be challenging, as calorie requirements and weight maintenance are a concern to most women. This is complicated by a confusing number of "miracle" diet and nutrition plans, which can be misleading and unhealthy.

As an active, athletic woman, your body often needs more nutrients than it receives. Most girls and women do not eat enough calcium and also have diets that lack enough iron, zinc, and vitamins D, E, and B, including folate. By knowing your potential deficiencies, you can correct them. You can design your own eating plan with a healthy balance of nutrients, vitamins, minerals, fluids, and adequate calories to enjoy the best food, health, and fitness.

Food Content

The building blocks of foods are carbohydrates, proteins, and fats; however, very few foods are "pure" carbohydrate, protein, or fat. Both natural foods, such as milk, and prepared foods, such as a cheeseburger, are combinations of protein, carbohydrate, and fat. Foods also contain vitamins and minerals, which function in the body as enzymes and regulators of organ and muscle function. Vitamins and minerals are in highest concentration and absorbed best by the body when eaten as they occur naturally in foods.

Balanced nutrition requires eating a wide variety of healthy foods to meet all your needs. Unfortunately, many prepared foods and meals are not well balanced and are high in fats or sugars and low in fiber, vitamins, and minerals. The nutrition profile of the average athletically active female is low in carbohydrates, milk products, red meat, fruits, and vegetables. Understanding the value of these foods or their nutritional equivalents will allow you to correct these deficiencies.

The body needs carbohydrates, proteins, fats, vitamins, minerals, water, and electrolytes on a daily basis to function most effectively. Amounts of carbohydrates, proteins, and fats are measured in grams; one gram is about the weight of a paper clip. Vitamins and minerals are measured in micrograms (mcg), milligrams (mg), or international units (IU). The Food and Drug Administration, through much nutritional research, has standardized Reference Daily Intakes (RDI). Formerly called Recommended Daily Allowances (RDA), these guidelines help to set standards for meeting your nutritional needs to optimize health.

Carbohydrates

Carbohydrates are the best fuel source for muscles, brain, and blood. They are broken down by the digestive system into glucose, which is either stored or released directly into your bloodstream to provide energy for the body. Sugars are the simplest forms of carbohydrates; simple sugars include glucose, sucrose, and fructose. More complex carbohydrates, including starches and fibers, are simple sugars that are bonded with each other. Fiber is an important carbohydrate nutrient; insoluble fiber is not digested but is essential for transporting waste out of the body.

Foods that are primarily carbohydrates include fruits and vegetables, breads, pasta, cereal, and "fat-free" desserts and candy. Reading the food label of a package gives you information about total grams of carbohydrates, including the breakdown of sugar and fiber content. Carbohydrates contain four calories per gram; one gram equals about a quarter teaspoon of sugar.

The Importance of Carbohydrates to Athletes

Glucose is stored in the liver and muscles as glycogen. When the body needs fuel and does not have enough glucose in the bloodstream, it converts this stored glycogen to glucose, which travels in the blood to where fuel is needed. Glycogen is always the first source of energy, and for athletes, is the optimal source of energy, especially during competition or an event. The glycogen-to-glucose breakdown is a simple, quick body process. To improve performance, athletes try to maximize the amount of glycogen their body has available. Glycogen storage can be increased before an event by "carbo-loading" (see Chapter 14, "Exercise Fuel"). The total body storage capacity of glycogen is about 1,500 to 2,000 calories (Kcal)—basically enough energy to live off of for one inactive day or to carry you through 60 to 90 minutes of intense aerobic exercise.

It is recommended that girls and women eat at least 55 percent of their calories as carbohydrates, which can be obtained from healthy servings of fruit, vegetables, bread products, and whole grains or beans. Dairy products also contain carbohydrates. Like all foods, however, there are best, good, and poor types of carbohydrates. Best types of carbohydrates are broken down to glucose more slowly and also contain healthy fiber.

Lately, high-carbohydrate diets have received bad press due to the popularity of "high-protein/low-carbohydrate" diets. This is unfortunate. Research in medicine, nutrition, and exercise physiology repeatedly shows that carbohydrates provide the best fuel for life and athletic performance. Diet plans have been compared, and over the long term, weight is best maintained with high-carbohydrate diets.

The Glycemic Index

Glycemic index, or GI, is an index given to mostly carbohydrate foods based on how quickly they raise blood sugar levels. The index is a number from 0 to 100; the higher the number, the quicker the food reaches the bloodstream as glucose. Sugar has the highest glycemic index (100); soybean one of the lowest (18). Foods with a high glycemic index are often processed, starchy, and sugary foods, although some natural foods, such as honey and watermelon, have high indexes. Foods that contain fat or fiber along with the sugar have lower indexes because the fat and fiber slow the release of glucose.

Athletes in particular can use the glycemic index of foods to determine which types of carbohydrates provide the best fuel before and during events and training. High glycemic index food products such as GU or Cliff Shotz or drinks such as Gatorload or Endurox provide quick sources of energy and are useful in long endurance events in which the body has depleted its glycogen supply. High glycemic index carbohydrates need to be eaten frequently during endurance events lasting more than two hours to maintain blood glucose levels and provide energy. Before competition, low to medium glycemic index foods are recommended to promote steady blood glucose over the next one to two hours (See Chapter 14: Exercise Fuel).

Research has recently suggested that people who regularly eat high glycemic index diets have a greater risk of diabetes, obesity, and heart disease due to a tidal wave of high and low blood sugar levels. High GI foods send a sudden flood of glucose into the blood, which causes the pancreas to release a large amount of insulin, the hormone that transfers blood glucose from the blood and into storage as glycogen or fat. The amount of insulin released corresponds to the amount of blood glucose; high levels of both glucose and insulin can be dangerous to body organs and increase the risk of diabetes. Also, there is a rebound of low blood sugar, which can cause sleepiness, moodiness, irritability, and, in diabetics, coma. Hunger is felt again sooner after high glycemic index foods are eaten due to this low blood sugar.

In contrast, low and medium glycemic index foods cause a slow release of glucose into the bloodstream. Normal amounts of glucose circulate and low amounts of insulin are released in a steady stream. This keeps blood glucose levels stable and protects the body and brain from the dangerous effects of unstable blood sugars. Mood is also stabilized, as brain glucose supplies are constant. In people at risk of diabetes, with a family history or a history of (gestational) diabetes in pregnancy, eating a low to moderate glycemic index diet will reduce the risk of developing diabetes later in life.

The Benefits of Low Glycemic Index Foods

Fewer hunger pangs	Stable energy levels
Steady blood sugars	Less fatigue
Stable mood	Less insulin requirements

Learning to prevent large swings in blood sugars to improve a sense of well-being and performance is a valuable lesson in nutrition. A food's glycemic index can sometimes be surprising: white flour, white bread, and white rice have a high glycemic index, but whole-wheat flour, whole-wheat bread, and brown rice have a lower index. Starchy foods such as white potatoes, corn, and carrots also have a high glycemic index, although sweet potatoes, peas, and celery do not. The best way to incorporate the glycemic index into your lifestyle is to purchase a book that lists common foods (refer to "Resources" at the end of this book). The glycemic index of foods can also be lowered by eating them with foods that slow their digestion, specifically fat, protein, or fiber. For example, eating corn with butter or potatoes with meat lowers the glycemic index. You can also lower glycemic index of pastas and rice by cooking them al dente (firm, not overcooked, and mushy). The following is a chart of some common foods. Basically, low glycemic index foods have GIs less than 55, medium are 55 to 74 and high are 75 to 100.

LOW GI FOODS	MEDIUM GI FOODS	HIGH GI FOODS
Oatmeal 46	Power Bar 58	Jelly beans 80
Yogurt, sweetened 34	Ice cream 61	French bread 95
Meat ravioli 39	Raisins 64	Waffles 76
Soybeans 18	Sweet corn 55	Short-grain white rice 76
Milk 30	White rice 60	Corn flakes 87
Black beans 31	Pizza 62	Baked potato 90
Grapefruit 26	Wheat bread 71	French fries 78
Apple 39	Macaroni and cheese 67	Corn chips 76
Sweet potato 46	Croissant 70	Donut 78
Sponge cake 47	Banana 56	Pretzels 85
Fettucini 34	Chocolate 51	Rice cakes 80
Orange 46	Oatmeal cookie 58	Sugar, honey, 100
Peanuts 15	Popcorn 58	Bagel 75
Thin spaghetti 47	Pita bread 57	Watermelon 75

Fiber

A high-fiber diet has been recognized for years for its health benefits. Dietary fiber content is very important to long-term health. In fact, it has been identified as a necessary diet nutrient by the Food and Drug Administration (FDA). Fiber is a natural plant product that helps slow digestion, lowering glycemic indexes of foods. Fiber has also been identified for its many health prevention benefits, particularly reduced risk of breast cancer, colon cancer, diabetes, heart disease, constipation, diverticulosis, stroke, hypertension, and obesity.

The Reference Daily Intake (RDI) for fiber, based on a 2,000-calorie diet, is 25 grams/day. This should be your minimum. Because large amounts of fiber, especially if your digestive system is not used to it, can cause bloating, stomach upset, and diarrhea, increasing the overall amount of fiber in your diet should be done gradually with fiber distributed evenly throughout meals and snacks. Products such as Beano can help with gas and bloating if that is a problem. Eating various sources of fiber daily—such as popcorn, fresh and dried fruits, vegetables, nuts, beans, and whole grains is also recommended. You should also drink plenty of water with fiber, because this will make your stomach feel full for longer. Because of the cleansing effect fiber has on the digestive tract and bowels, avoid high-fiber products the night before, morning of, and during events, unless your body is used to a high-fiber diet.

The Health Benefits of a High-Fiber Diet

Decreases breast cancer

Decreases colon cancer

Decreases cholesterol

Prevents and manages diabetes

Prevents heart disease

Prevents constipation

Prevents diverticulosis

Helps prevent stroke

Prevents high blood pressure

Helps prevent obesity

Helps you feel full longer

Proteins

Proteins are essential for the body to build and repair muscle and tissues and produce enzymes and hormones, which keep the body regulated. Proteins are made up of combinations of several of the 20 types of amino acids. Some of these amino acids can be reused by the body, but almost half of them must be eaten on a regular basis; these are called "essential amino acids." Although proteins are best used by the body as building blocks for muscle tissue and hormones, they can also serve as an energy source if glycogen levels are low. They provide four calories per gram.

Vegetarians, especially vegans (who do not eat dairy, eggs, or fish) tend to have lower protein in their diets, sometimes lacking essential amino acids. In order to fully meet their protein needs, they can obtain complete proteins by combining grains (corn and wheat) and legumes (nuts, beans, and seeds) in their diet. These foods have additional benefits of having cancer- and disease-fighting properties. Vegetarian diets are quite healthy if followed intelligently to make sure protein (and calcium) needs are not neglected. Vegetarians who do not eat fish, dairy, or eggs should eat at least two servings daily from each of these food groups: legumes, grains, and nuts and seeds.

Vegans Must Eat at Least Two Servings Daily of Each of the Following

Legumes—dried beans and peas, soybeans, tofu, peanuts, peanut butter

Grains—cereals, breads, pasta, corn, rice, wheat

Nuts and seeds—cashews, almonds, sunflower seeds, walnuts, pumpkin seeds

---

There are benefits to meat, poultry, and dairy sources of protein, as they have other valuable nutrients. Red meat is the most optimal source of iron, an essential mineral often deficient in active women. It also contains B vitamins, zinc, folic acid, and complete proteins. Actually, many of the nutrients in meat (iron, folic acid, vitamin B_6, and zinc) are the same that are lacking most in women's diets. Red meat and fish also contain creatine, a building block of energy molecules. Fish is an excellent protein, as it contains healthy omega-3 fatty acids, which reduce heart disease and stroke, and is recommended to be eaten twice weekly.

Good Sources of Protein

Red meat	Eggs
Poultry	Legumes, tofu
Fish	Nuts and seeds
Dairy products	Certain whole grains

There has been some controversy regarding contaminants such as hormones, antibiotics, and bacterial or viral diseases associated with meat, poultry, and fish sources of protein. Hormones are fed to some chicken and cattle to increase size and decrease fat, and antibiotics are used liberally to prevent diseases. There are no specific dangers to eating these foods in small amounts, but there are some theories that in large quantities they can lead to food allergies or interfere with growth in younger children. If you are concerned about these risks, purchase meats and dairy products labeled "organic"; these are required to be free of hormones and antibiotics. Many milk, egg, and meat products are now labeled specifically as hormone-free or antibiotic-free.

Fish, although one of the healthiest proteins, can also be harmful especially to women planning pregnancy. Certain types of large fish, including swordfish, tilefish, large tuna steaks, and mackerel should not eaten more than once monthly due to their higher mercury content, which interferes with brain development in unborn and young children. These fish should be avoided for the first year prior to planning a pregnancy. Raw fish and shellfish can also transmit parasites and hepatitis A.

Food preparation is another concern. Fully cooking meats is recommended to kill any potential bacteria or diseases and is always recommended when preparing poultry. Eating blackened food is not recommended, as the charring has been linked to stomach and intestinal cancer.

Most girls and women actually eat enough protein, as it is found in many sources other than meat or fish. Tofu, nuts, peanut butter, cheese, milk, yogurt, and dried peas and beans are good sources of proteins. Some whole-grain breads and pastas also have protein. Many food and energy bars now contain protein as well. Athletic and active women require 1.4g to 1.8g/kg/day (.7 to .9 g/lb/day) to make up 20 to 25 percent of the diet. For an average 140-pound woman, this equals 100 to 126 grams of protein daily. (A three ounce serving of chicken contains 30 grams.)

Because most women's protein needs are easily met, there is no need for protein or amino acid supplements. These are expensive, put a strain on the kidneys, and cause dehydration and bone loss. They are also often combined with other chemicals, which can be dangerous.

The Pitfalls of Protein and Amino Acid Supplements

Overload kidneys

Cause dehydration

Cause calcium loss

Are expensive

Are ineffective

Are often combined with other unhealthy ingredients

Fats

Fats are a necessary building block of nutrition and are broken down into fatty acids. The most essential fatty acids that must be supplied by foods are linoleic and linolenic acid, essential for transporting the fat-soluble vitamins A, D, E, and K. Fatty acids also help in energy production, the chemical balance of hormones, and nerve and brain function. In the body, fat cushions vital organs, including the eyes, liver, and heart, and also provides insulation against heat loss. Fat is also a very efficient long-term storage site for fuel, providing nine calories per gram.

Fat's bad reputation comes from its high calorie content, which can lead to obesity if eaten in large amounts. Saturated fats found in meat and poultry have a legitimately bad reputation because they contain harmful cholesterol. What contains "bad" cholesterol, however, seems to change almost daily. It used to be thought that eggs, high-fat cheese, and butter fats were very bad for the heart, blood vessels, and arteries. Now these products have been found to also contain healthy fatty acids that are beneficial when eaten in moderation (one egg and one or two servings of butter fat foods a day).

The greatest risk of "bad" fats are due to trans-fatty acids and saturated fats, which increase risk of cardiovascular (heart and blood vessel) disease and stroke. Trans-fatty acids found in stick margarine, shortening, and many snack foods are processed oils that become unhealthy in the chemical processing they go through. Saturated fats are found in high amounts in fatty meats, especially pork fat and rinds, beef fat and lard, and chicken fat and skin. Processed meats, including sausages, hot dogs, and pepperoni, should be avoided as much as possible, as they not only contain very high amounts of saturated fats, but also nitrates, a cancer-causing chemical.

Saturated fats can be avoided by choosing lean cuts of meat (sirloin and tenderloin), avoiding poultry skin and fat, and avoiding foods made with lard or beef, pork, or chicken fat. Full-fat dairy products should be eaten in moderation due to their higher content of saturated fats. Butter is somewhat controversial. Because it is a saturated animal fat, until recently, butter was considered unhealthy, and stick margarine was thought to be a healthier alternative. However, current research reveals that stick margarine is actually the worst type of spread (it is a trans fat). In contrast, butter has been found to contain conjugated linoleic acid, a healthy essential fatty acid. Therefore, eating a serving of butter a day is fine and is a much healthier choice than stick margarine. For those with high cholesterol and heart disease, using soft "buttery spreads" containing monounsaturated or polyunsaturated fats is the best choice, especially soft spreads containing plant products that assist in lowering cholesterol. (Take Control, Benecol, Smart Balance).

The most important research has shown that healthy fats, such as omega-3 fatty acids and monounsaturated and polyunsaturated fats, actually protect the heart from disease by raising the level of the good cholesterol, HDL. This makes certain fats some of the heart-healthiest foods. Heart-healthy fats include peanut butter, avocados, nuts, olive and peanut oil, and fish oil. Omega-3 fatty acids have also been shown to prevent some cancers.

Cutting all fats out of your diet is never recommended, especially for active athletic women, because fats are an essential part of hormone functioning, vitamin transport, and disease protection. Fats also promote a feeling of fullness and satisfaction from meals, reduce cravings for unhealthy foods, and allow carbohydrates to be digested more slowly, stabilizing blood sugar levels. Fat-containing foods such as meat, poultry, and dairy products provide natural sources of necessary nutrients especially important to women: iron, folate, and B vitamins in meats and calcium in dairy products. Fats should make up 20 to 30 percent of your regular diet.

Healthy Fats

CLASSIFICATIONS	EXAMPLES
Monounsaturated fats	olive, safflower, canola, peanut oils, nuts, seeds, avocados, olives, very lean meats and poultry
Polyunsaturated fats	cold-water fish sunflower, corn, soybean, safflower, flaxseed, grapeseed, cottonseed, sesame, walnut oils, soy products, wheat germ, whole grains

Healthy Fats That Are Good Sources of Omega-3 Fatty Acids

Soybean oil

Flaxseed oil

Flaxseeds

Walnuts

Walnut oil

Fish oil

Canola oil

Cold-water fish, including salmon, sardines, lake trout, tuna (albacor, bluefin), oysters, squid, mackerel, swordfish*

Omega-3 enriched eggs

*Sardines, large tuna steaks, mackerel, swordfish, and oysters contain higher mercury and PCB levels; in pregnancy, eat these no more than once a month. (Canned tuna, especially albacore, can be eaten twice a week.)

Unhealthy Fats That Should Be Eaten Sparingly

CLASSIFICATIONS	EXAMPLES
Trans-fatty acids	hydrogenated and partially hydrogenated oil, stick margarine, shortening
Saturated fats	lard, animal fat, full-fat dairy products, palm and palm kernel oil, coconut oil

Vitamins

Vitamins are organic nutrients that function as enzymes and regulators of important chemical reactions in the body. Vitamin deficiencies can result in diseases and problems with certain body structures and functions. Vitamins are either water or fat soluble. Water-soluble vitamins are not stored by the body, and, therefore, have less risk of overdose and more risk of deficiency. Because fat-soluble vitamins are stored (in fat), it is possible to overdose, causing liver damage. Studies have shown that athletic, active women do not get enough vitamins B, D, and E through their diet.

TYPE	VITAMIN	FUNCTION
Fat soluble	A	vision, skin, hormones
	D	bones and calcium
	E	prevents cell damage
	K	blood clotting
Water soluble	B	metabolism
	C	healing, connective tissues

Fat-Soluble Vitamins

The fat-soluble vitamins include A, D, E, and K. Vitamin A is important for night vision, skin, and hormone regulation and is found in milk, butter, and eggs. Beta-carotene is a building block of vitamin A that has cancer-fighting properties, but only when eaten from food sources. Beta-carotene supplements are not recommended as studies have shown that high doses may actually increase certain cancer risks. Healthy natural sources of beta carotene include leafy greens and orange-colored fruits and vegetables (cantaloupe, squash, carrots, sweet potatoes).

Vitamin D is essential to women because it acts as a hormone that aids in bone building and calcium absorption. Vitamin D can be made by your body cells through sun exposure; 15 minutes of direct sun (not through sunscreen or glass) on your face and hands daily will allow your body to make enough. Vitamin D is found in egg yolks, saltwater fish, and liver and is added to most milk and milk products.

Vitamin E is well known as an antioxidant that can prevent cancer and prevent cell damage including damage to blood cells and muscle tissue during exercise, so it is important to exercising women. It is found in vegetable oils, nuts, beans, and green leafy vegetables.

Vitamin K is important for blood clotting and also regulates calcium.

Water-Soluble Vitamins

Vitamin C is necessary for muscle, bone, and soft tissue health. It also helps wound healing and immunity and is an antioxidant that has cancer-fighting properties. Vitamin C is found in orange juice and citrus fruits, tomatoes, strawberries, and red, orange, and yellow bell peppers. Vitamin C aids the absorption of iron. At least 60 milligrams of vitamin C should be obtained through foods or drinks daily.

The B vitamins are important for energy metabolism. B vitamins are also known as the "stress" vitamins, because the body needs them for repair and higher function in times of stress or illness. Important B vitamins to women are folate, which helps prevent anemia and birth defects in pregnancy, and vitamin B_6, which is important to nerves, hemoglobin, and antibodies. B_6 can also improve mood and help with PMS. B_{12} is also important for nerves and blood cell formation. Thiamin, riboflavin, and niacin are involved in energy metabolism and are needed at higher doses also during times of high activity. It is common for active and athletic women to not consume enough B vitamins.

Minerals

Minerals are inorganic chemical nutrients that perform vital roles in the body. The important minerals for women include calcium, iron, magnesium, and zinc. Unfortunately, many women's diets are deficient in these important minerals. Other minerals required in much lower quantities include phosphorus, copper, selenium, manganese, and chromium.

Important Minerals and Their Function

MINERAL	FUNCTION
Calcium	bone building
Iron	carries oxygen in blood
Magnesium	muscles, nerves, bones
Zinc	metabolism, growth, immunity

Calcium is one of the most important minerals for women. It is essential not only for bone strength and health, but is also needed for heart, muscle, nerve, enzymes, and blood clotting. Calcium is required by the body as the building material for bones, and low dietary calcium is directly linked to osteoporosis. Because calcium is constantly needed to rebuild bone and also for other body functions, it must be replenished daily. The body loses calcium in nails, hair, skin, sweat, urine, and stool. Athletic women lose extra calcium through sweat, and women on high-protein diets or those who drink several carbonated beverages daily also lose calcium more quickly (see chapter 5, "Bone Health and Osteoporosis").

Unless you are a real dairy-product lover, it is tough to get enough calcium without eating calcium fortified foods or taking supplements. Other natural sources include almonds, broccoli, kale, canned salmon, sardines, spinach, and dried peas or beans.

Calcium is available as supplements in compound form, including calcium carbonate, found in antacids; calcium phosphate, found in cereals and food bars; and calcium citrate, the most efficient form of calcium supplement for your body and the type recommended if taken with iron. The recommended amount of calcium for women is 1,200 to 1,500 milligrams a day. This translates to at least four calcium-rich products a day such as yogurt, milk, cheese, or calcium-fortified food. If you are taking calcium supplements, try to take them in the evening in split doses (dinner and bedtime) to promote absorption. If you are taking iron supplements, choose calcium citrate instead of carbonate to improve absorption of both minerals.

It is very important to have a diet with enough calcium. Practical advice for all girls and women is to take one 600 milligram calcium supplement before bedtime to replace calcium-rich foods not eaten during the day. If dairy products are not eaten regularly, try to drink calcium-fortified juices or other calcium products (check labels for content). Calcium also has other added benefits, including easing symptoms of PMS, preventing muscle cramps, and improving weight loss success.

Iron

Iron is involved in all body cell functions. It plays the very important role of transporting oxygen throughout the body in red blood cells. Women are at greater risk of low iron levels due to menstruation; athletes also tend to have lower levels of iron because it is broken down with exertional exercise and lost through the kidneys, digestive system, and sweat. Women should get 18 milligrams of iron daily, and needs go up in pregnancy. The best sources of iron are meat, poultry, fish, eggs, fortified foods, and foods cooked in an iron skillet. Nonmeat sources include wheat germ, whole grains, green leafy vegetables, and dried fruits. There are also many iron-fortified cereals and foods available.

Iron supplements, other than those found in a multivitamin, should not be taken unless prescribed by a doctor. If you are required to take iron supplements, ask your doctor for a ferrous gluconate formula, as this tends to have less constipating and digestive system side effects. Iron absorption is improved when taken with a source of vitamin C and is made worse with caffeine products.

Magnesium

Magnesium helps regulate glycogen (thought to prevent diabetes), regulates body calcium, and aids in muscle, nerve, and body enzyme function, playing a role in preventing fatigue. Magnesium can help relieve muscle cramps and also helps with symptoms of PMS. Magnesium has also been found to prevent hypertension, hardening of the arteries, and can also help prevent migraines. Magnesium is found naturally in hard tap water, spinach, beans, whole grains, nuts, seafood, meats, and chocolate (it can help prevent chocolate cravings in PMS).

Zinc

Zinc helps metabolize nutrients and allows growth and immune function. It also affects hormones. Zinc is needed in higher doses during growth, pregnancy, and with athletic activity. Zinc is found in meats, seafood, and milk products, and absorption is inhibited by fiber; therefore, vegetarians are at particular risk of having low zinc levels. Women should get 12 milligrams of zinc per day.

Water and Electrolytes

Water is essential for life and activity. Water is necessary for transporting nutrients in the blood, digesting and excreting nutrients, providing the structure to your body cells, regulating temperature, lubricating joints and organs, and protecting the brain and spinal cord.

Water must be replaced in large amounts daily and is the number one nutrient needed to survive. Athletic and physical activity requires water; sweating requires more. Dehydration is the term used to describe low water levels in the body. Signs of dehydration include thirst, weight loss, weakness, fatigue, loss of appetite, dry mouth, small amounts of dark-colored urine, headaches, poor concentration, overheating, and, ultimately, whole body collapse.

Water or juices in plentiful amounts is the best fluid source for your body. Water can also be absorbed by the body in foods (soups, melons, and vegetables). It is recommended that at least eight, 8 ounce water or juice drinks are consumed each day, in addition to drinking that makes up for sweat lost during a workout. (For specifics on fluid recommendations during exercise, see chapter 14, "Exercise Fuel.") Caffeine, alcohol, and some stimulants found in "energy drinks" are diuretics and cause your body to lose water (resulting in more urination); therefore, these drinks should not be considered part of your minimum daily fluid needs.

Electrolytes

Because the blood is full of molecules, the correct ratio of molecules to water must be maintained in order to keep the blood flowing and allow for transport of nutrients in and out of cells. Much of this transport follows gradients across cell membranes. Electrolytes facilitate these gradients via chemical interactions between molecules; thus, electrolytes maintain proper body fluid levels and transportation of essential nutrients. Electrolytes are lost through sweat, urine, and digestion and must be replenished daily. Sports drinks are formulated to replenish electrolytes. The most important electrolytes are sodium and potassium.

Sodium is necessary for maintaining water in the blood and for regulating nerve and muscle activity. It is lost in sweat and must be replenished with exercise that lasts more than 60 minutes, or sooner if exercising in high temperatures. Low sodium levels can cause drowsiness, weakness, cramping, and confusion. Endurance athletes who drink water without sodium during long events can develop serious illness. Sodium is found in many natural and most processed foods.

Potassium also plays a role in muscle and nerve activation and also functions in glucose transport and glycogen storage. Potassium is lost in sweat; low potassium can cause muscle weakness and fatigue, and in severe cases, affect heart rhythm. Potassium is found in fresh fruits and vegetables.

Special Diets

Special dietary restrictions or limitations require greater attention to nutrition. Medical conditions or illnesses might also require special diets or supplementation. If you experience any of these, consulting a nutritionist is recommended.

Diabetes

Diabetes requires careful maintenance of blood sugar, through blood monitoring and controlled diet. Blood sugar monitoring should be done as recommended by your doctor and also during exercise, especially if the exercise is for more than 30 minutes. You should always have a high glycemic index food available in case you develop hypoglycemia (low blood sugar) and maintain your low to medium glycemic index diet with regularly scheduled meals. The best nutritionist for you is a certified diabetes educator. It is highly recommended you consult a nutritionist if you are diabetic, as your nutritional needs are beyond the scope of this book.

Illness

If you have an illness with fever, you will likely have to replenish the electrolytes potassium and sodium due to sweating. Similarly, gastrointestinal illness causing vomiting or diarrhea requires additional electrolytes; good ways to replenish are by drinking sports drinks. If you are taking antibiotics, increasing your daily intake of yogurt will help protect the normal bacteria in the bowels and prevent you from developing diarrhea. You must take a multivitamin during times of illness, as more vitamins are needed for the body's healing and stress response. An additional B complex and vitamin C can also be helpful. Avoid working out if you have fever, vomiting, or diarrhea.

If you regularly suffer from irritable bowel syndrome or frequent diarrhea, you need to consider replenishing your electrolytes and drink extra fluids. A higher-fiber, lower-fat diet with smaller, more frequent meals can help regulate you.

Lactose Intolerance

Lactose intolerance is the inability to digest lactose, the sugar that naturally occurs in milk and milk products. Babies are born with the enzymes necessary to digest lactose, but some adults outgrow it. With lactose intolerance, diarrhea and gas result after eating dairy products. Diarrhea can cause dehydration and loss of electrolytes, so these should be replenished. Lactose intolerance can be managed through pills that help digestion, such as Lactaid, or dairy products that contain the enzymes. If you cannot eat dairy products due to lactose intolerance you are unable to correct, make sure you are getting calcium through fortified foods and juices, or taking supplements to equal four servings per day. Soy milk is an alternative but is not usually as high in calcium as dairy products, so check the label.

Vegetarian Diets

Vegetarians must be very attentive to their diets, especially the amount of calcium and protein they take in. Although vegetarian diets are high in vitamins and fiber, they tend to be low in iron, calcium, and magnesium. Vegans, those who eat plant products only, must include two servings daily of beans or soy, grains, and nuts or seeds in order to ensure adequate protein combinations. They must also eat calcium-fortified foods or take calcium supplements to fulfill the 1,200 milligrams-a-day requirement.

Pregnancy

Nutritional needs increase in pregnancy. Folate supplements should be taken when planning a pregnancy to prevent birth defects that can develop early in the development of the fetus, even before a woman learns she is pregnant. Most prenatal vitamins contain 600 to 1000 micrograms of folate, more than the RDI of 400 micrograms a day. Calcium needs increase to at least 1,300 milligrams daily and iron to 30 milligrams a day. After the first trimester, calorie needs increase by 300 to 500 calories a day, and more if you are exercising. Protein needs also increase slightly. Fluid needs increase dramatically, and water should be always available (see chapter 15, "Pregnancy Fitness," for more information).

Weight and Percent Body Fat

Weight and BMI

Three values are commonly used to measure your body composition. Weight, the most common standard, is cheap, convenient, and fairly reliable, although it can fluctuate up to five pounds with body fluids. Weight and height are used to calculate the Body Mass Index (BMI), another common term. This differs only from weight in that it adjusts for height; BMI also varies with body fluids. BMI, measured in kilograms per meters squared, is an unreliable guideline; standards usually do not differentiate between men and women or allow for the difference in muscle or fat content. In athletic women, BMI is especially inaccurate because muscle weight is heavier than fat weight, making you seem "fat" by BMI standards. Essentially, Body Mass Index is a number value that has replaced height and weight charts. The number is even more confusing because the recommended numbers are similar to but slightly different from body fat percent. According to standard guidelines,

BMI over 30 is considered obese, under 18, extremely underweight, and between 18 and 25, normal.

Body Fat Percentile

Body fat percentile provides the most accurate estimate of body composition. Body fat percentile is an indication of the percent of your body that is made of fat. Normal body fat percent for women is 20 to 30 (for men it is lower). In women, below 17 is extreme low body fat; between 30 to 33, high body fat; and above 34, extremely high body fat or obese. The recommended healthy body fat percentiles increase slightly with age.

Body Fat Standards for Women Recommended by Age Group					
	20 TO 29	30 TO 39	40 TO 49	50 TO 59	69+
Very low	<16	<17	<18	<19	<20
Low	16–19	17–20	18–21	19–22	20–23
Optimal	20–28	21–29	22–30	23–31	24–32
Moderately high	29–31	30–32	31–33	32–33	33–35
High	>31	>32	>33	>34	>35

Body fat percentile measurement methods vary in practicality, cost and accuracy. The most accurate measurement is through DEXA, an expensive measurement done in a radiology lab or doctor's office; this is the same radiographic measurement used to determine bone density. The second most accurate method is water displacement, although this requires your body to be underwater in a special tank, even more impractical and expensive. One of the simplest, most common measures of body fat percentile measurement is skinfold measurements, in which a tester uses calipers to measure fat pinches at various sites on the body. This evaluation is very dependent on the tester's skills; if done by an experienced tester, it can be up to 3 percent accurate. The other common method is bioelectric impedence; this is a machine that looks like a scale and is common in many gyms and even available for home use. This can be a very unreliable measure, as it is highly dependent on water weight, temperature, electrolytes, blood flow, and other factors. Bioelectric impedence is even less accurate in athletes with a large amount of muscle.

All these measurements are interesting and can suggest health, but should not be the basis of an exercise or nutrition regime. Remember, if you are using weight as your guide, that muscle weighs more than fat. If you are increasing strength but not changing your weight, you are becoming leaner. The following are loose guidelines for healthy weights in athletic women. The lower numbers are for petite, small-boned, less-muscled frames; the higher numbers accommodate for large bones and bigger muscle size.

Healthy Weight Guidelines for Muscular, Athletic Women (BMI 18 to 25)

HEIGHT (INCHES)	RECOMMENDED WEIGHT (POUNDS)
4'10"	95 to 123
4'11"	98 to 128
5'	101 to 132
5'1"	105 to 136
5'2"	108 to 141
5'3"	112 to 146
5'4"	115 to 150
5'5"	119 to 155
5'6"	123 to 160
5'7"	126 to 165
5'8"	130 to 170
5'9"	134 to 175
5'10"	138 to 180
5'11"	142 to 185
6'	147 to 190
6'1"	152 to 196
6'2"	157 to 201

Weight Loss or Gain

The best weight changes are made slowly. The slower changes are made, the more likely your body will maintain the change, as it has a tendency to return to its "steady state," or the weight it has been at for the longest. A pound is gained by eating 3,500 calories more than your body burns. To lose this pound, 3,500 fewer calories need to be eaten or 3,500 more burned off. The best way to gain or lose is change your dietary calorie intake by 500 kcal a day. This should equal a one pound weight loss or gain per week. Keeping a food diary for seven days can make you more aware of your eating habits and strategize change in a healthy way. Nutritionists and support groups can be very helpful in reaching goals for weight changes. (See Chapter 4, "Weight Concerns and Body Image," for more on diets.)

Calorie Guidelines

Calorie counting can be a source of frustration and focus for many girls and women. Although formulas have been standardized, calories might need to be adjusted for each individual based on genetics, amount of muscle or fat, and other activity in addition to athletic activities. The amount of calories required to maintain weight for one woman can be more or less than for another; and, just like sleep, training, and other aspects of life, the amounts can never be exact, as all bodies are different. Still, estimates of calorie needs can provide helpful guidelines.

Nutritionists have devised various complicated formulas for estimating calorie needs. The standards are all in kilograms (kg) of body weight, which can be converted as 1 kg= 2.2 pounds. There are three formulas commonly used by nutritionists, the Harris Benedict, the Total Energy Expenditure Method, and Activity Factors. The first two formulas do not account for additional calories burned in exercise, and they should only be used as a guideline for basic calorie needs.

Harris Benedict Equation

Daily calories (kcal) = 447.6 + 9.2 (Weight in kg) + 3.1 (Height in cm) −4.3 (age) × 1.7

Total Energy Expenditure Method

Daily calories (kcal) = Weight in kg × 40 kcal/kg

To make it easier and more specific to your athletic activity level, measure your weight in pounds by the following numbers based on activity level. Light, for which you multiply your body weight by 13, implies 20 to 30 minutes total aerobic activity a day (heart rate at 65 to 80 percent). Moderate, a factor of 16, implies 45 to 60 minutes of aerobic activity a day. Heavy, a factor of 19, implies 75 to 90 minutes. Exceptional, a factor of 22, implies more than 2 hours a day.

Activity Factor
Daily Calories = Weight in lbs. × Activity Factor (AF)

Calories Required at Various Body Weights, Based on Activity Level				
WEIGHT POUNDS	LIGHT AF* = 13, LIGHT	MODERATE AF* = 16, MODERATE	HEAVY AF* = 19, HEAVY	EXCEPTIONAL AF* = 22, EXCEPTIONAL
115	1,495	1,840	2,185	2,530
120	1,560	1,920	2,280	2,640
125	1,625	2,000	2,375	2,750
130	1,690	2,080	2,470	2,860
135	1,755	2,160	2,565	2,970
140	1,820	2,240	2,660	3,080
145	1,885	2,320	2,755	3,190
150	1,950	2,400	2,850	3,300
155	2,015	2,480	2,945	3,410
160	2,080	2,560	3,040	3,520
165	2,145	2,640	3,135	3,630
170	2,210	2,720	3,230	3,740
175	2,275	2,800	3,325	3,850
180	2,340	2,880	3,420	3,960
185	2,405	2,960	3,515	4,070

Modern technology also makes it possible to have your baseline calorie burning rate measured. This test is now being done in some health clubs. It is done by monitoring breathing to measure oxygen used during a short time. This gives an estimate of your basal metabolic rate, or how many calories your body burns in a day of rest. Unless this testing is done in a specific physiology lab, the results can vary, and, just like the formulas on previous pages, should be used only as a guideline. The healthiest assessment of body composition, weight, and appropriate caloric intake and activity levels specific for you are made with the combined efforts of your physician and nutritionist. It is highly recommended to consult with both of these health professionals if you are seeking help with weight changes.

A Balanced Diet

The ideal diet for an active woman includes 50 to 60 percent carbohydrates, 20 to 30 percent protein, and 20 to 30 percent fats. To fulfill your vitamin and mineral requirements, a multivitamin is always recommended, and if you do not eat at least four servings of dairy or calcium-fortified foods a day, add a calcium supplement. The best brands are those made by reputable drug companies. (For information on the quality of your vitamin or supplement, see "Resources" at the end of this book.)

Essential Components of a Healthy Diet

50 to 60 percent carbohydrates

20 to 30 percent protein

20 to 30 percent fat

Enough calories

A daily multivitamin

Four servings of calcium-rich foods or supplements

To make it easy, the following chart breaks down the recommended calories and grams (in parentheses) of each nutrient required for a diet that is 55 percent carbohydrate, 25 percent protein, and 20 percent fat. These numbers are only guidelines, not strict dietary rules, and should be adjusted if you require extra carbohydrates for training (eat slightly less fats and proteins).

Guidelines for a Healthy Athletic Diet

TOTAL CAL/D	PROTEIN CAL(G)—25%	FAT CAL(G)—20%	CARBO CAL(G)/DAY— 55%
1,200	300 (75)	240 (27)	660 (165)
1,500	375 (94)	300 (33)	825 (206)
1,800	450 (113)	360 (40)	990 (248)
2,000	500 (125)	400 (44)	1,100 (275)
2,200	550 (138)	440 (49)	1,210 (303)
2,400	600 (150)	480 (53)	1,320 (330)
2,600	650 (163)	520 (58)	1,430 (358)
2,800	700 (175)	560 (62)	1,540 (385)
3,000	750 (188)	600 (67)	1,650 (413)
3,200	800 (200)	640 (71)	1,760 (440)
3,400	850 (213)	680 (76)	1,870 (468)
3,600	900 (225)	720 (80)	1,980 (495)
3,800	950 (238)	760 (84)	2,090 (523)

Food Labels and the FDA

Reference Daily Intake(RDI) and Percent Daily Value (%DV)

Food labels provide information on the nutritional value of food products and compares them to the standards established by the Food and Drug Administration (FDA). RDI is the number amount recommended for each nutrient in daily consumption. %DV represents the amount of the nutrients a food provides of the days total RDI. Food labels have recently been updated to have even more useful information regarding content. The label has everything important about the food—how big a serving is, how many calories, fats, saturated fats, carbohydrates including sugars and fiber, protein, and vitamin and mineral content it contains. The content is listed not only in gram amount, but also as a percent of the recommended amount (%DV) for an average 2,000-calorie diet based on 60 percent energy from carbohydrates, 10 percent from protein, and 30 percent from fats. (Note these are higher in fat content and lower in protein than the recommended athletic diet.) This 2,000-calorie diet is an established norm that is the basis for the RDI (formerly called the RDA), nutrient values recommended for the average American man and woman.

To compare the FDA's recommended diet with that recommended for you as a healthy athletic woman, as described in the previous section, you should double the amount of protein, lower the amount of fat, and increase the amount of calcium by half. Regarding vitamin and mineral recommendations, the FDA's RDIs are slightly low for folate, iron, and calcium. As is shown in the following chart, this can be corrected by taking a daily multivitamin. If you eat a well-balanced diet, a regular multivitamin will do fine, or you can choose from the many brands of multivitamins marketed for women, which have slightly more iron, folate, and calcium, or multivitamins marketed for "stress," or "performance," which have increased amounts of B vitamins. Being aware of recommended doses not only keeps you healthy, but also will prevent toxic vitamin overdoses.

Recommended Vitamin and Mineral Amounts for Active Women, Content of "Centrum Performance" Multivitamin, and Maximum Healthy Dose

		RECOM-MENDED	IN CENTRUM	MAXIMUM DOSE
FAT-SOLUBLE VITAMINS*	Vitamin A	5,000 IU	5,000 IU	10,000 IU
	Vitamin K	90 mcg	25***	****
	Vitamin E	30 IU (9 mg)	30 IU	1,000 mg
	Vitamin D	400 IU	400 IU	2,000 IU
WATER-SOLUBLE VITAMINS	Vitamin C	75 mg	60 mg	2 g
	Thiamin	1.5 mg	1.5 mg	****
	Riboflavin	1.7 mg	1.7 mg	****
	Niacin	20 mg	20 mg	35 mg
B VITAMINS	B_6	50 mg	2 mg	200 mg
	Folate	400 mcg	400 mcg	1,000 mcg
	B_{12}	50 mcg	6 mcg	100 mcg
	Biotin	300 mcg	30 mcg	10 mg
	Pantothenic Acid	10 mg	10 mg	10 g

MINERALS	Calcium**	1,000 mg**	162 mg**	2,500 mg
	Magnesium	600 mg	100 mg	****
	Iron	18 mg	18 mg	45 mg
	Zinc	15 mg	15 mg	40 mg

*Fat-soluble vitamins are stored by the body and can be overdosed (vs. water-soluble).
**The standards for calcium intake and content of Centrum are lower than the female athlete's needs.
***Do not supplement extra vitamin K.
****Not established.

Food Labels

Each food label includes the %DV (percent daily value), indicating the amount one serving contains of saturated fat, cholesterol, and sodium. It is always wise to be aware of amount of saturated fat and cholesterol in your diet, especially if you are at risk of heart disease or have high cholesterol. If you have high blood pressure, you also need to limit your sodium intake. As an exercising woman without risks of heart disease or high blood pressure, you probably do not need to restrict sodium intake, as it is lost easily through sweat, and you can be more liberal with fat and cholesterol.

The FDA has also set standards for foods that make claims to their fat-, calorie-, and sugar-free content. "Calorie-free" means less than 5 calories per serving, and "sugar-free" and "fat-free" mean less than .5 g per serving. For other common terms on food labels, see the following chart.

Labeling Terms

Low saturated fat = 1 g or less per serving

Low sodium = 140 mg or less per serving

Very low sodium = 35 mg or less

Low cholesterol = 20 mg or less and 2 g or less of saturated fat

Low calorie = 40 cal or less

Fat and Cholesterol Content of Meat, Poultry, and Seafood, per 100 g serving

Lean = less than 10 g total fat, 4.5 g or less saturated fat, less than 95 mg cholesterol

Extra lean = less than 5 g total fat, less than 2 g saturated fat, and less than 95 mg cholesterol

Other Common Labeling Terms

High = contains 20 percent or more of the %DV of a nutrient

Good source* = contains 10 to 19 percent of the %DV of a nutrient

Reduced/less/fewer = 25 percent less fat/sodium/sugar/calories than the regular product

Light = one-third fewer calories or half the fat or sodium in low-cal or low-fat product

Healthy = low in fat, cholesterol, sodium, and contain at least 90% of %DV vitamins A or C, iron, calcium, protein, or fiber.

*Beware of "good sources" of calcium. They only contain 100 to 190 mg each.

Calcium is a very important reason to read labels. Note that a "good source" is a very misleading term, as these foods are only required to contain 10 percent of the Reference Daily Intake, 100 mg. For active athletic women, the actual recommended intake of calcium should be at least 1,200 mg a day, so do not think that because you ate a "good source" of calcium that your calcium needs have been met. You would actually need to eat 12 "good sources" a day to meet all your calcium requirements!

Also, there are some food labels that claim that the food lowers risk of coronary heart disease. This means that the food is low in both overall and saturated fat and cholesterol and essentially qualifys as "extra lean." Food labels that claim to lower cancer risks include foods that are low in saturated fat and are also a "good source" of fiber or vitamins A or C. The FDA also has requirements for restaurants that make claims to have healthful foods, providing guidelines and standards for their meals. The U.S. Department of Agriculture (USDA) regulates meat and poultry products.

Supplements are not regulated by FDA; therefore, there are no requirements or standards to establish or measure safety, effect, or potency. You are more likely to find a safer supplement by buying a product made by a company that makes other FDA-regulated products (such as a large drug company) or has a USP label. The USP (United States Pharmocopeia) is a governing body that regulates the safety and efficacy of supplements. You can also go to www.consumerlab.com to see a safety rating on many supplements.

The best recommendation is to eat a minimum of four servings of fruits, four vegetables, four dairy, three protein (tofu, nuts, meat, fish), two whole grains, three fats, and four breads daily. You should drink at least eight, 8-ounce glasses of water, juice, or sport drinks. If you can do this, you will meet all your nutritional needs. Taking one multivitamin daily along with one calcium supplement will balance any nutrients you might have missed during the day. If you have questions or want to try to improve your nutrition, consult with your doctor and a nutritionist. Your efforts will be rewarded as you start to notice yourself feeling healthier and stronger, thinking clearer, and performing better. Your disease and cancer risks will go down. You will feel healthy and fit, inside and out!

CHAPTER FOUR

Weight Concerns and Body Image

Body image, or how you feel about the way you look, affects girls and women at all ages and in all aspects of life. If body image is positive, it improves confidence, performance, and success. If body image is negative, it can lead to low self-esteem, shaky confidence, and eating disorders causing poor health and poor performance. Maintaining a positive body image can be very challenging for many reasons.

Society plays a large role in girls' and women's unhealthy obsession with body image and weight concerns. Being female automatically subjects you to pressures to be thin and beautiful, thin and fit, or thin and successful. Athletic girls and women are also subject to athletic or performance pressures to be thin, especially those who are involved in activities such as skating, dance, and diving that are judged and require thin physiques. These problems usually start early in life and can be difficult to overcome. Most girls and women have struggled with weight concerns and body image problems at some time in their life.

Weight management can be a very difficult balancing act, because a desire to be as thin as possible combined with poor body image can lead to bizarre eating and exercise habits. Many active and athletic women struggle to achieve healthy yet nutritional lifestyles. Even elite athletes can tend to limit themselves from certain food groups, missing out on healthy fats, carbohydrates, and other essential nutrients. To have healthy eating habits, girls and women must develop an understanding of what their nutritional needs are and develop a realistic awareness and expectation of body shape. They need to understand that not everyone can be a size 6, and that this size is healthy for only a very small percentage of women. Striving for a healthy, well-muscled physique that performs at its best is the ideal goal. Fortunately, the popularity of women athletes such as Mia Hamm, Julie Foudy, Leila Ali, Jenny Thompson, Summer Sanders, Gaby Reece, and Lisa Leslie has made a strong, well-muscled female physique desirable. These women understand the strength and beauty of muscles and are role models for young girls. Their popularity is a tremendous breakthrough for girls and women.

Struggling with Weight and Body Image

Body Image

Body image is a term used to describe how you see your body. It is a state of mind that can affect confidence, not only in regard to how you look, but also how you feel about yourself, which can affect your physical and mental health.

Unfortunately, many women have poor body image; even those who have beautiful, thin, fit bodies can look in a mirror and criticize themselves for their imperfections (that are often out of proportion to how they look) rather than their strengths. In contrast, women who have positive body image are confident in knowing that, no matter what the weight on the scale, they are fit, strong, healthy, and beautiful.

To have a positive body image you must realize that the women on TV, in magazines, and in movies spend their entire life and savings on their looks. Some images are not even real, and have been altered by computers or airbrushed to hide natural imperfections. Many models and actresses have had plastic surgery, are buried beneath tons of makeup, are shot with flattering camera angles, and wear only clothes that look good on them. Some models and actresses admit that they often don't look like their photos in real life!

Also, many female movie stars and fashion models live unhealthy lives; many smoke or take pills to control their weight, eat restrictive diets, and have abusive exercise schedules. Most do not have any significant muscle and would perform terribly as athletes. A recent study found that one-fourth of Miss America contestants have a Body Mass Index less than 18—far below healthy weight limits. These women do not represent ideals of fitness or health.

Pressure to Be Thin

Pressure to be thin can come from many areas—standards of the sport or athletic activity, coaches, trainers, parents, friends, and magazines. Because of this constant pressure, many girls and women feel "fat," whether they are or not (most athletic girls are not). The statistics are frightening—70 to 80 percent of women feel they need to lose weight, one-fourth of college women have some bulimic behaviors, and up to 60 percent of girls and women have some components of eating disorders.

In fact, most young girls who are thin are not eating enough and begin dieting and restricting calories at an early age in order to conform to the pressures of a coach, parent, society, or themselves. By eating less than their body needs, they can stunt growth and prevent bone development. Between the ages of 8 and 13, healthy girls are growing 2 to 3 inches per year. Along with this growth comes healthy weight gain, at an average of 40 pounds. This is no time for dieting! A young girl's body needs fuel not only to be active every day, but to supply growing bones, muscles, and nerves.

Adolescence is the time when body image begins to develop, but it can be difficult to maintain a healthy body image as the body grows and changes so quickly, including gaining healthy weight. Unfortunately, this is the time that many girls begin to diet, trying to stop the changes on the scale. There are various ways dieting can be attempted—taking diet pills, skipping meals, eating low-calorie diets, avoiding certain foods, or eating artificial meal substitutes. Some very deadly habits and serious eating disorders can begin this way, interfering with normal development and decreasing metabolism. These bad eating habits make it difficult to maintain normal weight and good health and are especially destructive to athletic performance.

Dieting at a young age is the start of developing poor body image. Mood can become directly related to weight fluctuations and dieting success or failure. Dieting itself can delay puberty and cause stunted growth, depression, difficulty concentrating, frequent illness, and injury, including fractures, pain, poor skin, brittle hair and nails, and irritability. These symptoms can cause a rebound effect of even worse body image, leading to further dieting, eating disorders, or overeating. These problems can interfere with participation in activities and even lead to dropping out of athletic activities.

Evaluating Body Image

Body image is affected positively and negatively by many events, including getting weighed at the doctors; trying on skimpy clothes; seeing a picture of yourself; spending time with someone much thinner or heavier than you; a coach, peer, or friend's comments; eating a large or small meal; or doing a challenging workout or athletic event. As a woman, the ups and downs of weight are normal; there are times in life when we eat more and less. Events such as an important competition or social event might lead us to slim down temporarily, and a battle to keep this weight off can be difficult. Pregnancy can also cause weight changes that are difficult to reverse. All these variations and events can lead to frustration, especially if you weigh yourself every day.

Body image and weight management problems become serious when this affects other aspects of life, such as not wanting to spend time with others when eating is involved, regularly skipping social, family, or work activities to work out, or cancelling social engagements based on weight. Your role in life as athlete, friend, and family member will not be affected by more or less pounds. It will be affected by happiness and self-confidence. Feel good about yourself, and understand that occasionally questioning how you look is normal.

If you have body image concerns, as most girls and women do, review the following statements and allow yourself to consider how positive you feel about your body image. Starred statements suggest a higher risk of eating disorders.

Statements to Consider When Evaluating Your Body Image

I seriously worry about my weight on a daily basis.*

I want to weigh 10 pounds more or less than I do now.

I have been on more than one diet in the past year.

I have or have had an eating disorder.

People tell me I am "too thin," but I always feel fat.*

Even though I weigh less than I have in the past year, I feel fat.*

I weigh myself more than once a day.*

I get anxious if I can't exercise more than one hour each day.

If I gain more than one pound, I get anxious or depressed.*

I feel guilty when I eat foods that contain any fat.*

I would rather eat by myself than with family or friends.*

I don't talk about my fear of being fat, because everyone tells me I am too thin.*

I'm afraid I won't be able to stop eating if I start.

I get very upset when people urge me to eat.

Sometimes I think that my undereating or overexercising is not normal.*

*More serious signs that suggest components of an eating disorder

Agreeing with many of these statements is a sign that you might have an eating disorder. Be aware that even women with an overall healthy body image occasionally agree with some of these statements. It takes some discipline to be successful in weight management; the danger is in letting this get out of control and letting it control you. Being able to recognize behaviors consistent with eating disorders and knowing that you need to correct thoughts and actions out of line with positive body image are key to maintaining confidence, happiness, and health.

The Problems with Dieting

To function most effectively as an athlete, and in all roles of life, your body must have enough fuel. Food is fuel. Not having enough interferes with your performance. It also causes overall fatigue, mood changes, weak muscles, and poor health. Restrictive dieting can also lead to eating disorders, which can be lifelong, and, at times, life-threatening.

Risks of Restrictive Dieting

Temporary weight loss	Eating disorders
Rebound weight gain	Poor athletic performance
Slower metabolism	Impaired mental functioning
Serious health risks	Mood Changes

Restrictive dieting—in which you eat less than 1,200 to 1,500 calories a day (depending on height, muscle, and bone mass) and less than 1,800 to 2,000 calories a day if you are very active in athletics and fitness activities—ultimately results in mood and mind changes, including depression, loss of control, fatigue, difficulty concentrating, and poor sleep. Dieting also negatively affects exercise, including poor balance, overheating, poor endurance, earlier exhaustion, and muscle weakness. Other physical problems include headaches, light-headedness, fatigue, digestive problems, and bowel problems. High-protein diets can cause very serious problems with kidneys, cholesterol levels, and bone strength. Diet supplements can cause liver and heart failure. These health risks outweigh any health benefits of being thin.

Physical Problems of Restrictive Dieting That Interfere with Exercise	
Poor balance	Light-headedness
Overheating	Fatigue
Poor endurance	Digestive problems
Muscle weakness	Illness
Headaches	Injury

Chances are, you have been on at least one diet. Think about how you have felt while on a very limiting diet. Were you more likely to get angry, irritable, sad, and frustrated? Were you snippety, less patient, dependent on caffeine, and jittery? These mood changes try the patience of everyone around you and can even cause you to lose friends, jobs, or positions on the team. You probably lacked energy and lost steam halfway through workouts or competitions. Dieting does not allow your fuel stores to work effectively. Thus, if you are in a hard workout or competition, you run out of energy like a car without gas.

Mind and Mood Changes Common to Restrictive Dieting	
Unable to concentrate	Impatient
Irritable	Frustrated
Angry	Depressed
Exhausted	Sluggish

Your body needs fuel to run effectively. If it does not get enough fuel, your body will do everything it can to conserve energy and run at a lower metabolic rate, thinking you are in starvation mode, trying to stay alive. A lower metabolic rate is one that burns calories slower. This change in rate can stay around for longer than you are on the diet, causing you to quickly gain back the weight once you are off the diet. The healthiest and longest-lasting method of effective weight management is to avoid restrictive dieting altogether. This will allow you to avoid failure, rebound weight gain, slower metabolism, and health risks associated with limited food types, calories, and possible eating disorders. The slower you lose weight, the easier it will be to keep it off.

Diets: Bad, Fair, Good

Bad Diets

The diets listed here are unhealthy, especially for an athlete. These diets do not provide enough calories, nutrition, or the right kind of fuel. They strain body organs. Instead of improving health, they risk destroying it. The longer you are on these diets, the greater the risks become.

Low-Carb/High-Protein Diets

These diets, including the Atkins Diet, the Ketogenic Diet, the Zone Diet, and the Scarsdale Diet, are extremely popular because of the quick water-weight loss that occurs at the start of the diet. This water-weight loss is mistaken for fat loss, and it quickly returns as soon as the dieting stops. These diets make you look thin and trim because eating proteins is dehydrating, and causes large amounts of body water loss. Although bodybuilders might follow these diets to look more defined, they quickly gain the weight back after competition when they stop dieting. Aerobic athletes, dancers, and performance athletes cannot function effectively on these diets because protein and fats are a terrible source of performance fuel, and the body requires extra water and calories to break them down (see chapter 14, "Exercise Fuel").

High-protein, low-carbohydrate diets cause a state of ketosis, chronic dehydration, low appetite, bad breath, and also nausea and depression. These diets are especially dangerous for people with high blood pressure, heart disease, and kidney problems. They can also cause gout. High-protein diets also cause your body to lose calcium, increasing your risk of fractures and osteoporosis. In athletes, the oversupply of protein puts a tremendous strain on your kidneys, which are already stressed by the breakdown products of intense exercise and occasional dehydration; combining these two types of stress on the body can be very dangerous. Also, by missing out on healthy fiber and vitamins found in fruits, vegetables, and grains, you are putting yourself at greater risk of heart and blood vessel problems, digestive problems, and many types of cancer. Women who go off the diet in search of more normal eating tend to immediately gain back weight as the water weight returns. Also, studies have shown that these diets do not cause weight and fat loss any quicker than other types do over the long term. So why take the health risks?

The Dangers of Low-Carb/High-Protein Diets

Increased risk of kidney disease	Bad breath
Dehydration	Nausea
Increased risk of heart disease	Mood changes
Increased risk of cancer	Poor endurance
Increased bone loss	Digestive problems
May cause gout	Nutritional deficiencies

"Fat-Burning" or "Metabolism Enhancing" Products

Stay away, stay away, stay away from these diets, including Metabalife, Herbalife, Hydroxycut, Xenedrine, Trim Spa, Stacker 2, and many other diets with the words *thermo, lean, fat burner,* etc. They contain ephedrine (also known as ephedra or ma huang), a dangerous, addictive drug that is not only illegal in high-level athletes, but also potentially deadly because it can increase incidence of strokes, seizures, and heart attacks. They also act as diuretics and cause water loss and dehydration leading to heatstroke. They are even more dangerous when combined with caffeine or other herbs. Usually, once you stop the drug or product, you gain back the weight. These dangerous chemicals can also be found in teas and drinks. Some professional athletes, and many other unfortunate dieters, have lost their lives because of these products. It is hoped that the FDA will ban ephedra from the market.

Avoid These Products at All Costs!

INGREDIENTS AND WORDS	EXAMPLE PRODUCTS TO AVOID
Ephedrine	Metabalife
Ephedra	Herbalife
Ma huang	Hydroxycut
"Thermo"	Xenedrine
"Lean"	Trim Spa
"Fat burner"	Stacker 2

"No-Fat" Diets

No-fat diets become a problem in the long run because fats are necessary for life. Fats contain vitamins and essential fatty acids, which keep your body running smoothly. Women who restrict fat in their diet have hormone imbalances, fertility problems, and dry hair and skin. Your body also needs healthy fats to prevent heart disease and cancer (see chapter 3, "Nutritional Health").

Eliminating Foods

Unless you are diabetic, lactose intolerant, have a specific allergy, or have been diagnosed with some other medical problem that requires you to cut out certain foods, you should not eliminate entire food groups. Restricting yourself from many types of foods for fear of getting fat is a type of self-control that is similar to anorexia, especially if these limitations keep you from regularly eating a well-balanced diet.

Certain Foods Only

Very unhealthy eating habits come from diets such as the Cabbage Soup Diet, the Apple Cider Diet, and the Grapefruit Diet. These limit your eating to one type of food, restricting all the health benefits of other foods. They are not balanced and are usually so low in calories that your metabolism goes down and you do not have enough energy to function, much less work out. These diets often cause water-weight loss and leave you feeling deprived for normal eating. Any weight lost on these diets usually returns within a week.

Fair Diets

The following diets are not ideal because they are expensive, inconvenient, and do not allow for vacations or social eating. They are also quite low in calories and natural food nutrients. They often fail because once you return to eating foods that are not in the diet plan, the weight returns. This is not a realistic or practical lifelong eating plan.

Diet Products Diets

Eating only diet products, such as Slim Fast, Scan Diet, nutrition bars, or protein shakes, can be unhealthy not only because of the limited amount of nutrition but also because it can be very difficult to keep off the weight once the diet is over, as normal eating habits are not developed. Additionally, because these diets are usually very low in calories, they tend to slow down your metabolism. The lack of variety of food can result in nutritional deficits and prevent you from receiving the healthy benefits of natural foods. These diets also isolate you from social eating.

Packaged Meals

Diet plans that require packaged, purchased meals can be healthy but are unrealistic and it is difficult to maintain the weight loss once the diet is over. They can also be expensive. An example is Jenny Craig, although because this diet can also be followed eating foods you prepare yourself, it can fall closer to the "good" category.

Good Diets

The best "diets" are not really diets at all, but eating plans for life. Of course, the healthiest approach is to allow yourself all foods occasionally, but stick to these eating plans most of the time.

Low Glycemic Index Diet

Eating low and medium glycemic index foods minimizes sugary foods in the diet. This is a healthful and reasonable diet plan that you can follow for life and promotes weight loss by maintaining blood sugars and controlling hunger by stabilizing insulin levels. It is also a diet full of healthy vegetables, fruits, and fiber with balanced proteins and fats. This is not a calorie-restricting or nutrition-restricting diet. Eating low and medium glycemic index foods also can prevent diabetes, heart disease, and stroke. Andrew Weil, M.D.'s *Eating Well for Optimum Health* and Jenny Brand-Miller's *Glucose Revolution Life Plan* are examples.

Smaller Portions with Personal Support

Smaller portions and personal support are the foundations behind the success of Weight Watchers and plans like ediet. These are the most successful, sensible, healthy weight loss plans and are also reasonably priced. They are effective because they promote slow weight loss (one to two pounds per week) by eating regular foods in smaller portions. They are also very effective as a result of personal and group support, which encourages and promotes confidence in dealing with weight control issues. A recent research study found diet plans backed by personal support, whether by phone, in person, or by e-mail, are the most successful at keeping off weight.

Diet Plans: Bad, Fair, Good

	TYPE OF DIET	EXPLANATION
BAD Dangerous, unhealthy impractical, and strange. Athletes cannot function on these diets!	Low-carb/high-protein	Dangerous for athletes, causes bone loss, harmful to kidneys and body fluid status
	Metabolism pills and products	Addictive, expensive, dangerous
	Eliminating foods	Unhealthy, impractical
	No fat	Unhealthy
FAIR Mostly healthy, just difficult to maintain weight loss after diet is over	Diet products	Have to buy product, normal eating habits not established
	Packaged meals	Have to buy food, impractical, expensive
GOOD Very healthy, practical	Low glycemic index foods	Promotes healthy eating
	Balanced meals, smaller portions	Normal eating; smaller portions, support

Eating Disorders

Eating disorders are diseases in which weight control and eating behaviors have gone so far as to become life- and health-threatening. They can result from a diet taken too seriously, a hope to improve performance, a desire to please others, goals of becoming a model or making a weight class, or an extreme sense of perfectionism and even competition to be thinner than others.

Eating disorders are an actual medical classification in which food is limited or purged in order to be thin. They are classified as psychiatric disorders and are very serious. The driving force is always a poor and distorted body image, low self-confidence, and a drive for perfectionism. Eating disorders can result from peer pressure, although most girls and women with eating disorders isolate themselves from others. The psychological aspects of disordered eating stem not only from trouble with body image, but also from feeling a need for control. Eating disorders are common among girls and women who are type A personalities with a desire for perfection and an ability to obsess so much over their drive to be thin, that they neglect their body's need for food. Athletes with a tendency toward eating disorders include jockeys, dancers, skaters, gymnasts, aerobic or fitness instructors, swimmers, and divers. Because of these athletes' excellent ability for self-discipline, they are capable of going to great lengths to lose weight.

Eating disorders are identified as either bulemia or anorexia, although some can have components of both. Anorexia athletica is a newer classification that recognizes extreme exercise as a method of purging calories. Girls and women with eating disorders can recover but require much social, family, and counselor support along with lifetime eating habit and body image changes.

Bulemia

Bulemia is a vicious cycle of eating and purging. Eating can be bingeing but can also be a regular meal; purging is done in a variety of ways, although most commonly purging is by vomiting. Other ways to purge include the use of medications such as laxatives and diuretics or by extreme amounts of exercise. These are all very dangerous behaviors. Bulemia can result in erratic heart rates, loss of tooth enamel, and disturbances of electrolytes the body needs to regulate muscle, nerve, and heart function. Not only does it cause fatigue, dehydration, and poor body function, in athletes it causes poor performance and could lead to serious episodes of passing out. The worst possibility is a heart attack, which can be deadly. Bulemia is very common, with statistics suggesting one-fourth of college students exhibit some bulemic behavior.

Body Signs of Bulemia

Eroded tooth enamel	Dehydration
Chubby cheeks	Weakness
Scraped knuckles	Broken blood vessels in face
Bad breath	Stomach and bowel problems
Inability to hold down a meal	Coughing, lung problems
Easy vomiting	Irregular or missed periods
Irregular heartbeat	

Anorexia

Anorexia, the disease of restricting calories, is a very life-threatening problem. Anorexia is an extremely distorted body image of feeling fat while being grossly underweight. Unfortunately, many girls and women have died from this disease because the body simply cannot live without food. It might function for a while in "starvation mode," but there is only so much it can do for itself. All living creatures need food to exist; there is no way around it.

Girls and women with anorexia are starving themselves and are unhealthfully thin. They constantly feel tired and are unable to keep up in practice, school, or work. Their hair becomes dry and their skin scaly and even hairy as the body tries to keep itself warm because it has no fat. The heart rate slows but speeds up quickly with even small movements. Anorexia interferes with all aspects of life; it is as life-dominating as an addiction to drugs or alcohol. Anorexics are addicted to a quest for unobtainable, unrealistic, unhealthy thinness. If you have any of these symptoms, talk with your coach, trainer, friends, or parents. If that is too threatening, refer to the resources at the end of this book for help. Recovering from eating disorders takes professional help.

Eating disorders are more common than you think and should not be kept secret. Specialists in nutrition or psychology and doctors trained in eating disorders can provide supportive, effective help to return you to functioning in life at a healthy weight. Having the additional support of a friend, trainer, or family member can help you begin healing and returning to athletics and regular social activities. Seeking help will save your health and might save your life.

Body Signs of Anorexia

Dry skin	Erratic heartrate
Brittle nails	Protruding ribs and spine
Fine hair on face and body	Bruises
Hair loss on head	Cold hands and feet
Muscle weakness	Yellow tint to skin
Hollow facial features	Absent or irregular periods
Shrunken breasts	

Anorexia Athletica

Anorexia athletica is working out or exercising too much without adequate calories. This is a common problem among endurance athletes who overexercise while restricting calories to maintain low body fat. Highly active endurance athletes require an increase in daily calories between 2,000 and 3,000 calories a day more than women who do not work out at these levels. If these amounts of calories are not obtained, they can be classified as suffering from an eating disorder. Women who do more than six hours of intense aerobic exercise strictly for weight control (not playing a sport, hiking, or recreational activity) may be at risk of anorexia athletica. Anorexia athletica is usually associated with the female athlete triad.

The Female Athlete Triad

The female athlete triad describes a syndrome of eating disorder (anorexia), lack of a period (amenorrhea), and thinning bones (osteoporosis). The triad is common and becoming more and more recognized in girls and women who work out a lot and do not eat enough. Most frequently occurring in women with disordered eating and calorie restricted diets, it has also been noted in girls who do not eat enough protein or meat and also in girls who work out excessively without proper rest. One of the greatest risks to health is thin bones and stress fractures. The most reliable signs that an athlete has the female athlete triad include being extremely thin (body fat less than 18 percent) and a loss of regular menstrual period, particularly for longer than six months. Other signs include being obsessed with body weight, worsening performance, and constant fatigue. The female athlete triad must be addressed by a doctor as soon as possible to restore normal hormone balance, bone health, and healthy eating habits. It often is treated with a multidisciplinary team of nutritionists, psychologists, and doctors.

Body Signs of Anorexia Athletica and the Female Athlete Triad

Extreme thinness (body fat <18%)	Loss of appetite
Loss of regular periods	Constant pain
Stress fractures	Repeated injuries
Chronic fatigue	Poor endurance

Eating Disorders

Some athletic girls and women have milder forms of these diseases and are able to preserve their performance, although they are at risk of developing more severe forms of eating disorders. Being able to recognize the signs of anorexia (severe calorie restriction and limitation) and bulimia (bingeing and purging) can prevent development into a life-threatening disease, as treatment is more effective early in the course of the disorders. Often, these problems begin in junior high or high school, although younger girls can also feel pressures to be extremely thin.

Amenorrhea

Amenorrhea is the medical term for not having a period for more than six months. Most girls should be having regular (monthly) periods by age 14 to 16. Not having a period is a sign that the body is not cycling estrogen as it should. The reasons for amenorrhea are not fully understood, but low body fat and low calorie intake stresses the reproductive hormones to restrict their normal signals. Estrogen is necessary, not only for reproductive health, but notably for bone strength—just six months of not having a period leads to permanent bone loss. Amenorrhea can also be due to illness, overtraining, physical stress, psychological stress, low-calorie diets, low-fat diets, and low-protein diets. There are also some medical conditions that can cause this loss of regular periods.

Causes of Amenorrhea (Loss of Monthly Period)	
High exercise intensity	Low body fat
Recent weight change	Hormone imbalance
Dieting	Pregnancy
Stress	Illness
Poor nutrition	Low-calorie diet

Osteoporosis

Osteoporosis, the disease of thinning bones, is usually a disease of older women, but girls and women with the female athlete triad, overstressing the body by not eating enough or working out too much causes osteoporosis to occur more frequently and at an earlier age. Osteoporosis also leads to poor posture, loss of height, decreased breathing and lung capacity, and frequent stress fractures (see chapter 5, "Bone Health and Osteoporosis"). In younger women, it is linked to the loss of estrogen and can also be present secondary to consistently poor nutrition such as low-fat, high-protein, and low-calcium diets. Osteopenia, a medical term used to describe thinning bones that are more likely to develop osteoporosis, is also a sign of potential risk from the female athlete triad. Having Osteoporosis or Osteopenia at a young age is a risk factor for fractures throughout life, because bones are developing their greatest density between the ages of 12 and 30. If a female has an eating disorder during these ages and does not properly nourish her bones and body with enough calcium, calories, and fat, proper bone development and strength will not occur.

Positive Body Image

The best way to have a positive body image is to feel positive about yourself as a person. Stay active, exercise regularly, and feel strong and fit. Nurture your muscles, feed them healthy food, and maintain goals for your life and achievements. Wear clothes that flatter you; have friends who flatter you also.

Avoid uncomfortable situations and people who are negative about weight and being healthy. Remember that body fat is healthy and essential to life, fertility, and bone strength.

A positive body image allows you to feel attractive and strong through your life and also feel good inside and out. Being successful, loved, and stimulated by life allows distractions from obsession about weight and dieting. Some people suggest even putting away the scale to prevent the moodiness that comes with everyday weight fluctuations and using the fit of your clothes as a size guide instead. If you must weigh yourself regularly, remember that body water plays a large role in weight. Both glycogen, stored after a high-carbohydrate meal, and sodium, from salty food, cause water retention so the scale might read a few pounds higher after such meals.

If you are really struggling with your body image and weight maintenance, try yoga, meditation, pilates, or regular relaxation strategies. Some people meditate while walking, stretching, or doing yoga. This will help you feel less anxious about food and more positive about your body. Learn healthy ways to control your weight, and if you must lose a few pounds, do so by cutting back 500 calories a day. This can usually be done simply by cutting out unhealthy snacks, desserts, alcohol, or sugary drinks. You can also increase your water and healthy fluid intake, reduce the glycemic index of your diet, and increase your fiber intake. If you have overindulged in unhealthy, high-calorie foods for a few days, cut back your portions and desserts for the next week. Do not panic and starve yourself! Remember, extreme reduction in calorie intake only slows down your metabolism.

Healthy Ways to Control Your Weight

Make sure you eat enough calories (check chart in chapter 3).

Drink at least eight glasses of water a day.

Drink a glass of water before each meal or snack.

Eat a fruit or vegetable serving before each meal.

Do not deprive yourself of a food you crave for more than a week; eat a normal-sized portion of it.

Try to take small bites, chew several times, and put your fork down between bites.

Try to not skip meals.

Try to avoid sugary sodas, juice drinks, and sweets—these just contain empty calories.

Try to eat healthy fats such as nuts, peanut butter, olive oil, or fish to keep you full and healthy.

Control your stress so it does not cause you to eat more.

Do not allow people to pressure you to lose weight. If a parent or friend is pressuring you, tell them to stop or walk away when they do so. If you have a coach or trainer who criticizes you for your weight or weighs you frequently, do not allow this! Find another coach, and if this is a problem, speak to someone you can trust about it. A coach who pressures you when you are young can instill in you long-lasting attitudes and behaviors that are destructive to your body image and your health.

If you have a large shape and frame, take the pressure off yourself to look petite. Instead, focus on your strength. Focus on your health. Don't let people comment on your size, and if they do, thank them. Realize that big girls are stronger in all aspects—bones, muscles, and minds! Often just talking about these unrealistic expectations to be petite can help you put them into perspective. If you are feeling like you need to look like a super-skinny aerobics instructor, world-class figure skater, or supermodel, find a healthier looking inspirational role model. Look to competitive skiers, soccer players, basketball players, or women among your friends and family who are healthy, happy, and athletic at size 10, 12, or 14.

As a young athlete going through adolescence, changes in body shape, hormones, and flexibility might make sports activities temporarily more challenging. Consider changing sports if the one you are in requires you to be thinner than you can realistically be. A nutritionist or health-care professional can help you determine your healthiest weight and decide if the weight and body shape demands of the sport are realistic for you. Having an understanding coach is also essential. It is important to find sports and athletic activities that are easy for you; this will make it more likely that you will enjoy the activity and excel at it.

Remember, not everyone is built to be a figure skater. If you are not built small and light, you can switch to ice hockey, rollerhockey, skiing, or snowboarding. There are so many sports available to girls and women; you should find one that is just right for your body, that you feel comfortable with, and that you don't have to struggle with your body or diet to maintain. Finding a sport that allows you to excel at a healthy weight is best for your mind, body, fitness, and overall health.

Promoting Positive Body Image

Get involved in athletic activities with women of similar athletic builds.

Do not spend time with friends who make you feel bad about your size.

If coaches or trainers make you "feel fat," find new ones.

Remember that, as an athletic woman, you are stronger and healthier than most.

If you have trouble with self-criticism, find a nurturing counselor or therapist.

Choose relationships with people who make you feel good about yourself.

Try not to let weight rule your emotions; it is just a number, and it can change!

Wear clothes that flatter you.

Wear your favorite outfit on days that you feel low confidence.

Compliment those around you; they will give it back!

Get a nonathletic friend to exercise with you once in a while.

A healthy nutrition plan and realistic attitude toward body image will lead to optimum performance and confidence. Do not be discouraged if you fall into unhealthy habits occasionally; return to the healthy habits as soon as you can. In times of stress, give yourself some slack. Keep exercising regularly, and make sure you have the essentials of nutrition.

When you lose inspiration, think of your athletic or performance role model and her strength, health, and beauty. Focus on how good a workout feels. If you must diet, do so in moderation with a well-balanced eating plan. Remember, the slower you change your weight, the longer it will last. Do not deprive yourself of calories, nutrition, or the occasional "treat." Drink plenty of fluids, control your stress, and make yourself as happy as possible. Maintaining a healthy body image and weight requires work and patience, just like anything that is worthwhile. In time, you will feel great about how you look and, therefore, how you feel—every day!

CHAPTER FIVE

Bone Health and Osteoporosis

Bones are the supporting structure of our body, giving us our height, posture, stature, and strength. Strong, healthy bones are important to athletic activity, as they form the frame and skeleton for muscles. Having a solid skeleton allows better muscle strength and more efficient movement. Bone is a constantly changing tissue that grows and remodels; this process is known as "bone turnover." Bone turnover is regulated by hormones, which maintain the delicate balance of bone breakdown and bone rebuilding. The most rebuilding occurs early in life, as the body creates the strongest foundation of bones until age 30.

After age 30, there is a natural slowdown in buildup of bone. Over time, bones become naturally thinner. This process occurs much more dramatically in women. Unfortunately, being female is a risk factor for having weaker bones. There are also other risk factors that can compromise a woman's strong skeleton, making bones thinner and weaker.

Osteoporosis, the condition of thin, weak bones and increased risk of fractures, is known as a "silent disease" because it is sometimes not diagnosed until several fractures have already occurred. Thin bones can also occur in young, athletic girls and women, causing stress fractures, which can lead to muscle, tendon, and ligament problems and increase the risk of other fractures. Younger girls and women who have frequent stress fractures have a much greater risk of osteoporosis and associated dysfunctional posture and serious fractures later in life.

Women of all ages should make bone health an important concern to avoid the pain, fractures, and time lost from athletic and life activities that occurs with osteoporosis. Strengthening your bones will help guarantee a future of strength, mobility, and reduced hospital and doctor visits! It is very important to do the best you can to protect your bones. A preventive, proactive strategy as outlined in this chapter can help you meet this goal.

Osteoporosis

Osteoporosis is the medical term for the disease process of having bones that are fragile and more easily breakable. Osteoporosis bones look holey and thin under the microscope, similar to fragile sheer lace, rather than the tight-knit pattern of healthy bone (see figure 5-1). Osteoporosis bones have less dense structure with less hard strong calcium to hold them together and provide strength and stability.

The most common osteoporosis fractures are of the hip, spine, and wrist; these often occur in older women and can be debilitating, painful, and life-changing. Not only do the fractures themselves cause problems as immediate and sometimes ongoing pain and disability, but there can be other med-

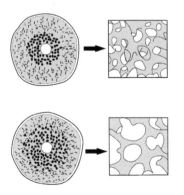

FIGURE 5-1A **normal, healthy, dense bone: left, slice through long bone; right, microscopic view.**

FIGURE 5-1B **frail, holey bone of osteoporosis: left, slice through long bone; right, microscopic view**

FIGURE 5-1 **Illustration of normal versus osteoporosis bone (slice through long bone on left and closeup of inner bone structure on right).**

ical complications as well, including blood clots, pneumonia, constipation, and impaired nerve function. The cost of treating fractures due to osteoporosis, including surgery, hospitalization, and medical complications, is high. Because bones in osteoporosis are so weak, fractures can also happen without falling. For these reasons, osteoporosis has become a serious issue for medical clinicians and researchers.

Common Areas of Fractures Due to Osteoporosis and Their Consequences

Wrist—motion and use might never be the same; two to four months to heal

Vertebra (spine)—very painful, can occur without a fall; two to four months to heal with long-term pain

Hip—requires surgery and hospitalization; can be very serious; full recovery takes 6 to 12 months

---

In addition to fractures, posture is impaired in osteoporosis. Because the bones of the spine lose their height, they collapse, causing a slumped posture. The ribs fall closer together, and the bottom ribs press on the pelvis, causing pain. This limits breathing capacity, as the lungs cannot expand, causing increased risk of respiratory diseases such as pneumonia and decreased endurance. Motion becomes more limited, as trunk rotation and shoulder motion are restricted. Neck and back pain is common, due to both the collapsing bones and the weakened, strained muscles.

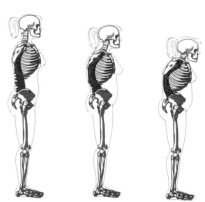

FIGURE 5-2 **Illustration of progressively hunching posture as older woman develops osteoporosis. A: healthy posture, B: moderate osteoporosis posture, C: severe osteoporosis posture. Note loss of height, collapsed ribs, decreased lung space, and protruding abdomen.**

Long-Term Negative Consequences of Osteoporosis

Fractures	Dysfunctional and painful posture
Surgery	Loss of lung volume and breathing capacity
Disability	Poor endurance
Pain	Medical costs
Loss of strength	Hospital stays
Loss of height	Other medical complications

Risk Factors

Osteoporosis is due to a combination of factors. Older age and female sex are significant risk factors; after menopause, the risk of osteoporosis becomes much higher. Osteoporosis is also more likely in people with family members who have osteoporosis, as well as in thin, Caucasian, and Asian women. Girls and women who have a history of eating disorders including frequent dieting and poor nutrition are more likely to get osteoporosis. High-protein and low-calcium diets along with other bad lifestyle choices such as smoking and drinking excessively contributes to osteoporosis as well. Also, women who are inactive or do not participate in regular weight-bearing and resistive exercise are more likely to develop osteoporosis. Having a diagnosis of osteoporosis means your risk of fracture is four times greater than if you do not have it.

Risk Factors for Osteoporosis Fractures

(Charts adapted from the National Osteoporosis Foundation)

PERMANENT	MODIFIABLE
Having a fragility fracture* as an adult	Cigarette smoking
A close relative with a fragility fracture*	Not having a period for more than six months
Caucasian or Asian race	Diet low in calcium
Postmenopause	More than two alcoholic drinks per day
Female gender	Falling, poor balance
Lifelong history of absent periods	Low levels of activity
Bad eyesight (increasing fall risks)	Frail health
Early menopause (before age 45)	Weak muscles

Lifelong history of eating disorders	Hormone imbalance
Chronic health problems	Low-calorie or poor nutrition diet

*Fragility fracture = a fracture occurring from a fall from standing height or lower

There are also certain medical conditions that make osteoporosis more likely, due to both the underlying disease and also due to side effects of medications for treatment. The most common medications that directly affect bone health are corticosteroids, often used to treat asthma, arthritis, and immune disorders. Women with hormone imbalances such as Cushing's disease, hyperparathyroidism, hyperthyroidism, and genetic sex hormone deficiency are also at higher risks. Also, diseases that cause disabilities to limit walking such as multiple sclerosis and spinal cord injuries can lead to thinning bones.

Risk Factors for Osteoporosis That Cannot Be Changed

FACTOR	EXPLANATION
Older age	With age, bone density decreases. 15 percent of women in their 50s have osteoporosis; 50 percent of women in their 80s have it.
Female sex	Women have a much greater risk than men. Women have thinner lighter bones, less muscle mass to protect them, and are hormonally more susceptible.
Family history	Genetics pre-programs a body to be susceptible to certain things such as osteoporosis and greater rate of fractures.
Small size	Small, thin people are more at risk. Muscle and fat protect and strengthen bones.
Other medical risks	Certain medical problems such as hypothyroid and hormonal imbalances lead to higher risks of osteoporosis.

Risk Factors for Osteoporosis That Can Be Changed

FACTOR	HOW
Low activity level	Those less active and less on their feet have weaker bones. Bones get stronger the more they are used.
Low-calcium diet	Calcium is necessary for bone formation; it is the basic substance of bones.

Smoking, excess alcohol	Excess alcohol and tobacco interfere with bone formation.
Not having periods during reproductive years	Estrogen is needed for the delicate balance of hormones to form and maintain bones.
High-protein diets	High-protein diets interfere with calcium absorption.

The Role of Hormones

Estrogen is important to the bones' ability to absorb and retain calcium, maintaining structure and protecting bones from becoming weak. A regular menstrual period is the result of estrogen circulating through the body; therefore, women who do not get their periods regularly are at increased risk of having osteoporosis secondary to decreased estrogen levels. After menopause, estrogen levels decrease as well, contributing to the increased risk of osteoporosis. This is one reason estrogen supplements have been prescribed after menopause (other reasons include reducing uncomfortable side effects of menopause such as hot flashes). However, estrogen supplements only prevent osteoporosis and risk of fractures, they do not treat it. Although women who take estrogen after menopause actually do develop less fractures, the Women's Health Initiative, a groundbreaking study concluded in 2002, revealed that after five years of continuous treatment with hormone supplements, women can have slightly higher risks of breast cancer, blood clots, stroke, and uterine cancer. Therefore, prescribing estrogen supplements for postmenopausal women is no longer the treatment of choice. (If you are taking estrogen supplements after menopause, they should be at the lowest doses possible and taken along with progesterone to preserve a more natural body hormone balance; also, try not to take them for more than five years.)

Testing and Diagnosis

Testing is easy, painless, and risk-free, as only minor levels of radiation are used; the greatest risk is not having it done. A true diagnosis of osteoporosis can only be made after a bone density test has been done, specifically the DEXA test, as mandated by the World Health Organization. This is the "gold standard" test for bone mineral density. It is a safe test that uses very low-dose radiation— much less than a standard x-ray. It measures density at the hip, spine, and wrist.

Testing is ordered by a medical doctor and is usually done by a technician; insurance covers the test every two years in women who have reached menopause and in women who have had stress or multiple fractures.

Currently, 40 percent of post-menopausal women in the United States have osteoporosis; the number might actually be greater if more women were tested.

Ask your doctor for a bone density test if you have reached menopause or have had more than three fractures over your lifetime (not due to a serious accident).

Terms and Fracture Risk Increase

Osteoporosis = four times greater risk of fracture

Osteopenia = two times greater risk of fracture

Bone density testing establishes the strength and density of your bones, predicting future risk of fractures. It can also be used to monitor bone lost or gained after one or two years of treatment. Bone density test results are translated into a "T" score, which is a number that compares your bone density to the recommended normal. A T score lower than −2.5 is diagnostic of osteoporosis; between −1 and −2.5 is diagnostic for osteopenia. In young women, the Z score, a T score that is adjusted for age, is a more accurate number.

World Health Organization Classifications of Osteoporosis

TERM	DEFINITION	WHAT IT MEANS	RECOMMENDED TESTS
Osteoporosis	T score less than −2.5	Bones are four times more likely to fracture	Bone density testing two years after medications and treatment started
Osteopenia	T score between −1 and −2.5 SD	Thin bones are heading toward osteoporosis	Bone density testing at least every three years

DEXA testing is recommended at least once for all women after menopause and at all ages for women who have had more than one fracture not due to an injury. You should always have your bone density testing done at the same facility, as different machines can give different results. Standard follow-up is done one to two years after treatment begins, and every two to three years if you have osteopenia. For those with normal bone density measurements, repeat testing should be done at least once after three to four years. Other types of testing, such as heel ultrasound or wrist or finger screening, are less expensive, take less time, and have less radiation, but are much less comprehensive and do not allow for accurate evaluation of overall body bone density. These other types of testing are not recommended for women with risk factors, unless DEXA testing is not available.

Tests to Evaluate Bone Health

TYPE OF TEST	HOW IT IS DONE	PURPOSE
DEXA	A scan is taken of your body	The gold standard for bone density; it measures density at your spine and hip and establishes a diagnosis of osteoporosis
PDXA	A scan is taken of your wrist, finger, or heel	Bone density at specific site tested; does not necessarily correspond to hip or spine
QUS (Quantitative Ultrasound)	An ultrasound scan is taken of the heel and shin	Determines bone density of the heel, which corresponds closely to the hip. Used as a convenient, quick screening tool
X-ray	A picture of your bones is taken	Evaluates fractures and other bone problems; not a screening tool for osteoporosis
Bone scan	Dye is injected into your blood; hours later, you have a scan taken	Evaluates a possible stress fracture or other problem with the bone; not a screening tool for osteoporosis
MRI, CT scan	A scan is taken (MRI more comprehensive)	Evaluates whether you have a stress fracture or other problem in your bone; not a screening tool for osteoporosis
Blood tests	Blood is drawn	Evaluates hormones and indicators of bone turnover helpful to understand cause
Urine test	Urine sampled	Measures calcium lost in urine
Bone biopsy	A needle is put into the bone	Evaluates abnormal bone

Doctors who diagnose and treat osteoporosis can have medical degrees in various specialties; this is a reflection of the many aspects of health that thin bones can affect. For more complicated cases and when frequent stress fractures or fall fractures occur in younger girls or women, referral to an endocrinologist (hormone specialist) is recommended, as these are medical specialists who are most qualified to evaluate and treat osteoporosis. If you are in your teens or reproductive years and have had more than three fractures or absent periods, a bone density test should be done to screen for osteoporosis or osteopenia. If there is evidence of decreased bone density, it is recommended that you go to an endocrinologist to evaluate and correct the problem now to prevent future problems. For osteoporosis after menopause, your primary care doctor, gynecologist, orthopedist, physiatrist, or rheumatologist may manage your treatment.

Treatment

The ultimate goal of diagnosis and treatment of osteoporosis is to reduce the number of fractures. Because bone density is the most reliable measure of osteoporosis, treatment is focused on increasing bone density. Bone strength is directly related to density, and ultimately, the stronger the bone, the less likely it will fracture. Bone strength also improves with proper diet and exercise. Hormones and genetics also influence bone strength. Treatment of osteoporosis is most effective using a combination of medications, calcium, vitamin D, weight-bearing exercise, and lifestyle and dietary modifications.

The most effective osteoporosis medications to date are the bisphosphonates, marketed as Fosamax and Actonel. Taken once weekly, these drugs are the most likely to increase bone density, decrease fracture risk, and reduce bone breakdown. Bisphosphonates function by interfering with the natural process of bone resorption and have been shown to reduce spine fracture risk by 30 to 50 percent and hip fracture risk by 24 to 50 percent. Estrogen supplements can prevent the development of osteoporosis and some fractures but are not recommended specifically for treatment, nor are they recommended for more than five years after menopause. Other types of drugs that are also used are described in the following chart. Consult with your doctor if you are taking some of the less-effective medicines, especially if you have a definite diagnosis of osteoporosis.

Medications Used to Treat and Prevent Osteoporosis, in Increasing Order of Effectiveness

DRUG TYPE (COMMON NAME)	FUNCTION	SIDE EFFECTS	EFFECTIVENESS
Calcitonin (Miacalcin), nasal spray; also can be injected	Helps bones absorb calcium; also helps with pain of vertebral (spine) fractures	Itchy or runny nose, pain from injection	More effective five years after menopause; minimal effect on bone density or strength
Estrogen, oral or patches (Estraderm, Climera, Premarin) cyclic estrogens with progesterone (Premphase), estrogen with progesterone (Prempro, Femhrt, Activella)	Allows bones to absorb and retain calcium better	Blood clots, stroke; some women at greater risk of breast cancer; mood changes, depression, weight gain, breast tenderness	Prevention only: although the number of hip and spine fractures are reduced, these are not recommended for treatment of osteoporosis
Selective estrogen receptor modulator, (SERM) Raloxifene, "Evista"	Tissue-specific estrogens used in women who have had breast cancer or other risk factors with estrogen; prevents breast cancer in some women	Similar to estrogen side effects	Recent studies do not show that these reduce the risk of hip and other fractures; more preventive than treatment
Bisphosphonates, Fosamax (Alendronate Sodium), Actonel (Risedronate Sodium)	Decreases bone breakdown	Irritation of the esophagus; needs to be taken first thing in the morning with a full glass of water; remain upright for 30 minutes	Extremely effective; reduces all fractures vertebral (spine) to fractures by 30 to 50 percent and the the incidence of hip fractures by 24 to 50 percent
Parathyroid hormone, Forteo (teriparatide)	Increases bone formation and decreases resorption	Needs to be injected daily; will often be used in combination with drugs; may cause cancer	Potential to increase bone formation and reduce fractures by 60 percent; not yet widely available or tested

Nutrition is very important, as bone growth and strength cannot occur without calcium, the building block of bone. Vitamin D and magnesium also play an important role. Vitamin D helps the body retain calcium and prevents it from being excreted out of the body via the kidneys. Bone specialists recommend taking 1,300 to 1,500 mg of calcium in two or three divided doses with two of the doses taken in the evening (one with dinner, one before bed). A multivitamin containing 400 IU of vitamin D should also be taken with the evening meal. There are also other trace minerals involved in bone formation, including magnesium; these are covered by taking your multivitamin daily, a recommended habit for everyone.

When totaling your calcium and vitamin D intake, include food and drink sources so you do not overdo the amounts. Adding your total calcium milligram is easy by reading labels—add a zero to the percent daily value of calcium listed on the food label to easily calculate the mineral content. Supplement to total 1,500 mg. For example, if you have eaten three servings of dairy products, each containing 30 percent the "daily value" (%DV) of calcium (such as milk, cheese, and calcium-fortified orange juice), your total calcium intake through foods is 900 mg. So on this day, you only need to take one 600 mg supplement of calcium. Daily vitamin D needs are covered in your multivitamin and the milk products you have consumed. It is not recommended to take more than 2,000 mg of calcium or 800 IU of vitamin D daily. Also, do not take vitamin A supplements if you have osteoporosis; this has been shown to increase fracture risk.

In women who have osteoporosis, excess salt, high-protein diets, alcoholic drinks, and carbonated drinks should be kept to a minimum, as these can interfere with the body's calcium absorption and retention. Caffeine can also increase calcium loss, but this effect is minimal, unless you are also a smoker. Smoking is detrimental to the bones and should be stopped!

Exercise improves bone strength, just as it improves muscle strength. Our bodies work as hard as possible to positively respond to the healthy stress of exercise, resulting in not just stronger muscles and lung and heart function, but also stronger bones. The proven way to strengthen bones is with weight-bearing exercise, brisk walking, mountain biking, stair climbing, soccer, basketball, racket sports, and hiking. The greater the weight-bearing impact, the greater the effect. (Gymnasts and runners tend to have very strong bones, despite their thin frames.) Resistive weight training has also been shown to positively stress bones and make them stronger.

It is recommended to use a combination of these weight-bearing exercises for the most effective increase in bone strength, ideally doing weight-bearing exercise for at least 20 to 30 minutes each day, along with upper body strength training three times a week for 20 minutes. Lower body strength training should be done if your exercise program is not weight bearing such as swimming, cycling, or kayaking. Be aware that exercise can also be overdone, causing bones to negatively respond to the excess stress with stress fractures; therefore, impact or intense weight training is not recommended for more than one hour each day, unless you are a highly trained athlete.

Prevention

The good news is that for most women, osteoporosis can be prevented. The best things you can do to prevent osteoporosis is do regular weight-bearing and resistive exercise; eat a healthy diet with at least 1,200 mg calcium daily; limit carbonated drinks, salt, and excess protein; and don't smoke. Additional preventive measures are limiting alcohol to no more than 10 drinks a week and having a bone density test if you have had more than three fractures in your life or have gone through menopause. If you are of reproductive age, make sure you are having regular periods.

Calcium Intake

> Research suggests that 90 percent of American women do not get enough calcium.

Calcium is a mineral your body needs in daily supply, because it cannot be made by the body and is cycled out of the body through nails, hair, skin, sweat, urine, and stool. Unless you are a person who loves dairy products and regularly eats four servings a day of milk, cheese, or yogurt, or regularly eats calcium-fortified foods (see chapter 3, "Nutritional Health"), you must take supplements. Most women must make a conscious effort to eat 1,200 to 1,500 mg calcium a day, because the majority of American women's diets do not even contain half the recommended amount! The bonus: Calcium eases symptoms of PMS, prevents muscle cramping, and has also been found to help with weight management.

Daily Recommended Calcium Intakes*

AGE	AMOUNT MG/DAY
Birth to 6 months	210
6 months to 1 year	270
1 to 3	500
4 to 8	800
9 to 13	1,300
14 to 18	1,300
19 and over	1,200
Pregnant and lactating	1,300
Athletic girls and women	1,500

*Adapted from the National Osteoporosis Foundation

Calcium Supplements

Calcium, a mineral element, is only available to our body in combination with other substances called calcium compounds. The best compounds are those found naturally in dairy products and certain foods, such as broccoli, almonds, and canned salmon. Supplements are usually one of three compounds: calcium carbonate, calcium phosphate, or calcium citrate. The RDI, or daily recommended milligrams of calcium, refers to the amount of calcium in the supplement compound (not total milligrams of compound), also called "elemental calcium." When reading labels, be sure to look for the amount of "elemental calcium" in the supplement compound. Another way to determine the actual calcium of a food source is to take the "percent daily value" (%DV) listed on the food label and add a zero (the FDA's recommended daily intake of calcium is 1,000 mg). For example, one cup of milk has 30%DV of calcium; this equals 300 mg elemental calcium.

The type of calcium compound and the ease of its breakdown by the digestive system affects how well it reaches the bones. In order for calcium to become available to the bones, it must be absorbed; this occurs best in a chewable or liquid form. Calcium is also absorbed best when taken in smaller doses of 500 mg or less at a time. The two most common compounds are calcium citrate and calcium carbonate. Calcium carbonate is found in stomach-soothing tablets such as Tums and offers a cheap and tasty way to get your calcium supplement. Calcium carbonate is best absorbed with food. Calcium citrate can be taken at any time and is recommended for women who also take iron supplements, as carbonate can interfere with iron absorption. (Otherwise, the calcium and iron supplements should be taken separately.) Try to take "purified" forms of calcium, rather than "natural" ones. Oyster shell, bonemeal, or dolomite preparations or many "natural" preparations are not recommended, as they can contain high levels of lead, magnesium, or aluminum, which can be dangerous.

Because of the inconsistencies of the amount of calcium that actually gets absorbed by the bones, it is recommended to slightly exceed the recommended dose and aim for 1,500 mg daily. This is especially true for active athletic girls and women, as calcium is lost through sweat. If your diet is rich in calcium, taking one 300 to 600 mg supplement or taking a multivitamin that contains calcium daily is still recommended. Vegetarians and women who do not eat dairy must take supplements or eat calcium-fortified foods to total at least 1,200 mg a day.

> To test absorption of your calcium supplement, place one tablet in a glass of half vinegar, half water. If it dissolves within 30 minutes, it is recommended as an easily absorbed supplement.

Tips to Help Your Body Absorb Calcium Most Effectively

Divide your total dose if you need to supplement more than 600 mg; take half with dinner and half before bedtime.

Make sure it is an absorbable form (see above).

Do not take it with iron unless you are also taking vitamin C or calcium citrate.

Calcium carbonate should be taken with food.

Take calcium with or after a snack or meal.

Tips in Selecting a Calcium Supplement

Avoid "natural," aluminum, oyster shell, or bonemeal supplement types.

Look for "purified" on the label.

Select a chewable or liquid form.

Experiment with different flavors to find one you like.

———

The importance of maintaining and developing maximum bone strength is clear. Living a healthy, physically active life with a diet rich in calcium is the best thing you can do to take care of your bones. Continue your activities, making sure you are doing weight-bearing exercises and strength training if your sports activity is not impact. Take an extra calcium supplement or two if you are not sure you ate enough foods, and make sure you are having regular periods or have had a bone density test if you are in menopause. Do not smoke and avoid excessive alcohol, carbonated drinks, and high-protein diets. As with anything, if you have concerns, and especially if you have had multiple fractures, see your doctor.

PART II

The Musculoskeletal System: Understanding and Improving Movement and Strength

CHAPTER SIX

The Neck

For many reasons, neck pain is very common in women. Active girls and women can get neck pain as a result of activity, injury, stress, and even sleeping in one position. There are many locations of neck pain— one sided, both sides, at the base of the head, and between the shoulders. Neck pain can also travel to the scalp, face, middle back, shoulders, arms, and hands. It can be associated with headaches, stiffness, and disturbed sleep. Because neck pain is so common, and is often a dull and achy pain, it is frequently ignored until it limits activities or sleep. Not treating these symptoms when they begin can lead to neck pain becoming chronic, which is harder to resolve.

Neck trouble can occur from injury in contact sports such as boxing, hockey, or soccer; from jolting motions in sports such as pole vaulting or power lifting; in sports that require repetitive motion such as swimming; or held postures such as cycling or yoga. Muscle spasms, neck sprain, and tight knots can also occur for no reason and are worsened by stress. Diagnosis of the cause of neck pain should be made by a doctor who is best trained to assess possible weakness or nerve damage and rule out serious injury. An early diagnosis leads to appropriate treatment and quicker return to normal activities and a pain-free life.

Functional Anatomy

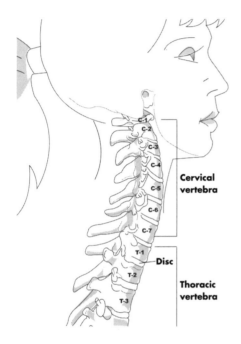

FIGURE 6-1 **Side view: Cervical and upper thoracic spinal column, with numbering of vertebral bones. Bones are separated by discs.**

The neck, known as the "cervical spine," holds up the head, surrounds the spinal cord, and supports and protects the nerve supply to the body as it leaves the brain. The neck is composed of seven vertebral bones, numbered C1 to C7, starting at the skull. These numbers correspond to the level of the pair of nerves that leave the cord in the spaces between the two vertebrae. The vertebrae are separated by cartilage discs to cushion and lend support (see figure 6-1). Discs are made up of the "annulus," the outer lining, and "nucleus pulposus," the inner, cushy gel center (see figure 6-2). The stacked vertebras and discs are the central weight-bearing structure of the spine; behind it is the spinal canal, where the spinal cord is contained. The bones form a strong scaffolding around the spinal cord and are held in place by muscles and ligaments. Through these layers, roots of the spinal cord leave to form the nerves that supply the arms.

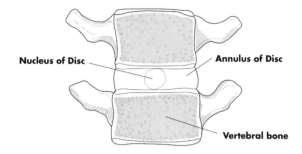

FIGURE 6-2 **Front view: Two vertebral bones cushioned by a disc (cross-sectioned to show annulus and nucleus).**

Nucleus of Disc

Annulus of Disc

Vertebral bone

Pairs of nerve roots leave at each level of the spinal cord to the left and right. Each nerve root merges with other nerve roots in specific patterns to form the larger nerves in the head, neck, shoulder, arm, and hand, innervating both sensation and strength. This pattern forms a map, allowing doctors to figure out the source of nerve problems.

Muscles

The cervical spine is supported and surrounded by ligaments and muscles that allow the neck to move in rotation (turning), flexion (bending) forward and sideways, and extension (arching). The closest muscles to the neck bones are the paraspinals (see figure 6-3.). These are layered muscles that connect and move the neck and spine. The sternocleidomastoid muscles are located on the side of your neck to turn your head; the trapezius muscles cross your neck and shoulder joints and go into your upper back (see figure 6-4). Muscles that surround your shoulder blades, including the upper, middle, and lower trapezius, levators, and rhomboids can also contribute to or be affected by neck problems (see figure 6-5).

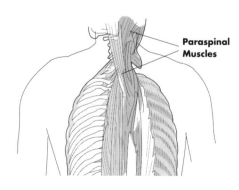

Paraspinal Muscles

FIGURE 6-3 **Back view of deep paraspinal muscles, connected at several levels.**

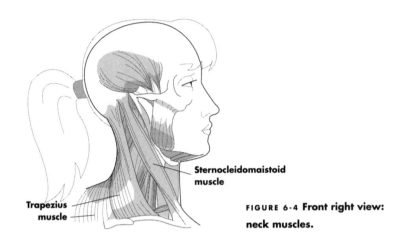

Sternocleidomaistoid muscle

Trapezius muscle

FIGURE 6-4 **Front right view: neck muscles.**

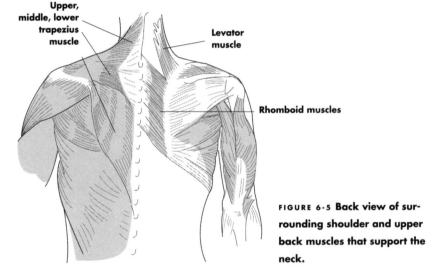

Upper, middle, lower trapezius muscle

Levator muscle

Rhomboid muscles

FIGURE 6-5 **Back view of surrounding shoulder and upper back muscles that support the neck.**

Pain and Injury Patterns

Neck pain and injuries can sometimes be very serious because of the close proximity to the spinal cord and nerve roots. The following are the most common pain and injury patterns, listed in order of descending frequency.

Sprain

Neck sprain is the most common cause of neck pain. Pain is usually achy and tight either in the middle or off to one side; muscles can feel very sore, and movement can cause pain. Whiplash, in which the head gets quickly thrown back in an accident, fall, or contact injury in sport, is a common cause of severe neck sprain. A "stiff neck" is also usually due to neck sprain, caused by muscle spasms that occur while sleeping, working in one position, or lifting too much. You might have woken up with this pain or started noticing it at the end of the day. Occasionally, the onset of neck sprain can be related to an increase in or change in position or activity such as a new computer position at work, a period of lifting or carrying heavy objects, a new baby, repeated motions in sports training such as "heading" practice in soccer, or having to be in one position for a long time such as "head up" swimming in a triathlon.

Causes of Neck Sprain

Whiplash injury	Overuse of neck muscles
Stiff neck while sleeping	Lifting
Holding a posture or position too long	A fall
Looking down for long periods of time	Hitting your head

There are many reasons why neck sprain can be so painful. If the pain began after an injury, there might be small tears in the muscles with underlying weakness. To protect the neck from further damage, the body reacts by tensing or tightening up, further limiting movement and causing more spasms and weakness. The head can feel heavy and the muscles very stiff.

Although neck sprain does not lead to any permanent or serious nerve damage, occasionally there can be associated pain or tingling into the arms due to nerve irritation from spasms of the neck and surrounding muscles.

Symptoms of Neck Sprain

Tight, stiff muscles

Soreness to touch

Trouble turning the head

Difficulty getting comfortable

Heavy head

Neck sprain often causes pain and tightness into the surrounding muscles of the upper shoulders and upper back. Sometimes there can be tight bands of muscles that are "knotty," painful, or swollen. Massage often relieves the pain of the knots but sometimes can make the knots more painful and irritated. These can turn into "trigger points," or tight bands of muscle that, when pressed, send pain shooting down the arms.

Neck sprain is also closely related to stress; stress can cause neck pain, and neck pain can cause stress. Usually they occur together and make one another worse. Neck pain is particularly stressful if it limits activities. Often doctors and therapists will tell you to refrain from exercise, which can make stress, and neck pain, worse! Stress and pain often result in hunched or shrugged shoulders, causing more spasms and tightness. This vicious circle can be very hard to treat. The pain cannot only limit athletics and sports performance, but also interfere with work and sleep.

The best treatment of neck sprain is movement—stretching, slow rotations, and shoulder rolls. This loosens up the muscles, releasing tightness and also increasing muscle strength. Massage and heat are other ways to loosen muscles and increase movement. The worst thing to do is hold the neck stiff; soft neck collars or braces are *not* recommended. Although they might feel good in the short term, all that results from these braces is further tightness, limited movement, spasms, and weakness. If you have been given a soft collar and feel it gives you relief, wear it no more than two hours a day, at the end of the day when muscles feel weak and tired, or while sleeping to help position your head and neck more comfortably. "Old school" medicine includes using rest and bracing to recover from pain, but for the active woman, rest will only make muscles stiffer and weaker and make healing time longer.

"Old School" Medical Advice You Should **Not** Take If You Have a Neck Sprain

ADVICE	REASON NOT TO FOLLOW ADVICE
Wear a soft collar	Leads to further muscle spasms, pain, and weakness
Stop exercising	Leads to increased stress, stiffness, and weakness
Try not to move it	Increases spasms and weakness
Take painkillers regularly	Addictive and should only be taken for severe, excruciating pain as needed

> PERFORMANCE TIP **If you have a neck sprain, avoid the use of soft neck collars, which limit movement and cause stiffness and weak muscles. Instead, start gentle movement and stretching as soon as possible.**

Disc Bulge, Herniation, and Degeneration

Disc pain can be severe and shooting at times from a sudden jerking motion or injury, but it can also occur without injury. Discs can put pressure on the ligaments, causing pain, or pressure on the nerves, causing weakness, numbness, and shooting pain. Disc injury can also cause symptoms similar to sprain with achy, tight stiffness. Some people are genetically prone to disc problems, or they can also be a result of activity done earlier in life.

There are three major types of damage to discs that cause pain in the neck: disc bulge, disc herniation, and disc degeneration. If the disc is protruding from its normal space between the bones of the spine but is retaining its nucleus, it is called a bulge. If the disc is torn and the nucleus is squished out, this is called a herniation. If the disc has lost its nucleus due to an old herniation, wear and tear, bad genetics, or over time with age, this is called degeneration.

All these conditions can be associated with various intensities of pain. Having a disc problem does not necessarily mean you have to limit activity, but it does mean you need to take care of your neck by avoiding jolting activities, including contact and aggressive play in sports. An athlete might be taken out of sports for a while, depending on the severity of the disc herniation and whether nerves are involved. Routine stretching and strengthening of the surrounding muscles will also help prevent the disc problem from becoming worse. Medications and injected steroids can help relieve the inflammation that contribute to pain and nerve symptoms. Herniations are the most likely reason people undergo surgery for neck pain, although this is only necessary in fewer than 5 percent of cases.

Pinched Nerves

"Pinched nerve" is a common term used to describe neck pain that is usually on one side and sends pain down the arm. Medical terms for this condition include "nerve compression" and "radiculopathy." This is caused by abnormal pressure on the nerve, preventing it from sending its signals fully, causing numbness or weakness, causing it to send abnormal signals, or causing pain, burning, or tingling. These symptoms can occur all the time or when the head is turned certain ways.

There are a few problems that can lead to a pinched nerve. The most common cause of radiculopathy in a young, active female is a disc herniation. Nerves in the neck can also be pinched from fractures and arthritis. Occasionally, tight muscle knots can also lead to symptoms of a pinched nerve.

A "burner" or "stinger" is a temporarily pinched nerve due to a fall or forceful pull of the arm or neck. These occur most commonly in field sports and last between a few minutes to a few days. They feel like a sudden, sharp, burning, stinging, or shooting pain that travels from the neck down into the arm and hand. Burners and stingers are the symptoms of a stretching nerve injury that causes small tears in the nerves' protective sheath. Usually, the body repairs them within a week, but sometimes they can cause longer-lasting symptoms.

Most Common Causes of Pinched Nerves in the Neck Area

Disc herniation

Arthritis, stenosis, degenerative disease

Burner/stinger

Arthritis, Stenosis, and Degenerative Disease

Arthritis, stenosis, and degenerative disease are due to both aging and wear and tear. Like a rusty joint, the neck bones become irregularly shaped and collapse, decreasing movement. Usually associated with stiffness in the morning, occasionally these conditions can be associated with arm numbness and weakness as the collapsing, irregular bone can pinch nerves. Certain positions, most often tilting the head to one side or back, can make the neck and arm pain worse. Unfortunately, these conditions are not reversible and can lead to chronic neck pain.

Fractures

Fractures to the cervical spine occur because of injury and are usually severe. The most serious risk of cervical spine fracture is damage to the spinal cord, as fracture leads to instability of the spinal column, leaving the spinal cord unprotected. If there is pressure on the spinal cord or nerve roots, the body usually cannot heal this, resulting in paralysis and long-term disability. Due to this risk, after a severe injury or fall on the head, the injured person should not be moved until emergency medical personnel stabilize the neck with a board or brace and x-rays can be taken. Fractures of the cervical spine are treated very seriously and often require surgery to stabilize the spine, followed by eight to twelve weeks of bracing to allow it to heal. Fractures will take an athlete out of play for several months to one year. If there is associated spinal cord injury, the athlete might become permanently disabled.

WARNING **After any serious fall or hit on the head, do not move the shoulders, head, or neck of the injured person; have her lie as still as possible, and call 911 immediately.**

Evaluation and Treatment

Evaluation

Because of the importance of the nerve supply, injuries to the neck should always be evaluated by a doctor if there has been a serious injury, the pain has lasted more than one week, or the pain is accompanied by arm pain or numbness, tingling, or weakness. Sharp neck pain or achy pain that limits activities should also be seen by a doctor, because the sooner treatment begins, the sooner healing will occur.

Reasons to See a Doctor If You Have Neck Pain

A very jolting injury	Pain that keeps you from sleeping
Loss of feeling	Pain that is worse in different positions
Loss of strength	Pain that lasts more than one week

The doctor should examine your posture, alignment, and movement; feel for areas of tenderness; and test reflexes, sensations, and strength. In anyone who has had an injury, especially women over 35, it is likely that x-rays will be taken, although on the initial visit they are not always necessary. If the pain continues or is accompanied by the more serious signs of weakness or numbness, an MRI is usually recommended to evaluate the discs and nerves. Sometimes, a nerve conduction test/EMG is ordered to evaluate amount of nerve damage.

Treatment

Because most neck pain is not associated with any serious permanent damage, most treatment includes medications, exercises, stretches, and avoiding activities that make the pain worse. As with all injuries, everyone is a little different and treatment should be tailored individually to you. Most neck pain takes one to three months to resolve. Keep in touch with your doctor or health-care professional to make sure you are doing the right things. You should be feeling a little better every week.

If you have been evaluated and treated by a doctor for your neck pain but do not feel you are getting better, ask your doctor to refer you to a physical therapist to help alleviate pain and restore motion and strength to the area. Traction can sometimes relieve pressure on the disc and nerve. Under no circumstances should the physical therapy sessions make you feel worse.

Medications alleviate the pain, inflammation, and spasms. This allows more normal movements and prevents developing weakness. Medications used for neck pain include painkillers, steroids, nonsteroidal anti-inflammatories, muscle relaxers, and antidepressants. Painkillers are mostly narcotics, which are addictive and should only be used if the pain is excruciating. Steroids can be prescribed for a short time to break the inflammation cycle in the body and shrink the irritated inflamed tissues. Nonsteroidal anti-inflammatories, the most commonly prescribed pain medications, also break the inflammatory cycle in the body to decrease stiffness. (See chapter 13, "Exercise Problems and Injuries," for more on anti-inflammatories.) Muscle relaxers are medications used essentially for back and neck pain that relieve the feelings of tightness and stiffness. These also allow for increased movement and decrease weakness and discomfort. A common side effect of muscle relaxers is drowsiness. Other types of medications include anti-convulsant medications and antidepressants. These types of medications target nerve pain and tend to be used when the neck pain is more chronic, lasting between three to six months.

Sometimes injections can help. Trigger-point injections are injections of cortisone, lidocaine, or saline into the tight, tender muscle knot. This breaks up the muscle spasms, scar tissue, and tightness that can develop with neck pain. Trigger-point injections can be repeated every week or two, but should not be done for more than two months if not effective. Epidural injections are steroid injections into the spine. These decrease the inflammation in a focal area of nerve pinching, reducing pressure and pain on the nerve. Epidurals can be repeated if pain symptoms persist, but more than three are not recommended, due to soft tissue weakening effects of steroids. The doctor's skill level is directly related to the success and lowered potential complications of cervical epidurals.

In cases of a fracture, surgery is usually required to fuse the unstable spine, followed by bracing for up to three months to allow the bones to heal. In neck pain caused by problems other than fracture (specifically disc damage), fewer than 5 percent of cases actually require surgery to remove the pressure on the nerve from disc or bone. Fusion is a very serious procedure with risks of decreasing neck movement and perhaps continued neck pain. If an anterior fusion is done, swallowing difficulties can sometimes result. If there is no fracture, surgery should only be performed if there is weakness, loss of sensation, or incurable pain. If you have doubts about your need for surgery but it has been recommended, seek a conservative second opinion, and even a third! Spine surgery has serious risks—and no definite guarantee of complete success.

Stretching and gentle neck, shoulder, and upper back strengthening exercises will relieve pain, restore normal motion, and strengthen the area to prevent a feeling of heaviness and ache. Doing stretches regularly will not only make the pain go away quicker, but also prevent it from coming back. These exercises should feel good and not cause increased pain. Strengthening muscles in the back of the neck and shoulders also helps protect the spine and keep it upright. (Strengthening and stretching exercises are described at the end of this chapter.)

Posture and positioning is very important. Avoid activities that cause you to have your head tilted forward, back, or turned to one side for more than a few minutes, and never hold your head in a position that causes you more pain or symptoms. Sleeping position also can make a big difference. There are many types of neck pillows available. Use the one that is most comfortable for you.

Alternative medicine techniques are very popular methods of relieving neck pain. These include chiropractic care, acupuncture, and various forms of massage. Prior to seeking alternative treatment, it is in your best interest to have a medical doctor's evaluation of the cause of the pain first to make sure there are no precautions for proper healing of your neck condition. Quick thrusting chiropractic manipulations are not recommended in cases of disc herniations, neck misalignment, fractures, or severe arthritis, as it can make these conditions worse. Both acupuncture and massage are safe and effective treatments that work for many neck pain sufferers by increasing circulation, decreasing pain response, and promoting muscle relaxation. Massage is particularly well tolerated and effective, and there are no risks. In athletes, massage is recommended to maintain muscle flexibility and maximum pain-free movement.

Exercises and Stretches

Exercises and stretches are an essential part of restoring normal movement and strength and decreasing pain. If you have had an injury or accident recently, make sure you do not have a fracture or serious disc herniation before doing these exercises. Also, if any of these exercises cause pain or symptoms down your arms, you should not do them.

These exercises should feel good. They should be done at least every other day and will prevent neck pain, sprain, and injury if done regularly. Because the neck muscles function to hold the head steady, neck strengthening exercises involve small movements and held positions. Stretches are very important to the neck to release the tightness caused by held postural motions of daily and sports activities.

Be aware that neck pain tends to come back if you do not continue the stretches and exercises on a regular basis. Try to do the stretches at least once daily, if not several times a day, and the strengthening exercises at least two to three times per week.

Exercises for the Neck and Postural Muscles

The following strengthening exercises should be done standing or sitting up in sets of 10 on each side, alternating sides between sets. Perform the movements slowly, and hold at the farthest position for a slow count of three. Do not push through pain. If there is discomfort, try the exercise with less motion, less (or no) weight, or fewer repetitions. If there is still discomfort, skip the exercise and try again in one week. As you become stronger, increase each set to 15 repetitions. Your goal should be at least two sets, but as they become easier you can work up to three. Weights should start light, beginning with ½ to 2 pounds, increasing slowly; no more than a one-pound increase every two weeks is recommended to a maximum of five to eight pounds. Follow the exercises with the stretches described at the end.

Common Household Light Weight Equivalents

½ pound = a can of tuna

1 pound = a can of beans

2 pounds = a 32 oz. bottle of Gatorade

Note: At two pounds or greater, it is recommended to purchase weights, as they are better designed to be held without wrist strain. (The resources appendix at the end of this book list locations to order equipment.)

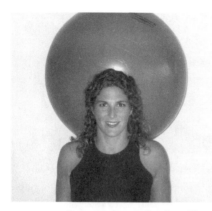

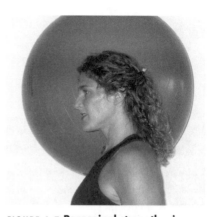

FIGURE 6-6 **Extensor strengthening:** Sitting up or standing with your back toward a wall, place an exercise ball (or two pillows) behind your head. Keeping your chin down, gently press the back of your head into the ball without moving your neck, and hold for a slow count of 10. Release.

FIGURE 6-7 **Paraspinal strengthening:** Repeat above with your side to a wall and a ball between the side of your head and the wall. With your chin neutral, not tilting your head, gently press the side of your head to the ball for a slow count of 10. Release.

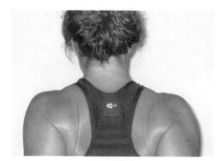

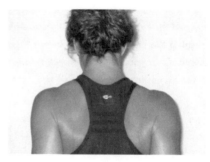

FIGURE 6-8 **Shoulder blade squeezes:** Standing or sitting up, squeeze your shoulder blades together (A), hold for three seconds; then relax (B). Make sure you keep your shoulders down (not shrugged).

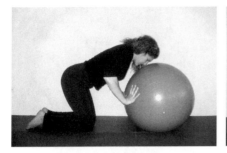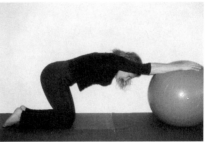

FIGURE 6-9 **Roll-outs (advanced): On your knees with your hands on a ball, palms down, (A) roll the ball out until your arms are straight while slowly counting to three (B). Pull ball back in, slowly counting to three, holding your head straight.**

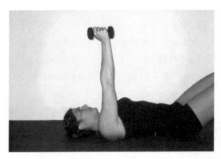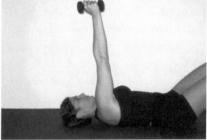

FIGURE 6-10 **Scapular strengthening: Lying on your back, with one arm straight up toward the ceiling, holding a light weight (A), lift your shoulder blade off the floor, pushing the weight up a few inches (B). Hold for a slow count of three, then slowly lower. Keep your head and neck relaxed. (You can do this exercise with both arms at the same time.)**

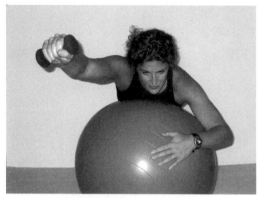

FIGURE 6-11 **Lower trap exercises: Lying on your stomach with your upper chest on an exercise ball (or two pillows or a bench), extend one arm overhead and slightly out to the side, palm down, holding a light weight. Slowly lift your arm up toward the ceiling about six inches. Hold three seconds, then slowly release.**

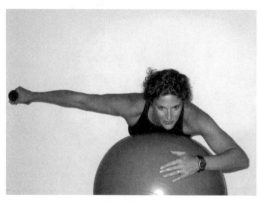

FIGURE 6-12 **Middle trap: Repeat above with arms directly out to side.**

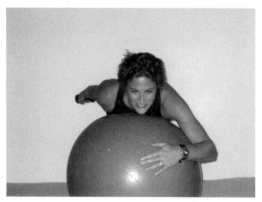

FIGURE 6-13 **Upper trap: Repeat above with arms below shoulders and slightly away from the side of your body.**

Loosening Exercises and Stretches to Be Done Throughout the Day

Try to do these loosening exercises and stretches three to five times daily in sets of three to five each. Hold each stretch for a slow count of five. Do not stretch to discomfort; you should feel a gentle pull then release. You can do these sitting or standing.

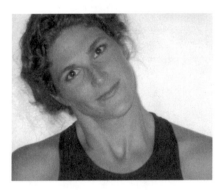

FIGURE 6-14 **Neck rolls: Starting with your right ear to your right shoulder, slowly roll your head forward so your chin is to your chest, your left ear to your left shoulder, and gently tilt your head back for a full roll. Keep shoulders down. Repeat five times to right, then reverse five times to left.**

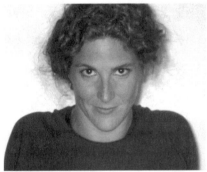

FIGURE 6-15 **Shoulder rolls: Keeping your shoulders relaxed, roll your shoulders back 10 times slowly and 10 times forward slowly. You may also do this exercise one shoulder at a time to increase movement.**

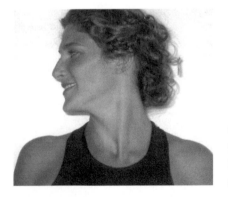

FIGURE 6-16 **SCM Stretch: Gently turn your head as far as you can to one side, holding for 5 to 10 seconds. Repeat on other side.**

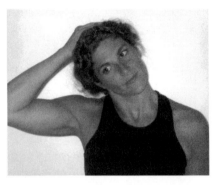

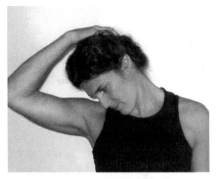

FIGURE 6-17 **Trap stretch: Tilt your right ear toward your right shoulder, gently pulling the top of your head down with your right hand, keeping your left shoulder down. Hold for 5 to 10 seconds. Slowly release and switch sides.**

FIGURE 6-18 **Combined stretch: Repeat previous exercise while holding your chin down into your chest.**

Neck pain is common, especially to active women who also do deskwork or take care of children. Although some neck pain can be serious with risks of nerve injuries, most neck pain is due to muscle sprain and spasms, especially if there are no symptoms in the arms or hands. Careful attention to daily posture and sleeping position and quickly addressing any tightness or spasms will help prevent neck pain from becoming chronic. Regular neck stretching and strengthening of the upper back and surrounding muscles will help maintain posture and mobility and prevent pain.

CHAPTER SEVEN

The Shoulder

The shoulder joint is important for all upper body movements. It is a unique joint in that it provides nearly 360 degrees of motion to the arm, but it must also provide a stable base of support to the arm. The shoulder is designed to be strongest with motion in the front of the body; applying force or repetitive motion in a direction behind the body or overhead as is part of many sports and activities can cause weakness and pain. Because of this, the shoulder joint is subject to all kinds of overuse, injury, and pain syndromes. Movement problems can result from either too much flexibility or too much stiffness, making healing a challenge. Sports in which athletes tend to develop shoulder problems include swimming, martial arts, weight lifting, rock climbing, kayaking, softball, racket sports, volleyball, and basketball.

Because shoulders are necessary for everyday activities, they tend to take more time to heal because complete rest is not always an option. Treatment can also be difficult, especially if the athlete is involved in a sport like swimming, which involves repetitive motion. In most cases, however, these problems can be prevented with strengthening and by using proper technique. As with all musculoskeletal and pain patterns, identifying and treating the cause of pain and dysfunction is essential to the quickest return to sports and daily activities.

Sports with Risks of Shoulder Injury

SOME RISK	HIGH RISK
Skiing	Martial arts
Snowboarding	Weight lifting
Windsurfing	Bodybuilding
Sailing	Rock climbing
Bowling	Hockey
Cycle sports	Swimming
Yoga, exercise classes	Kayaking
Canoeing	Racket sports
Rowing	Softball
Basketball	Rugby
Cheerleading	Volleyball
Golf	Gymnastics

Functional Anatomy

The shoulder joint is an intersection of three bones—the scapula (shoulder blade), the humerus (upper arm bone), and the clavicle (collarbone) (see figure 7-1). The scapula is the central bone, providing leverage and counterweight of the arm. The humerus is the strongest part of the arm on which all the muscles that control shoulder and arm movement attach. The humerus has a round "head" that fits into a cup in the scapula, forming the ball and socket joint that allows the multidirectional movement of the shoulder.

Bones are cushioned and their movement directed by cartilage, ligaments, and tendons. An important cartilage structure in the shoulder is the labrum, which, along with the tendons and ligaments that surround it, form the shoulder capsule. This capsule is where the head of the humerus sits in

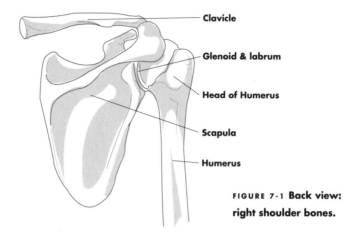

Clavicle

Glenoid & labrum

Head of Humerus

Scapula

Humerus

FIGURE 7-1 **Back view: right shoulder bones.**

the glenoid (socket) of the scapula. The shoulder capsule is angled forward slightly to allow greatest strength and movement in front of the body. There are many ligaments in the shoulder joint; one common area of injury in athletes is the acromioclavicular (AC) ligament. This ligament connects the clavicle, or collarbone, to the scapula, or shoulder blade. Tendons important to the shoulder joint include the rotator cuff tendons and the bicep tendon. The subdeltoid/subacromial bursa is a fluid-filled sac that allows the tendons to move smoothly over the joint (see figure 7-2).

The rotator cuff muscles hold the humerus close into the scapula; they function together to allow movement in different directions of rotation. These thin muscles can be subject to tearing, even without injury. The tendons of the rotator cuff muscles blend together to form the rotator cuff, which holds the humerus in the glenoid of the scapula. The most commonly torn rotator cuff muscle is the supraspinatus.

The bicep muscles have two tendons that also support the rotator cuff (see figure 7-3). The larger supportive muscles that contribute to arm and shoulder movement in front of the body include the upper trapezius, deltoid, pectoralis, and bicep muscles (see figure 7-4). The triceps, middle and lower trapezius, latissimus, and posterior deltoid contribute to shoulder and arm movements in the back. Smaller muscles in the back that control the scapula are the rhomboids, levators, and teres (see figure 7-5).

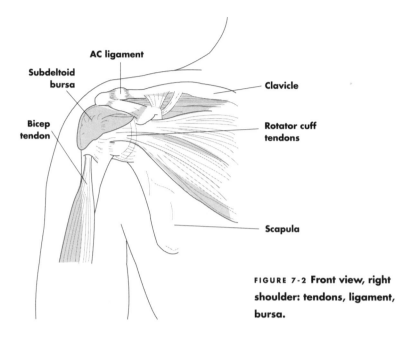

FIGURE 7-2 Front view, right shoulder: tendons, ligament, bursa.

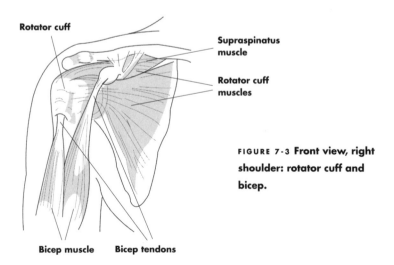

FIGURE 7-3 Front view, right shoulder: rotator cuff and bicep.

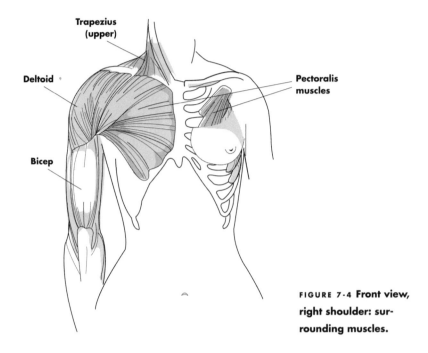

FIGURE 7-4 Front view, right shoulder: surrounding muscles.

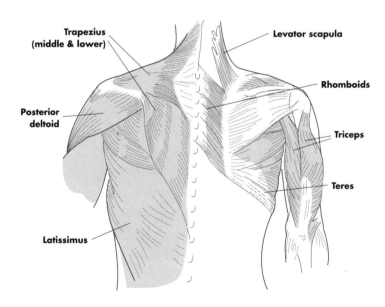

FIGURE 7-5 Back view, both shoulders: larger shoulder and upper back muscles on left; deep muscles on right.

Pain and Injury Patterns

Bursitis

Bursitis is common in women and athletes who engage in activities with repetitive shoulder motions. The pain can be dull at rest and sharp with movement, becoming worse with laying on the shoulder, rotation, and overhead motion. The shoulder is often stiff in the mornings and sore at the end of the day. Bursitis is an inflammation of the subdeltoid bursa and often causes pain in the deltoid muscle and difficulty raising the arm. There can also be tenderness and warmth over the shoulder. Bursitis is often treated with a steroid injection, anti-inflammatories, ice, and therapeutic exercises.

Tendinitis

Tendinitis has symptoms similar to bursitis, and the two syndromes can occur together. Many athletes tend to ignore this pain, because it is often a dull ache that can become less bothersome as the athlete warms up. Pain is greatest with rotation activities such as reaching behind the head or back. The tendons that are inflamed in tendinitis can be those of the rotator cuff muscles or the biceps. Rotator cuff tendinitis is very common in swimmers, kayakers, and pitchers. Biceps tendinitis can occur in weight lifters, bowlers, and rowers, due to stress to the shoulder with poor positioning, overuse, or overload. Nonathletic activities can also result in both tendinitis and bursitis due to a sudden increase in lifting or repetitive rotation motions. Chronic tendinitis, lasting more than three months, can lead to weak tendons, which can strain the muscles enough to tear them.

Impingement

Impingement causes a sharp pain in certain positions, usually with rotation or reaching overhead or behind the body. This pain can stay in the shoulder or shoot into the arm and is a result of inflammation of soft tissue structures that lie close together in the shoulder joint—when muscles, ligaments, joint capsule, or tendons are irritated or pinched underneath bones and tendons. Impingement is an overuse injury, often occurring after an increase in activity or amount of repetitions or weight. It can be common in athletes who do overhead motions such as swimmers or basketball players; those who bear body weight in their hands, including cyclists, gymnasts, and yoga enthusiasts; and athletes who perform repeated swinging motions such as golfers, tennis players, and pitchers.

Rotator Cuff Tear

This is a painful condition that makes overhead lifting and rotation activities difficult, with symptoms similar to tendinitis but with more weakness. The pain can be shooting, burning, and aching. It usually is painful to sleep on the side of the tear. In athletes, a rotator cuff tear can occur because of an injury, overload, or overuse. Rotator cuff tears are also common in women over age 45 due to "wear and tear" over a lifetime. They can develop after chronic tendinitis or impingement. A tear is usually diagnosed on MRI. Surgery is often required, with several months healing time.

Instability

Instability describes a joint with excessive motion. Often, athletes will complain of clicking or popping and a general feeling of looseness. There might be a fear of the shoulder "popping out." Pain is not always present. The problem with instability is that the risk of dislocation increases and predisposes to shoulder muscle weakness that usually results as shoulder structures slide and stretch out the tendons and muscles. Some women feel a "clunk" in the joint with certain motions and are able to make their shoulders pop out of joint. Instability is common in swimmers, gymnasts, waterskiiers, and athletes who have had dislocation or stretching injuries. Instability needs to be rigorously strengthened to prevent worse pain, weakness, and severe dislocations. Athletes with instability should try to avoid popping their shoulder out and refrain from motions that make the joint feel unstable. Occasionally, surgery is required to tighten the joint and reduce dislocation risk.

Dislocation

When a shoulder comes out of its socket it is painful, appears deformed, and cannot be moved. If a shoulder dislocates for the first time, it should be evaluated by a doctor immediately to make sure that no other structures are damaged. (Some girls and women have repeated dislocations with only mild discomfort and are able to relocate the shoulder themselves.) Dislocations can occur due to a loosened or torn labrum and capsule. Sometimes, a sling must be worn to allow the capsule to tighten up; surgery might also be necessary. As with all shoulder injuries, disciplined strengthening needs to be done once the dislocation is stabilized. Also, maintaining activities within the "safe zone" (see figure 7-6) is important to prevent reinjury.

Labral or Capsule Tear

This type of tear occurs either as an overuse injury typical of boxers and pitchers, or after a trauma or fall. A tear of the capsule that makes up the socket of the joint, it can cause clicking and even a feeling of locking with pain in certain motions. Labral tears can heal on their own, or can require surgery. The capsule and labrum can also be stretched, resulting in instability or dislocation, as described above.

Separation

This is a tear of the AC ligament most common after a fall directly on the shoulder or on an outstretched arm, often accompanied by a pop and sharp pain. Separation causes pain and swelling in the front of the shoulder. Because this can result in an unstable shoulder with trouble carrying or bearing weight, shoulder separations sometimes need surgical repair.

Arthritis

Arthritis causes stiffness and pain with motion. Arthritis usually occurs later in life or after a severe injury. It can limit motion and thereby lead to weakness. This dull pain can be throbbing, worse in the mornings, aggravated in bad weather, and severe after use.

Frozen Shoulder

A frozen shoulder occurs most commonly in older women who are less active. Frozen shoulders sometimes begin as bursitis or tendinitis, causing a woman to restrict use of her arm in order to avoid pain. The limited motion leads to a stiff, "frozen" shoulder, resulting in greater pain and limited motion. The treatment for frozen shoulder is to increase motion as much as possible with aggressive stretching and strengthening. This therapy is painful but essential to restore normal shoulder function; strong pain medications are often required to allow stretching to be more effective. Occasionally, surgery is needed to release the capsule.

Fractures

Fractures occur most often to the clavicle, humerus, and acromion, a connecting part of the scapula. Depending on the type of fracture, a sling or surgery can be required to stabilize the bone while it heals.

Shoulder and Neck Pain

Because of overlapping muscles crossing both the neck and shoulder joints, neck pain can cause shoulder pain and vice versa. There can be tight knots of muscle and a sensation of pain shooting down the arm on one side. Sometimes, there can be numbness or tingling down the arm due to a pinched nerve at a high level of the neck. This is usually associated with underlying muscle weakness (see chapter 6, "The Neck").

Evaluation and Treatment

If you develop shoulder pain, rest for a few days by avoiding any irritating sports or activities, including sleeping on the opposite side, avoiding overhead lifting, and limiting rotation and reaching across and behind you. Apply ice or cold packs to the shoulder two or three times a day for 10 minutes. If you can, take an anti-inflammatory medicine such as ibuprofen (Advil) or naproxen (Alleve) as directed for those days. If your shoulder is feeling better, keep icing and gradually return to normal activities with a focus on maintaining your full motion. Begin strengthening exercises. If your pain does not resolve within one week, or if you have limited motion, see a doctor as soon as possible, as shoulder pain has a tendency to quickly get worse and is easiest to treat early in its development.

Evaluation

The doctor will ask questions with regard to your symptoms of pain or history of injury or change in activity. The exam will focus on your strength, motion, and painful activities, with possible x-rays to look at the bones. If tears in the tendons, muscles, or ligaments are suspected, you might be sent for an MRI to evaluate these structures.

Treatment

Your doctor will likely treat you with medications for pain and inflammation and prescribe exercises to restore motion and strength. Icing after exercise is recommended to reduce inflammation. Physical therapy can be helpful to speed healing, restore motion, and make sure the exercises are done properly and are most effective.

If the pain is persistent, a cortisone injection given into the joint can reduce inflammation directly at the site of irritation. Sometimes, these are repeated in follow-up visits, but more than three cortisone injections are not recommended, as they can increase the risk of tendon tear. For pain that does not resolve with these treatments, arthroscopic surgery, done through small incisions, might be necessary. If there is severe damage to tendons, ligaments, or to the capsule, surgery must be done through a larger incision. Sometimes after surgery a sling must be worn to limit use and movement to allow full healing. Physical therapy or a regular exercise and stretching program as recommended by your surgeon is always important after shoulder surgery to ensure optimal return to motion and strength.

Modifying Activities

An important part of recovery from pain and injury and preventing a flare-up is changing behaviors that contributed to the problem in the first place. The "safe zone" describes the area of motion that a shoulder can safely go through without risk of injury or pain. This is the zone in which your shoulder muscles work most effectively and where you are strongest and least subject to injury. In sports, this is also your area of greatest strength; turning your body to open up the shoulder is an essential component of a strong tennis serve, pitch, and swimming stroke. Learning proper technique can correct shoulder straining positions or motions. Proper technique in sports always incorporates the most forceful movements into the safe zone. This zone is identified as the area in front of the plane of your body, between your arms stretched out to your sides and below your arms overhead (see figure 7-6). You can check to see if you are in the safe zone if you are standing with your head facing forward but you are still able to see your hands in your peripheral vision (without shifting your eyes or your head). Once you lose sight of your hands, you lose the safe zone.

In impingement, bursitis, or tendinitis, reducing the irritating activity is key to reducing the inflammation. These syndromes commonly return if you are not careful, so it is important to be aware of the pain- and inflammation-causing activities. These include proper positioning.

When lifting, your hands should start closer to your body with your elbows bent. When pressing or bearing weight (push-ups, road biking), your hands should be just at or outside of shoulder width. Position during sleep is a common irritant of shoulder problems; avoid sleeping on one side all night, and especially avoid sleeping on an arm stretched overhead. Most important is a gradual return to activities, particularly those that irritated your shoulder, after your shoulder pain is resolved, making sure you do not do "too much, too soon." Allow yourself to rest from these activities if your shoulder pain flares up, and make a habit of applying ice for at least 10 minutes after irritating activities or at the end of the day.

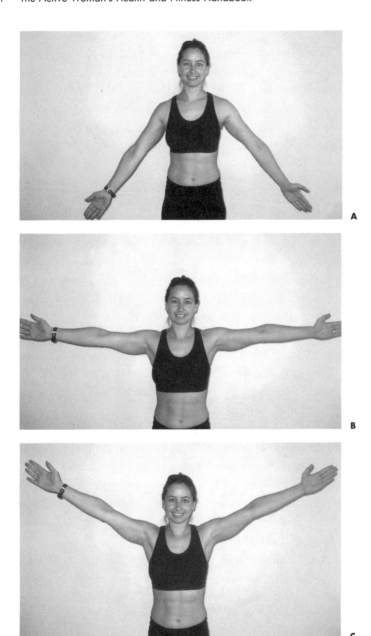

FIGURE 7-6 A through G: The safe zone is the area in front of the plane of your body, where you can always see your hands when your head is forward. A through D: front view; E through G: side view.

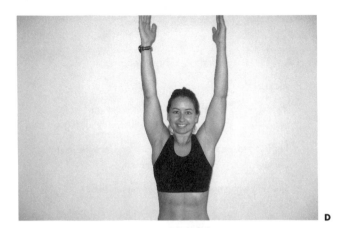

D

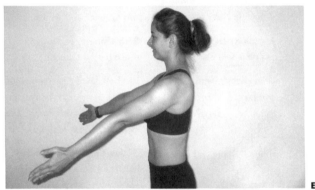

E

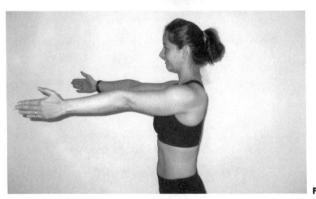

F

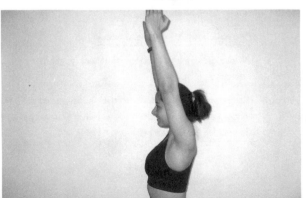

G

Correcting Activities That Irritate Shoulder Problems

	ACTIVITY	CORRECTION
Bringing movements into the safe zone	Putting on your coat	Painful side arm in first and reach around with good side.
	Reaching to the side for an item	Turn and face the item to grab it.
	Sleeping with your arm over your head	Break this habit!
	Putting your bra on with a hook in back	Fasten in front and spin the bra around.
	Reaching behind you to put on a seat belt	Rotate your upper body to reach for the seat belt.
Decreasing shoulder irritation	Lifting heavy items overhead	Use both hands, keeping your hands close to your body with your elbows bent; lift only light amounts; or ask for help.
	Lifting children	Sit down and lift from sitting; hold child close to your body.
	Carrying a heavy purse	Wear a backpack or lighten your load.
	Driving and turning a steering wheel	Hold steering wheel on bottom half (4 and 8 o'clock).
	Sleeping on the painful side	Sleep on your back, front, or opposite side.

Correcting Sports and Gym Movements That Irritate Shoulder Problems

SPORTS ACTIVITY	CORRECT MOVEMENT BY . . .
Throwing or serving a ball	Turn body sideways and keep arm in front of plane of body.
Swimming	Increase body roll and bend elbow.
Cycling	Widen grip on handlebars; adjust seat height to lessen weight on arms.
Yoga (downward dog, inversions)	Keep arms directly under shoulders, not stretched out beyond head; keep your shoulder muscles active; bear weight more in your legs; use a wall to support inversions.

Golf	Rotate from your hips to finish swing.
Weight training	Avoid lifting heavy weight overhead and behind your body.
Chest presses	Avoid curved chest press bar. Use spotter to prevent bar from dropping too close to your chest. Your hands should be slightly out from shoulder width.
Chest flys	Make sure your arms start in front of the plane of your body, not behind you.
Push-ups	Widen your hands; do not drop your body as close to the floor.
Tricep dips	Limit depth of dip.
Pull-ups	Start the next pull-up before your arms are fully stretched out. Turn palms facing toward you.
Lat pull-downs	Never pull down behind your head.

Shoulder Exercises

Unless you have had a recent dislocation or surgery, the following exercises are recommended for everyone to strengthen the rotator cuff and shoulder-stabilizing muscles. While doing each exercise, motion should be within a pain-free range. For all exercises, remember that, compared to larger, upper body muscles, the rotator cuff muscles are very small muscles and require only light weights to strengthen. Where you might normally use 10 or 15 pounds for biceps or triceps, rotator cuff muscles often do not require more than 2 to 5 pounds, and even less if you are injured. Each motion should be for a slow count of three on the up motion, hold for a slow count of three, and lower for a slow count of three. For all exercises, try to do two sets of 10, rotating through the circuit of exercises for one set, then repeating them all for the second set. This allows each muscle to rest. As you become stronger, and if you feel you must increase the exercise intensity, change only one of the following factors per week: increase the weight one pound every two weeks up to a maximum of eight to ten pounds (many can receive full benefits at five); increase your set to 15 repetitions; add a third set. Do not increase all these factors at once.

Start with the first three exercises listed and try to do them three to five times in the first week. If they are easy, progress to the next set of exercises listed. If you have pain, reduce repetitions, range of motion, or weight amount. If you feel achy afterward, apply ice for at least 10 minutes after exercise to decrease inflammation and pain. Some exercises may be done with both arms at the same time, if you are comfortable with the motion. These exercises are indicated by an asterisk*. It is a good idea to work both shoulders, as the body tends to have symmetrical weaknesses.

Be careful of some exercises at the gym: pull-ups, chin-ups, flys, and pecs should only be done after you are virtually pain-free. Safe upper body strengthening exercises include bicep arm curls, upright rows, tricep curls with arms in front, and lat pull-downs with arms pulling down in front. Remember, if an exercise causes pain, modify it by reducing weight, motion, and repetitions. You might have to skip the exercise and try again in a week when your strength has improved.

Exercise Tip: If an Exercise Causes Pain, Try One or All of the Following:

1. Decrease the weight.

2. Make the motion smaller (just holding a position improves strength).

3. Decrease the repetitions.

4. If there is still pain, stop the exercise and try again in a week.

5. Apply ice for 10 to 15 minutes afterward.

Rotator Cuff Strengthening Exercises

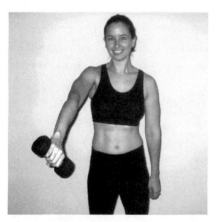 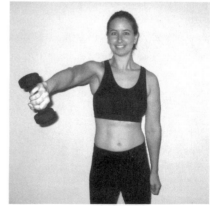

FIGURE 7-7 **Supraspinatus: With your straight arm over the outside of the front of your thigh, hold a weight with your pinky-side up (A) and slowly lift your arm to just below shoulder level (B).***

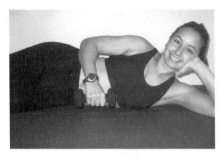
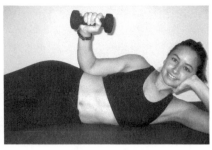

FIGURE 7-8 **External Rotation (right shoulder): Lie on your left side, holding your right elbow into your body with your elbow bent at 90 degrees (A). Keeping your elbow steady at your side, slowly rotate the weight up (B). Slowly lower back to starting position.**

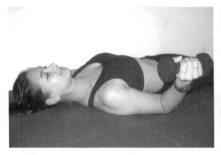
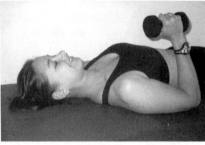

FIGURE 7-9 **Internal Rotation: Lie on your back, with your right elbow bent to 90 degrees at the side of your body. With your palm up toward ceiling, keeping your elbow bent and in at your side (A), rotate the weight up (B) and slowly lower back down.***

Strengthening Larger Surrounding Muscles in Front

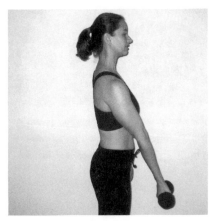 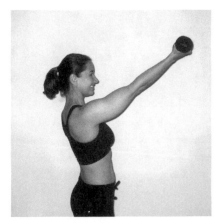

FIGURE 7-10 **Anterior Deltoid: With your arm straight down in front of your thighs, palm up, (A) lift the weight straight up within a pain-free range (B). Slowly lower***

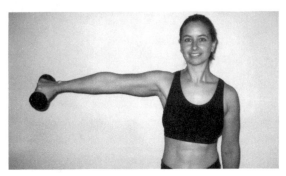

FIGURE 7-11 **Lateral Deltoid: Begin with your arm at your side, elbows straight, palm down. Slowly lift the weight out to your side to just below shoulder height. Slowly lower.***

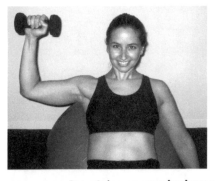 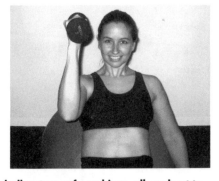

FIGURE 7-12 **Pecs: Lying on your back on a ball or two sofa cushions, elbow bent to 90 degrees and out to side but still in front of the plane of the body, (A) bring your arm toward the front (B). Slowly lower arm back to starting position.***

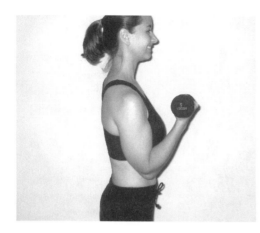

FIGURE 7-13 **Biceps: Keeping your elbow in front against your body, bend your elbow up, holding the weight with your palm up. Slowly lower.***

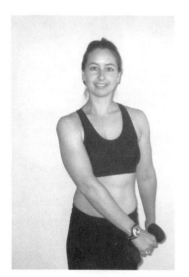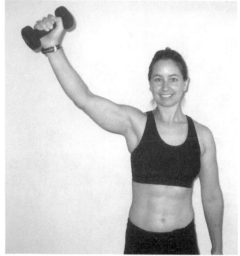

FIGURE 7-14 **Cross Body Reach: Starting with your right arm on your left thigh, holding the weight with your palm down, (A) slowly raise the weight up and across your body overhead on the right, keeping your elbow straight and your arm in front of the plane of your body (B). Slowly lower.**

* = These exercises may be done with both arms at the same time.

Strengthening Larger Muscles in Back

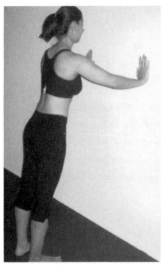
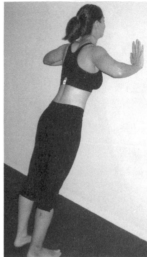

FIGURE 7-15 **Push-Ups: Basic push-ups off the wall. Stand about two feet from a wall, hands slightly wider than your shoulders, with palms flat against the wall (A). Slowly lower your body toward wall for a slow count of three (B), then slowly press back.**

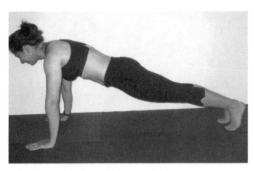

FIGURE 7-16 **Push-Up: Push up with your arms off the floor starting with your arms straight, slightly wider than shoulder width apart. Slowly lower to bend elbows so your face is several inches away from the floor. Keep your stomach sucked in, your body straight, and straighten your elbows back to start position.**

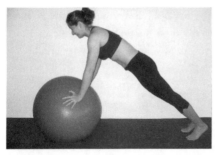
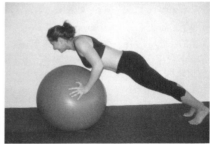

FIGURE 7-17 **Advanced Push-Up on Ball: Push-ups on a stability ball (A, B).**

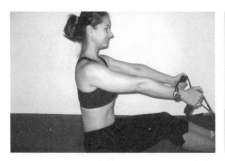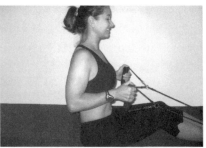

FIGURE 7-18 **Rows: Sitting, loop a stretch cord or band around a stable object and hold one end in each hand with your arms straight out in front (A). Squeezing your shoulder blades together first, bend your elbows and pull your shoulders back to pull your hands into the sides of your body (B). Slowly release your arms straight out in front. GYM VERSION: Upright row machine.**

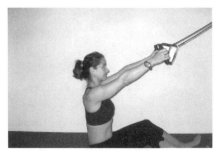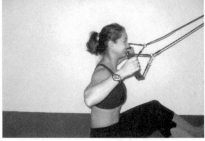

FIGURE 7-19 **Lat Pull-Downs: Using a stretch cord or band, loop it around a stable object overhead and in front (such as a door hook or curtain rod) and hold one end in each hand with your arms overhead and out in front of you with your palms facing out (A). Squeeze your shoulder blades together first, then bend your elbows and pull your shoulders down and back arms so hands come just in front of your chest (B). Slowly release back to start with your arms overhead and in front. GYM VERSION: Lat pull-down machine.**

Stretching

Hold each stretch for a slow count of five, repeating three to five times for each stretch session. Stretches are shown for the right side and should be done in equal repetitions on the left.

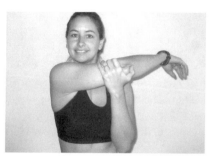

FIGURE 7-20 Tricep and Rear Shoulder Stretch: Reach your right arm across in front of your body. Pull your right arm across with your left hand behind your right elbow.

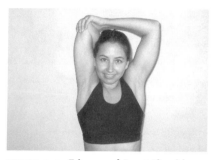

FIGURE 7-21 Tricep and Front Shoulder Stretch (right): Reach your right arm overhead with your elbow bent and gently press backward with your left hand behind your right elbow.

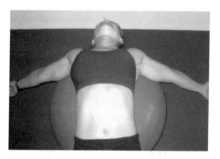

FIGURE 7-22 Pec Stretch: Lying on back on a ball or large sofa cushions, let your arms fall to your sides. (Note: This is outside the safe zone, but because it is a stretch without weight or movement, it is okay.)

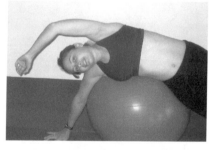

FIGURE 7-23 Side stretch: Lying on the left side of a ball, reach your right arm over your head and allow it to fall to the left side overhead.

Pain and injuries to the shoulder are common and can be quite painful and even disabling. With the exception of falls or traumatic injuries, overuse injuries can be prevented with appropriately positioned sports and daily activities. Strengthening exercises protect the shoulder joint and prevent weakening of the rotator cuff muscles. These exercises are important to all women, as shoulder pain and problems are common to both athletes and nonathletes. Rotator cuff and shoulder strengthening should be incorporated into a regular strength training routine to prevent pain and injury syndromes.

CHAPTER EIGHT

The Elbow, Wrist, and Hand

Because of the many directions of motion and constant use, the elbows, wrists, and hands are particularly at risk for pain and injury due to repetitive motion. Most of the pain problems are related to overuse and have commonly known names related to sports such as tennis elbow, golfer's elbow, and skiier's thumb.

Athletes who commonly suffer elbow and wrist injuries include racket sports players, golfers, baseball and softball players, and rowers. Mountain climbers, boxers, basketball players, and team sports players can also be subject to finger injuries. In falls, the hands and wrists are often the first to suffer, as they hit the ground first. Nonathletic activities frequently causing elbow, wrist, and hand pain include computer use, cleaning, and gripping or twisting activities. Because elbow, wrist, and hand problems often cause trouble with day-to-day functions in addition to fitness activities, avoiding overuse and injury problems is to your advantage. Early diagnosis, treatment, and prevention is important.

Functional Anatomy

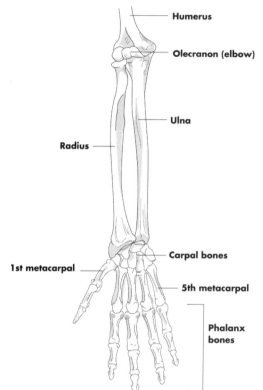

Humerus

Olecranon (elbow)

Ulna

Radius

Carpal bones

1st metacarpal

5th metacarpal

Phalanx
bones

**FIGURE 8-1 Palm view:
right hand bones.**

The elbow joint is made up of three bones: the humerus, radius, and ulna. The wrist has eight small carpal bones. The hand is made up of five metacarpal bones; the finger bones are called phalanx bones (see figure 8-1). Movement at the elbow and finger involves bending and straightening; the wrist bends as well as rotates.

The bones are connected by ligaments, and the muscles attach to the bones via tendons. There are many tendons connecting the muscles that control fine finger motion. These are bundled together by fibrous tissue in the small area of the wrist, creating two areas of possible pain in the hand and wrist, which are named after their location in the wrist: carpal tunnel syndrome and DeQuervain's tendinitis. The small muscles between the fingers that control finer movements are called intrinsic muscles. Finger muscles are named for their function: Abductors bring the thumb and fifth finger away from the hand, flexors bend the fingers, and intrinsics bring the fingers together and apart (see figure 8-2).

The larger muscles that control the fingers and hand attach to the forearm around and just below the elbow. They are named for their function in the palm down position: Wrist extensors bend the wrist back; flexors bend it down (see figure 8-3). Rotation of the wrist is controlled by the pronators and supinators. The medial (inside) and lateral (outside) epicondyles of the humerus are where the extensors, flexors, pronators, and supinators attach. These are common sites of inflammation and pain. Elbow movement is controlled by the large bicep and brachioradialis muscles, which bend the elbow, and the triceps, which straighten it (refer to figures 7-4 and 7-5, page 128).

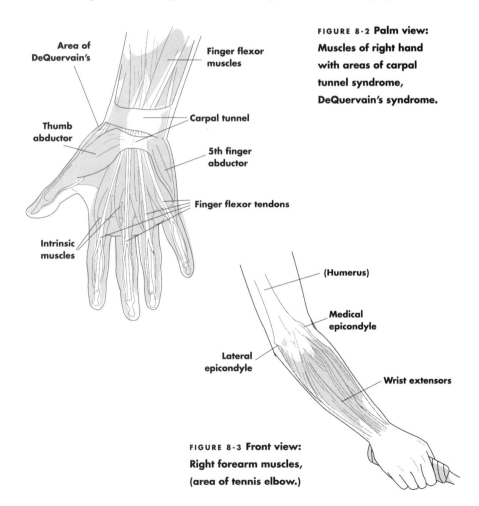

Area of
DeQuervain's

Finger flexor
muscles

FIGURE 8-2 **Palm view:
Muscles of right hand
with areas of carpal
tunnel syndrome,
DeQuervain's syndrome.**

Thumb
abductor

Carpal tunnel

5th finger
abductor

Finger flexor tendons

Intrinsic
muscles

(Humerus)

Medical
epicondyle

Lateral
epicondyle

Wrist extensors

FIGURE 8-3 **Front view:
Right forearm muscles,
(area of tennis elbow.)**

Pain and Injury Patterns

Pain and injury patterns are listed in descending order of frequency. Tendinitis is described first, as this is by far the most common and tendinitis is often a component of other injuries.

Tendinitis

One of the most common injuries, tendinitis causes pain and stiffness with movement at various sites at the elbow, wrist, and hand. It is caused by inflammation of the tendons due to overuse and strain. Pain can be sharp at times with aching dull pain at the end of the day and stiffness after rest. If the inflammation is at the point where the tendon attaches to bone, it can also cause pain in the bone. Because motion is painful, weakness often results. The most common types of tendinitis are tennis elbow, pain on the outside of the elbow, and DeQuervain's syndrome, or pain on the thumb side of the wrist. These develop either through frequent repetitive motion or through improper grip or wrist position that strains the tendons.

Golfers, racket sports players, rowers, climbers, and weight lifters often develop wrist or elbow tendinitis. Skiers can develop tendinitis in the thumb and wrist due to improper poling; water-skiers can get wrist tendinitis also. Although tendinitis is mostly an overuse injury, a fall or injury can result in chronic pain and weakness that develops into tendinitis.

Techniques to Avoid Tendinitis

Ensure proper form, technique, equipment, and grip size.

Decrease rotation and twisting motions.

Stop the activity if there is sharp pain.

Apply ice after activity if there is soreness or pain.

Rest until the pain goes away.

Stretch the wrist and elbow muscles several times daily.

Do the strengthening exercises at the end of this chapter.

Resting inflamed muscles and tendons by wearing a splint is helpful. The splint can also be worn while sleeping, to prevent unintentionally moving in irritating positions. Tendinitis also improves with icing, stretching, and strengthening activities; however, there is a fine line between strengthening and rest. The use of anti-inflammatory medications or steroid injections as recommended by your doctor can also be very helpful. An essential component of recovering from and preventing recurrence of tendinitis is to learn better technique in your sport or activity.

Tennis Elbow

The most common variation of tendinitis at the elbow is tennis elbow, medically termed "lateral epicondylitis" (see figure 8-3). Tennis elbow occurs in nonracket sport activities also, such as painting, computer use, or lifting. Tennis elbow causes pain over the outer side of the elbow with striking the ball, carrying, rotating, and gripping.

Relief comes from rest, icing, stretching, and strengthening. Anti-inflammatory medications are helpful as well. Sometimes, a cortisone injection is needed to resolve the inflammation, although this should not be repeated more than twice. For racket sports players, learning proper technique, decreasing amount of wrist motion, hitting the ball in front of the body, and having proper grip size and string tension can help resolve symptoms and keep the pain from returning. An elbow strap can also help. For those who develop tennis elbow without playing racket sports, treatment is similar and includes repositioning the keyboard or mouse, making grips easier to hold, decreasing lifted loads, and a gradual return to use of that hand and wrist. Strengthening exercises should continue indefinitely to prevent the problem from returning.

Tips to Avoid Tennis Elbow

Proper racket grip size

Lower string tension

A low-vibration racket

A lighter racket

Hit the ball in front of, not behind you

Do not flick your wrist when hitting

Loosen your grip on the racket

Golfer's Elbow

Golfer's elbow is similar to tennis elbow, but causes pain on the inner side of the elbow. It is treated with similar exercises as tennis elbow. Techniques in sports that help alleviate the pain include gripping the racket, club, or bat less tightly; having a properly sized grip; using low-tension equipment; and reducing wrist motion.

DeQuervain's Tenosynovitis

Pain over the thumb side of the wrist with gripping and pinching activities is called DeQuervain's tenosynovitis. It can occur in women who do paddle water sports, use clubs or rackets, lift weights, box, or do a lot of hand positions in yoga. This is also a common office pain syndrome. Curing DeQuervain's tenosynovitis requires modifying position and technique, as well as changing activities done throughout the day to lessen stress on the thumb side of the wrist. A brace that controls thumb movement is often helpful.

Locking Elbow

A locking elbow joint can occur in softball pitchers, catchers, gymnasts, and throwing track and field athletes. This can indicate either a bone chip, scar tissue, or thickened tendon that gets stuck in the joint. The condition can improve with rest and stretching. Bone chips might need to be surgically removed with minor orthopedic surgery done through a small scope.

Finger Dislocations and Jams

Finger dislocations and jams are also a very frequent sports injury. They are common in field and court sports. They can be problematic, as they are often quite painful, and if not splinted right away, fingers can heal in a bent or crooked position. It is recommended that finger injuries get evaluated by a hand specialist as soon as possible if there is a lot of swelling, pain, or trouble with movement. Referral to an occupational therapist is often recommended for this injury in order to maximize your chance of having full motion and use.

Nail Injuries

Nail injuries are also common. These include bruises under the nail bed, the nail bed filling with blood, or avulsions, in which the nail can get torn off. If these injuries affect more than half the nail, they should be seen by a doctor. To avoid these injuries, nails should be kept short in field and contact sports. Jewelry should be left in the locker room to avoid catching on clothes or fingers, which might lead to more injuries.

Ligament Injuries

Tendon or ligament injuries in the wrist and hand can cause a clicking sensation, pain, instability, and weakness. These can be due to severe injury or overuse with weakness that causes the tendon or ligament structure to become unstable and tear. These are treated with a splint, rest, and gradual return to activity. Ligament tears in the fingers are common as overuse injuries in rock climbers or due to falls and injuries. Skiier's thumb is a ligament tear at the base of the thumb due to a fall or caught pole. Ligament injuries are usually immobilized to allow healing, but sometimes, if they interfere with function, tendon and ligament tears might require surgery. It is highly recommended that you see a hand specialist if you suspect a ligament injury due to the essential, yet delicate, structure and function of the hand and wrist.

Ganglion Cysts

Cysts are quite common in the wrist, particularly over the base of the thumb. These tend to occur in people who use their hands and wrists a lot— climbers, golfers, rowers, tennis players, and computer users. Sometimes, they will resolve on their own. They can be drained with a large needle or surgically removed if they affect motion or cause pain.

Fractures

The most serious injuries are fractures. Usually, they require casting to limit motion while healing takes place, which can take between six to eight weeks. Casting can cause swelling of the fingers, wrist, or hand. (If there is also numbness or color change, call your orthopedist.) To reduce swelling, keep the arm elevated as much as possible and try to move and stretch the fingers, wrist, elbow, or shoulder joint above and below the casted area several times a day. This maintains motion at the healthy joints to prevent them from becoming stiff and painful.

PERFORMANCE TIP—CASTS To prevent swelling, keep the casted area elevated above the level of the heart as much as possible. Also try to move and stretch the fingers, wrist, elbow, and shoulder at least three times daily to prevent healthy joints from stiffening up and becoming weak.

After the cast is removed, there is often stiffness, limited motion, and weakness because the muscles have not been used. Gradually increasing the amount of movement and weight carried over the following month will reduce discomfort. Sometimes, there will be more hair growth where the cast was; this will eventually go away. Also, the skin can be very dry, flaky, and itchy. Frequent use of lotions and moisturizer will resolve this. Fractures in the elbow, wrist, and hand tend to lead to problems regaining full motion, so aggressive stretching is essential to restore your normal motion and function. If you cannot stretch the area yourself, or if there is a lot of pain, weakness, and stiffness, ask your doctor to refer you to an occupational therapist. Over the next three months after cast removal, you should gradually return to normal motion and function. You can begin your return to sports when you have 80 to 90% normal motion and strength.

Stress Fractures

In gymnasts, rowers, and people who bear a lot of weight through their upper extremities, stress fractures can occur at the wrist and forearm bones. Stress fractures cause deep, aching pain that develops either slowly or suddenly. Usually, stress fractures are not related to injury but often occur soon after an increase in the amount or intensity of training. Stress fractures tend to become areas of chronic pain. In young athletes, they can interfere with bone development (see chapter 5, "Bone Health and Osteoporosis"). Avoiding carrying, lifting, or bearing weight for four to six weeks from diagnosis is an essential part of the treatment. Bone density testing is recommended if you have repeated stress fractures.

Numbness and Tingling

Numbness and tingling in the fingers or part of the arm are signs of a pinched nerve. Although this pinching can be due to a herniated disc in the neck, more commonly it is related to pinching at the elbow or wrist. The two most frequent nerve "impingements" are cubital tunnel at the elbow and carpal tunnel at the wrist. They are named for the narrow bony and fibrous areas the nerves pass through. Nerve impingements can also result from injury if a sudden jolting or quick motion puts pressure on the nerve. Weight lifters and cyclists tend to get these injuries most often, due to weight strain combined with repeated motion and stretching of the nerves. Golfers, batters, bowlers, and racket sports players can also develop these problems. Desk workers, chefs, carpenters, and artists can develop these syndromes even more frequently. Often, when these nerve entrapments develop, symptoms are made worse by other activities done during the day such as typing, painting, or lifting.

Cubital tunnel syndrome is under the elbow and feels as if you are hitting your funny bone. It causes tingling or numbness into the fourth and fifth fingers. Often, relieving pressure on the elbow by limiting frequent bending and avoiding leaning on the elbow will help resolve this. Sleeping with the elbow bent aggravates cubital tunnel syndrome.

Carpal tunnel syndrome is common in people who use their wrists repetitively; less frequently due to athletic activities, carpal tunnel syndrome can occur in people who write a lot, cut or clip items, paint, or sleep with their hands curled in. This can also occur in pregnancy for no reason at all and in new mothers who use their hands frequently. Carpal tunnel syndrome tends to cause numbness and tingling in the thumb to middle fingers along with weakness and wrist pain. Wrist splints, anti-inflammatory medications, stretching, and decreasing repetitive activities are the most effective treatment. Vitamin B_6 at 100 mg daily can help with the numbness and tingling symptoms of this and other types of nerve irritation. (During pregnancy, consult with your doctor before taking extra vitamins.)

Bicyclists frequently develop numbness and tingling in the wrist and hand because they place a lot of weight on their hands in bent positions while riding. Often holding up their upper body with their wrists, there is a lot of stress on the joint and nerves as they are stretched and pressed on across this area. The numbness tends to go away after the ride is over but can become longer lasting if pressure and position are not adjusted through long rides. Gel or cushioned gloves are recommended to relieve pressure on the joint and nerves. Adjusting handlebar shape and position to lessen pressure on the wrists, changing position frequently, and making sure that the wrists are held straight rather than cocked to one side, avoiding any irritating positions are recommended to prevent possible nerve impingements.

Ways to Avoid Nerve Problems

Reduce wrist motion.

Make sure your wrist is straight, not bent, when doing activities.

Change position if you are feeling tingling or numbness.

Stop the activity if you have the tingling or numbness for more than 10 minutes.

See a doctor if the problem occurs during other activities.

Try a splint during activities and at night to reduce irritating motion.

Wear gel cushioned gloves for biking and lifting.

Take 100 mg vitamin B$_6$ daily.

Evaluation and Treatment

If you have any pain, weakness, or numbness in your elbow, hand, or wrist lasting more than one week, see your doctor for an evaluation. She will perform an examination that might include x-rays. Other tests she might order include a nerve test if there are nerve symptoms or an MRI if the pain does not resolve with simple treatments.

When a diagnosis is made, a splint might be recommended to rest the area and allow for healing. Changing positions or activity type to reduce pain is part of treatment and prevention. For pain and inflammation, treatments include medications and icing the painful area for 10 minutes a few times daily. If the pain is severe or persists, referral to an occupational therapist is recommended. She will work with you to decrease pain, increase strength, and restore normal motion.

Also, if you experience frequent numbness or tingling, to promote nerve healing, you should take a B complex vitamin including vitamin B$_6$ in addition to your multivitamin, avoid smoking, and drink alcohol only in moderation (no more than one drink per day). Wrist or elbow splinting can also help prevent stress to the nerve by reducing joint movement. Wearing the splint at night can help with treatment, as many people sleep in positions that stretch and irritate nerves.

Elbow and Wrist Exercises

Exercises to prevent and treat elbow and wrist injuries are simple and require light, one-half- to two-pound weights, because these muscles are small. All exercises should be done 10 times per set, two sets daily. Preferably, do the exercises as a "circuit," performing 10 reps of each exercise, then moving on to the next until it is time to repeat them again. If you are treating tendinitis or injury, ice for 10 to 15 minutes following exercise. Do not continue an exercise if it causes pain despite lowering the weight, decreasing the motion, and decreasing the number of repetitions. If you feel ready to increase the exercise intensity, you may increase the weight by a half pound weekly, or one pound every other week to a maximum of five pounds. You might also want to increase the repetitions in a set to 15, or add a third set. It is always a good idea to do the exercises on both sides to prevent problems on the opposite side.

Exercises and Stretches to Prevent and Treat Tennis Elbow

Perform each exercise slowly. These exercises can be done on both sides at the same time, but only after you have recovered from your injury and are comfortable with the exercise technique.

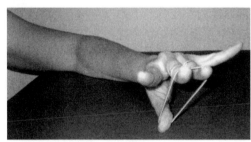

FIGURE 8-4 Rubber-Band Exercise: Wrap a thick rubber band around the ends of your thumb, middle, and fourth fingers. Holding your thumb stable and down, extend your third and fourth fingers up. Slowly release.

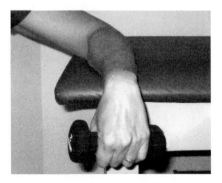 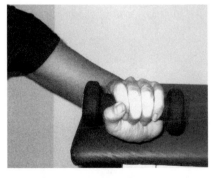

FIGURE 8-5 Bent Elbow Wrist Extension: With your elbow bent on a table or your lap, hold a weight palm facing down (A). Curl the back of your hand up (B). Slowly lower.

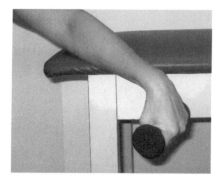 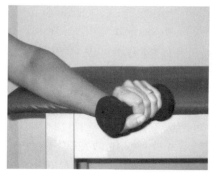

FIGURE 8-6 Straight Elbow Wrist Extension: Repeat above with your elbow straight on table or lap (A, B).

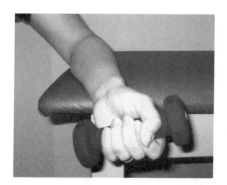 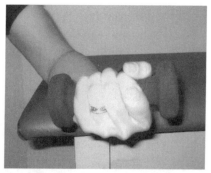

FIGURE 8-7 Bent Elbow Wrist Flexion: With your elbow bent on a table or your lap, hold a weight palm facing up (A). Slowly bend your palm up toward you (B). Slowly lower.

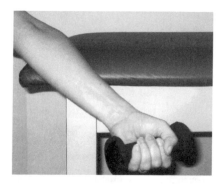 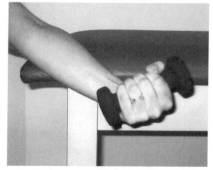

FIGURE 8-8 Straight Elbow Wrist Flexion: Repeat above with your elbow straight on a table or your lap (A, B).

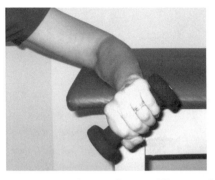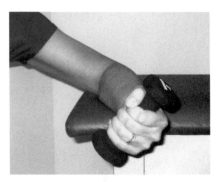

FIGURE 8-9 **Wrist Rotations: Holding a weight with your elbow bent on a table or your lap, palm down (A), rotate your wrist so your palm turns up (B). Slowly rotate back the other way.**

Stretches

Hold each stretch for a slow count of five. Repeat each five times, several times a day. They should feel comfortable, as a gentle, not painful, stretch.

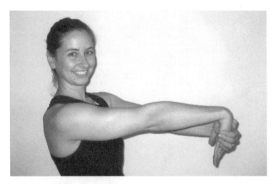

FIGURE 8-10 **Straight Elbow Wrist Flexion Stretch: Hold your arm straight out, pull your wrist down with your opposite hand to a bent wrist position with your fingers down.**

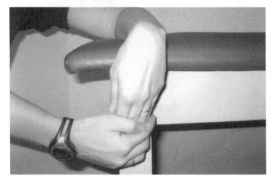

FIGURE 8-11 **Bent Elbow Wrist Flexion Stretch: Repeat above stretch with your elbow bent.**

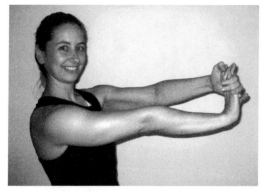

FIGURE 8-12 Straight Elbow Wrist Extension Stretch: Hold your arm straight out, pull your wrist up and back with your opposite hand.

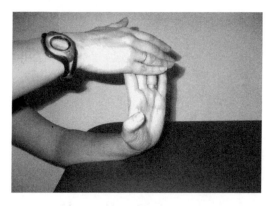

FIGURE 8-13 Bent Elbow Wrist Extension Stretch: Repeat above with your elbow bent.

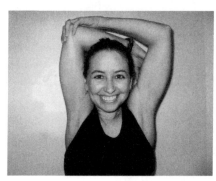

FIGURE 8-14 Overhead Tricep Stretch (right): Reach your right arm up and overhead, your elbow bent and your hand behind your head. Press your right elbow back with your left hand.

Exercises for Surrounding Elbow Muscles
May use three pounds more than at the wrist

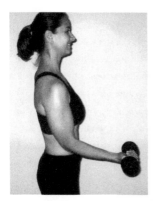 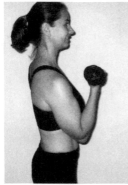

FIGURE 8-15 Bicep Curls: With your elbow fixed at your side, hold a weight palm up (A). Slowly bend your elbow (B). Lower slowly. Make sure your wrist is lined up straight with your arm. GYM VERSION: Pulley bicep curls and bicep machine.

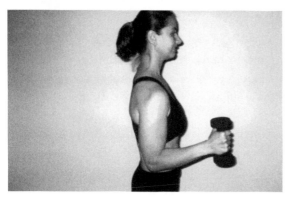

FIGURE 8-16 Hammer Curls: Repeat above, holding a weight with your thumb pointing up.

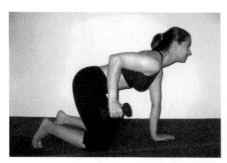 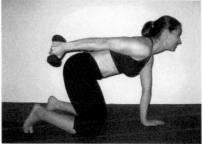

FIGURE 8-17 Triceps: On your hands and knees (or leaning on a table or chair), hold a weight with your elbow bent and in at your side (A). Slowly straighten your elbow, pushing your hand away, keeping your elbow and arm close to your body (B). GYM VERSION: Tricep pull-downs with pulley or tricep machine.

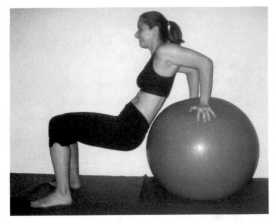

FIGURE 8-18 **Advanced Tricep Dips (avoid if shoulder pain): With your hands on a stability ball (chair, or bench) in sitting position, begin with your elbows straight and slowly lower to bend elbows 90 degrees (as shown). Press up to starting position with your elbows straight. GYM VERSION: Tricep dip bars and gravitron.**

Elbow, wrist, hand, and finger injuries, if not due to trauma, can be managed with rest, modifying equipment or activities, changing techniques, splinting, icing and anti-inflammatory medications, and strengthening and stretching exercises. These exercises should be done indefinitely to prevent the pain from returning, as most of these injuries are due to overuse. Because of the important function of these joints and their requirement for everyday activities, persistent pain, numbness, or weakness should be evaluated by a doctor if these symptoms last more than one week.

CHAPTER NINE

The Back and Abdomen: "The Core"

The back and abdomen form the "core" of the body. Like the trunk of a tree, the core supports our entire structure, protecting our internal organs and the essential spinal cord, which controls all movements and sensations. The supporting structures include the bones of the spine and ribs, the cushioning cartilage discs, the strengthening ligaments, and the moving muscles. All these structures can develop pain or injuries.

In athletes, back pain occurs commonly in gymnasts, dancers, divers, rowers, bowlers, and golfers. Impact activities such as running, horseback riding, tennis, and field sports can occasionally cause back problems due to the jerking motions and constant impact inherent in these sports. Back pain can also occur from injury or falls in field and court sports. Overuse injuries from repetitive activities or overtraining are also common. Sometimes, pain can develop after too much rest, bad posture, or poor positioning.

Back pain is the second most common reason people go to the doctor; it is a major reason for missed work and decreased activity. There are many health-care fields devoted to the treatment of back pain, including both traditional and alternative medicine. The options can be confusing. Fortunately, most back pain can be prevented and treated fairly easily.

Functional Anatomy

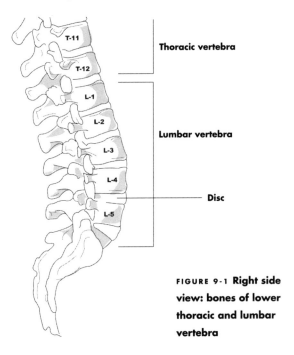

FIGURE 9-1 **Right side view: bones of lower thoracic and lumbar vertebra**

The bones of the spine are made up of vertebrae. These are the building blocks of support that carry the weight of the body. They are numbered by the area they are in: The middle back is made up of 12 thoracic vertebrae; the lower back made up of 5 lumbar vertebrae (see figure 9-1). The base of the spine is the sacrum, and the tailbone, or tip, the coccyx. The lower (lumbar) spine attaches to the pelvis and hips through the sacrum, the middle (thoracic) spine connects to the ribs and at the top is connected to the cervical spine, or neck. As the stable framework between the upper and lower body, the spine forms the base of support for all body motion and function.

The vertebral bones are connected to one another by ligaments and muscles, and cushioned by (intervertebral) discs. One of the most important functions of the vertebra is to support and protect the spinal cord and support the spaces for the nerve roots that leave at each level to supply the abdomen, thorax, pelvis, and legs. If a disc is herniated, it can press on a nerve root, sending pain or symptoms into the area supplied by that nerve. Most commonly, damage occurs between lumbar vertebras L4, L5, and S1 (see figure 9-2).

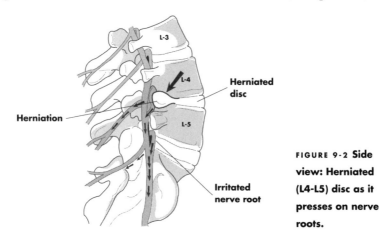

FIGURE 9-2 **Side view: Herniated (L4-L5) disc as it presses on nerve roots.**

The muscles surrounding the spine allow flexion (bending), rotation, and extension (arching). There are several layers of muscles, with small muscles connecting two vertebra and larger bands of muscles connecting several vertebra. These muscles are called paraspinal muscles and erector spinae, and they can become injured just as muscles can throughout the body. They help to support posture and motion (see figure 9-3).

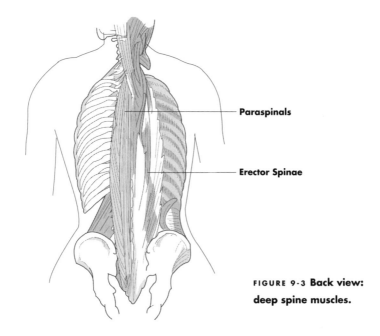

FIGURE 9-3 **Back view: deep spine muscles.**

The abdominal muscles are made up of four groups—the rectus abdominus, which go up and down, the transverse abdominus, which go across, and the internal and external obliques, which go diagonally. These provide support to the entire trunk, allow bending and rotation movement, and also maintain posture by opposing the paraspinals. The intercostal muscles connect the ribs and assist in breathing (see figure 9-4).

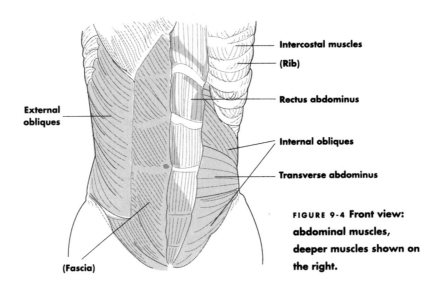

External obliques

Intercostal muscles

(Rib)

Rectus abdominus

Internal obliques

Transverse abdominus

FIGURE 9-4 Front view: abdominal muscles, deeper muscles shown on the right.

(Fascia)

Types of Back Pain

Back pain causes and syndromes are listed in decreasing order of frequency. Sprain is described first, as it is the most common cause of back pain and is a component of many other back pain syndromes.

Sprain
The most common cause of back pain, sprain causes pain that can be both sharp with movement or constantly achy, either in the middle or only on one side. Severe sprains can be extremely painful because the large muscles of the back can be very sensitive to a stretch, mild tear, spasm, or inflammation. In milder back sprains, muscles often feel very tight and stiff with initial movement causing pain, and lessening as movement continues. Sprain is

often due to an underlying muscle weakness, and as the muscles work harder to compensate for the pain, they go into spasm, the reason for stiffness. This can or cannot be associated with injury; occasionally, lumbar sprain can occur during sleep or after sitting or standing with poor posture. Although this does not lead to any permanent nerve damage (the greatest risk of back pain), it can cause enough discomfort to make you want to limit your activities.

Sciatica

Sciatica is the term for back pain that travels into the buttock, back of thigh, and legs. It generally means that there is an irritation of the sciatic nerve—the main nerve formed from the branches of the lumbar spine nerves. The nerve is located deep in the buttock muscles located close to the pelvis (see figure 9-5). When the sciatic nerve is irritated, by either bone, discs, ligaments, scar tissue, or inflamed and tight muscle, it causes pain, and in more serious cases, sciatica can also cause numbness or weakness. There are many causes of sciatica, described as the following syndromes: severe muscle spasm or sprain, pinched nerve, disc disease, arthritis, stenosis, and spondy. Sciatica can also be due to problems in the pelvis, including sacroiliac joint pain and piriformis syndrome (see chapter 10, "The Pelvis, Hip, and Thigh").

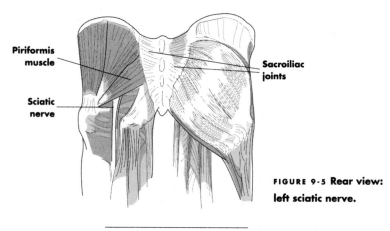

FIGURE 9-5 Rear view: left sciatic nerve.

Various Causes of Sciatica

Muscle spasm	Spondy joint
Pinched nerve	Sacroiliac pain
Herniated disc	Piriformis syndrome
Arthritis/stenosis/degenerative disc disease	Fractures

Pinched Nerve/Radiculopathy

When sciatica is due to a pinched nerve, the medical term for this is radiculopathy. A nerve can get pinched as it leaves the spinal column to supply the legs. This causes a shooting, sometimes burning pain down one leg. If it is severe and has serious consequences, it can also result in weakness or numbness of the leg and foot. Pinched nerves can be caused by disc problems, arthritis, stenosis, spondy, and occasionally, severe muscle spasm or fracture.

Disc Problems

Disc pain can cause various types of back pain, due to herniation, bulge, tear, or degeneration. Disc pain is usually more on one side than another, and in its worse case, a herniation, it might cause a "pop" sensation with sudden severe pain shooting down a leg due to pressure on the nerve (see figure 9-2). Both bulges and (annular) tears cause localized back pain and can lead to herniations. The worst complications of disc disease include thigh, leg, or foot numbness; burning; weakness; and other symptoms of a pinched nerve. Herniations are the most likely reason people undergo surgery for back pain, as continuous pressure on the nerve can result in permanent damage. However, most disc injuries and the nerves they press on heal with careful activities and abdominal strengthening and stretching, along with medications or steroid injections, if needed.

Disc degeneration occurs in time after a bulge or herniation, as the disc loses its inner cushion and collapses. This is less likely to cause sudden back pain, but presents with stiffness, achiness, and symptoms similar to arthritis. In cases of multiple sites of degeneration, it is called degenerative disc disease.

Arthritis, Stenosis, Degenerative Disc Disease

Arthritis, stenosis, and degenerative disc disease are described together, as they cause similar symptoms of stiffness and pain, have related causes, often occur together, and are treated similarly. Unless there has been a previous traumatic injury to the spine or you have a strong family history of early arthritis, these conditions occur later in life, usually after age 50, due to both aging and wear and tear. Occasionally, arthritis, stenosis, and degenerative disc disease can be associated with leg pain or numbness and weakness. Unfortunately, this condition is not reversible and can cause chronic back pain.

Strengthening the spine and abdominal muscles and keeping the hamstring and gluteal muscles flexible helps manage the discomfort. Anti-inflammatories can also be helpful for both conditions. Often, impact activities such as running and jumping can make the pain and disease worse. Swimming, cycling, and walking are preferred activities.

Spondy

"Spondy" is a shortened term for two conditions of spine instability causing pain with arching the back and also with twisting or other irritating spine maneuvers: spondylolisthesis occurs when one vertebra slips forward or backward on another; spondylolysis occurs when this slippage is associated with a fracture. Spondy is common to dancers, divers, gymnasts, and high jumpers who are required to arch their back repeatedly. In severe cases, bracing or surgery is necessary to stabilize the fracture and any instability. In milder cases, it can be treated more conservatively by modifying activities, avoiding extension (arching), spine and abdominal muscle strengthening and stretching, and posture reeducation.

Pelvic Causes of Back Pain

Sacroiliac joint pain causes very low back pain or buttock pain usually on one side. Actually a problem of the pelvis, it often mimics low back pain or sciatica. Most commonly, it is due to inflammation and instability of the joint formed by the sacrum and pelvis; later in life, this joint can also develop a type of arthritis called "sclerosis."

Piriformis syndrome causes focal buttock pain usually on one side that can be sharp, aching, or burning. This is a condition in which the piriformis muscle, located under the gluteus muscles, becomes inflamed and irritated. Because it lays beneath the sciatic nerve, it often can contribute to feelings of sciatica (see figure 9-5) (see chapter 10, "The Pelvis, Hip, and Thigh").

Bone Problems

Bone problems include contusions (bruises), fractures, and tumors. Fractures can cause severe pain, especially when they occur in the vertebra or coccyx. Stress fractures can also occur in any of the bones of the spine or pelvis and usually cause a dull, aching pain that gets worse with activity. The pain of fractures is usually located in one specific area but can also press on the nerves and cause pain into the legs. Vertebral fractures are common in women past menopause who have osteoporosis. Fractures can also occur in the pelvis either due to injury, weak bones, or a long-standing stress fracture; these can occur in athletes who are overtraining or not eating enough (see chapter 5, "Bone Health and Osteoporosis").

Coccyx (tailbone) contusions, dislocations, or fractures can occur because of an accident or trauma involving a hard landing on the rear, or after delivery of a baby. Coccyx injuries can be very painful, especially fractures, and can take up to one year to fully heal. A pressure-relief donut allows more comfortable sitting.

Scoliosis

Scoliosis, or curvature of the spine, results in crooked and imbalanced posture, putting stress and strain on muscles, ligaments, and bone. This does not always cause pain, but when it does, it can be difficult to treat. Scoliosis screenings should be performed in elementary school or by a growing girl's pediatrician for early detection and treatment with exercise, bracing, and sometimes surgery. Occasionally, scoliosis can develop later in life. Exercises (in extension and neutral) and stretches to prevent scoliosis from worsening are essential and should be done daily. Swimming is an excellent exercise to prevent and treat scoliosis.

Menstrual Pain and Internal Organ Problems

Crampy, achy back pain associated with menstruation known as "dysmenorrhea" usually occurs on the first few days of the flow. This condition usually improves with heat and anti-inflammatory medications. Endometriosis, fibroids, an ovarian cyst, pelvic inflammatory disease, or ectopic pregnancy can also cause feelings of back pain. Other internal organ problems causing back pain include kidney infections and bowel problems such as constipation. Any back pain that wakes you from sleep or is associated with fever or pain with urination, discolored or foul-smelling vaginal discharge, or unusual bleeding should be evaluated by your doctor as soon as possible. In severe cases of fever, bleeding, or pain, go to an emergency room if you cannot see your doctor immediately.

See a Doctor as Soon as Possible for the Following Symptoms

SYMPTOMS	POSSIBLE MEDICAL PROBLEM
Weakness, numbness, or pain in the leg(s)*	Pinched nerve, spinal cord damage
Trouble urinating or moving your bowels*	Nerve damage
Pain with urination	Urinary tract infection
Fever, chills, achy pain	A virus or the flu
Fever, chills, sharp pain in lower back on one side*	Kidney infection
Fever, chills, severe one-sided pelvic pain, pain with sex, vaginal discharge*	Ruptured ectopic pregnancy, pelvic inflammatory disease
Heavy vaginal bleeding and pain with cramps	Miscarriage, fibroids, endometriosis
Cramping, fullness, not moving bowels	Constipation or bowel obstruction
Cramping, diarrhea	Infection, irritable bowel syndrome

*If you have these symptoms but cannot see your doctor right away, go to an emergency room.

Abdominal Muscle Injuries

These are indicated by sharp pulling pains over the abdomen or ribs. The pain is usually in one area, tender to touch, and painful with deep breathing or twisting. Abdominal muscle injuries are usually due to a strained, torn, or pulled muscle resulting from sudden, quick motion or repeated activity. These can occur in tennis and volleyball players, horseback riders, or kickers. They usually resolve with a little rest, ice, and time. As the muscles heal, gentle stretching and strengthening exercises, increasing gradually in resistance, will prevent further injury or weakness.

Evaluation and Treatment

Abdomen or back pain that lasts more than a few days; is accompanied by other symptoms, especially leg numbness and weakness; or pain that keeps you from daily activities, including sleep, should be evaluated by a doctor. A proper and timely medical diagnosis with treatment will stop the pain problems from becoming worse and decrease the likelihood for the pain to return. Also, the sooner treatment begins, the sooner the pain will resolve.

The doctor's exam should include evaluating your posture, spine alignment, movement, areas of tenderness, reflexes, sensations, and strength. X-rays might also be taken, although on the initial doctor visit they are not always necessary. If the pain continues or is accompanied by the more serious signs of weakness or numbness, an MRI is usually recommended to evaluate the structures not seen on x-ray including discs and nerves.

Medications are often prescribed to alleviate the pain, allow more normal movements, and prevent further spasms and weakness. These medicines include painkillers, nonsteroidal anti-inflammatories, steroids, muscle relaxers, antidepressants, and anticonvulsants. Ask your doctor if the painkillers are narcotics, which can have many side effects, including drowsiness, stomach upset, and addiction; these are recommended only if the pain is excruciating. Nonaspirin pain relievers like Tylenol do not have addictive potential and have the least side effects. Steroids can be prescribed for a short time to break the inflammation cycle in the body and shrink the irritated and inflamed tissues. Steroids should be used sparingly, at low doses and for short periods of time (a week to 10 days), as they have the greatest amount of side effects, including elevated blood sugars and risk of stomach ulceration. Antidepressants are used in cases of chronic pain lasting longer than six months. Anticonvulsants are used to treat burning nerve pain, sometimes a symptom of chronic back pain.

Nonsteroidal anti-inflammatories decrease the inflammation and pain cycle in the body. There are many types of nonsteroidal anti-inflammatories; lower doses of some can be purchased without a prescription (Advil, Aleve, Motrin). These drugs are very effective for types of pain due to injury, overuse, or poor positioning.

Muscle relaxers are medications used essentially for back and neck pain and relieve feelings of tightness and stiffness, increasing comfortable movement. Increasing movement reduces muscle spasms, pain, weakness, and time for healing. As they tend to relax more than just the muscles, muscle relaxers can also cause sleepiness.

The two most common types of medications prescribed for low back pain include nonsteroidal anti-inflammatories and muscle relaxers, as these can be taken without worry of addiction, are usually inexpensive, and have low side effects. All types of medications have different levels of effectiveness and different side effect profiles in each individual. If you are taking medications but have stomach trouble, drowsiness, or other questionable side effects, and especially if you are still experiencing pain, ask your doctor for a different prescription.

Drugs Commonly Used to Treat Back Pain

TYPE OF DRUG	FUNCTION	EXAMPLES
Nonsteroidal anti-inflammatories	Decrease inflammation and pain	Advil/Motrin, Alleve, Celebrex, Vioxx, Bextra, Naprosyn, Diclofenac, Orudis
Steroids	Decrease inflammation	Medrol, Prednisone
Muscle relaxers	Decrease muscle spasm	Flexeril, Soma, Skelaxin, Robaxin, Zanaflex
Pain relievers	Decrease pain	Tylenol, Ultram
Narcotic painkillers	Decrease pain (addictive)	Darvocet, Vicoden, Percocet, Tylenol 3
Antidepressants/ anticonvulsants	Chronic pain lasting greater than six months or severe burning pain	Elavil, Pamelor, Zoloft, Paxil, Neurontin

Alternative medicine techniques are very popular methods of relieving spine pain. These include acupuncture, massage, chiropractic, and holistic healing methods. Acupuncture and massage can be very effective and have essentially no risk of side effects. It is recommended to have a medical doctor's evaluation of the cause of the pain prior to chiropractic treatment to make sure there are no movement precautions associated with your diagnosis. High-velocity chiropractic manipulations are not recommended, especially in cases of disc herniations, spondylosis, fractures, or severe arthritis, as it can make these conditions worse.

In most cases, back pain improves within three to six weeks and might return occasionally but does not cause permanent damage. Some women are more prone to repeated episodes of pain because of their type of work, athletic activity, repeated lifting activities, or family history. Still, fewer than 1 percent of individuals with back pain truly require surgery to relieve pressure on the nerve from disc or bone. Nonsurgical management is very effective at both treating and preventing back pain. Back pain is much less likely to return with regular preventive exercises that strengthen the abdominal and surrounding muscles to help protect the spine and keep it upright. Stretching hamstring and buttock muscles is also important to maintain flexibility and prevent muscle spasms.

Exercises and Stretches

Exercises and stretches are an essential part of restoring normal movement, strength, and decreasing pain. They also prevent back pain. Exercises are categorized by the direction they focus on: flexion (bending), neutral (straight), and extension (arching). Your doctor or therapist can help determine if your initial exercises and stretches should be in the direction of flexion or extension. With the exception of fractures (flexion should be avoided), spondylolysis (extension should be avoided), and stenosis (extension should be avoided), most exercises can be done if they do not cause pain. Neutral exercises, when done correctly, can be done for all types of pain.

Exercises should be done with slow motions. Count slowly to three with the up motion, hold for a slow three count, then lower for a slow three count. The abdominal muscles should be kept as tight (sucked in) as possible throughout each exercise to support the back. Aim for 10 repetitions, moving through the exercises to work as a circuit. Begin with two sets daily; these can be done all together as one session or divided into a morning and evening session. If these are easy, increase to 15 repetitions per set and gradually add a third set. If pain occurs with each attempt to do an exercise, it should be eliminated from your program. If it occurs only after a certain number of repetitions or occasionally, you should reduce the number of repetitions you do to avoid pain. You should feel better after exercise, not worse.

You might have good and bad days, where exercises can be quite comfortable on one day but cause pain on another. Skip painful exercises for a week, try again with a smaller range of motion or less repetitions, and gradually you should be able to do all the exercises comfortably. If you are currently having back pain, try to do the stretches every day and the exercises three to five days a week. Do the advanced exercises only when you are fully recovered and pain-free.

Flexion Exercises (Bending Forward)

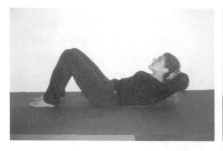 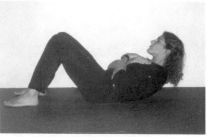

FIGURE 9-6 **Crunch: Lying on your back, knees bent, feet shoulder width apart, hands behind your head (A) or hands folded across your stomach (B). Suck in your stomach tight, and slowly curl up, lifting your head and shoulders about 10 inches off the floor, to height shown. Hold here for slow count of three; slowly lower for count of three.**

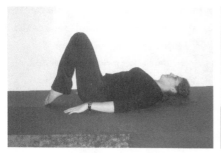 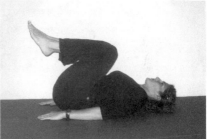

FIGURE 9-7 **Reverse Curls: Lying on your back, knees bent together, and feet tucked in as close to your buttocks as possible (A), suck in your stomach and curl both legs up to your chest with knees remaining bent and tucked in (B). Hold for a slow count of three, then slowly release to lightly touch toes on mat. If this exercise is uncomfortable, try it with one leg at a time, leaving the opposite leg on the mat.**

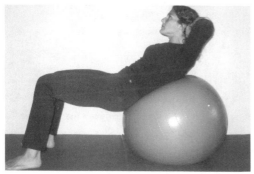

FIGURE 9-8 **Crunches on Ball: Sitting on large stability ball, slide down the ball so your upper back is on the top of the ball. Do crunches from this position.**

Neutral Exercises

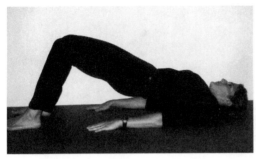

FIGURE 9-9 **Bridges: Lying on your back with your knees bent, feet shoulder width apart, suck in your stomach and lift your pelvis and hips up off the mat. Hold for a slow count of three and slowly lower. Work toward bringing your hips and pelvis up higher as you get stronger.**

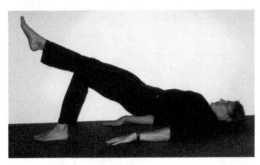

FIGURE 9-10 **One Legged Bridge: On your back in the above position, extend one leg out straight. Lift your pelvis up as high as possible, hold for count of three, and lower while keeping leg up. Repeat 10 times, keeping leg extended, then lower and switch sides.**

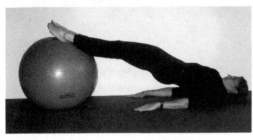

FIGURE 9-11 **Advanced Bridge: Lying on your back with your feet on a ball, suck in your stomach and lift your pelvis up, hold for slow count of three, then lower.**

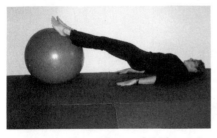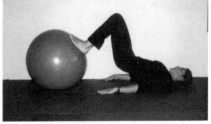

FIGURE 9-12 **More Advanced Bridge: Lying on your back with your feet up on a ball, as above, lift your pelvis up. Bend your knees, pulling your feet and ball in toward your body (B). Slowly roll your legs out to the starting position, keeping your hips up for the next repetition.**

Extension Exercises

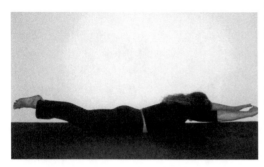

FIGURE 9-13 **Superman: Lying on your stomach with your arms straight out in front and overhead, legs straight back, and toes pointed, raise both hands and feet off the floor. Hold for slow count of three and release for count of three. If this is difficult, try lifting either just your hands or just your feet.**

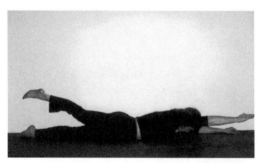

FIGURE 9-14 **Swimmer: Lying on your stomach with both arms straight out in front, legs straight out in back, with toes pointed, raise your right hand and left foot, keeping your legs and arms straight, and hold for count of three, then lower and switch hands and feet.**

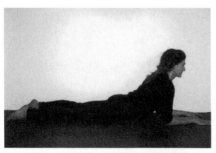
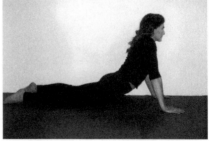

FIGURE 9-15 **Cobra: On your stomach, toes pointed down, arch your back to come up onto your elbows (A). Hold for three. Advanced Cobra: Come up onto straight arms (B).**

Upper and Lower Back Strengthening

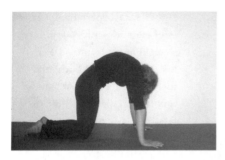 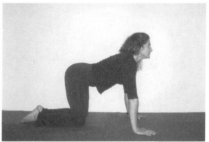

FIGURE 9-16 Cat and Cow: On your hands and knees, round your back with your head down and your chin to your chest (A). Reverse the curl with your back arched and head up (B).

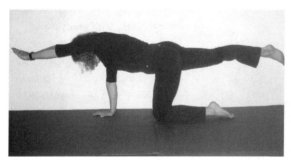

FIGURE 9-17 Hands and Knees Trunk Stability: On your hands and knees, lift your right arm up and left leg straight out behind you. Hold with back straight for slow count of three. Switch sides.

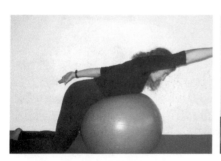 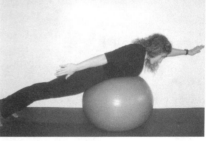

FIGURE 9-18 Swimmer on Ball (Upper Back Strengthening): On your knees, your stomach on large stability ball, alternate one arm out in front and one to back, then alternate arms (A). More advanced: Do above exercise with legs straight (B).

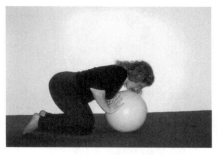
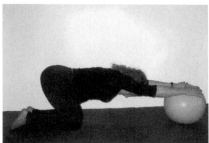

FIGURE 9-19 **Ball Roll-Outs: On your knees, with your elbows bent, hold a medium stability ball in front (A). Extend your arms to roll the ball out (B). Roll ball back in.**

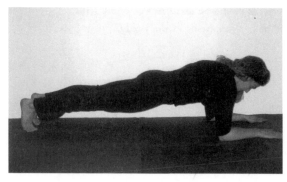

FIGURE 9-20 **Plank: On your stomach in push-up position, lift your hips off the mat and push your upper body onto bent elbows and hold in plank position with your stomach sucked in tight and your spine straight. Hold for a count of 10.**

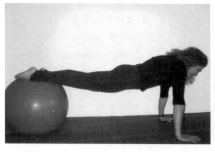
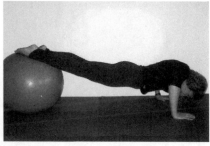

FIGURE 9-21 **Advanced Plank with Push-Up Ball: Both feet on a large stability ball, hands on floor, body straight in plank position (A). Keep your stomach sucked in tight. Do 10 slow push-ups (B).**

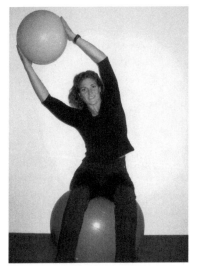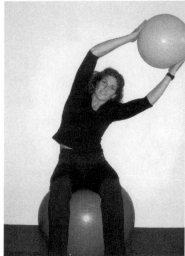

FIGURE 9-22 Double Ball Obliques: Seated on a large stability ball, with arms overhead holding a small ball, reach the ball from right (A) to left (B).

Stretches

All stretches should be held for a slow count of five, and then repeated five times.

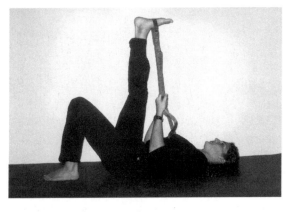

FIGURE 9-23 Hamstring Stretch: Lying on your back, wrap a strap (rope, belt, or long towel) around your foot and pull your leg with your knee straight in toward your body until you feel you're about to bend your knee.

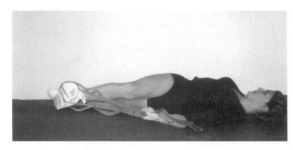

FIGURE 9-24 Outer Hip Stretch (right): From hamstring stretch above, pull your right straight leg across the left side of your body, using a strap or your left hand on the outside of your right calf.

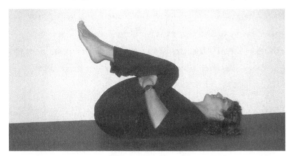

FIGURE 9-25 Buttock and Lower Back Stretch: Lying on your back, bend both knees and pull them toward chest, holding behind your knees.

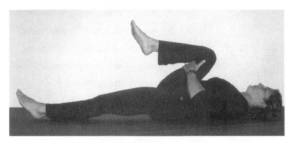

FIGURE 9-26 Buttock (Glut) Stretch: Lying on your back, bend one knee and pull it toward your chest, holding behind your knee.

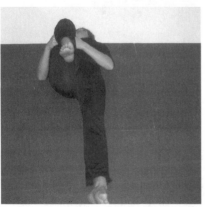
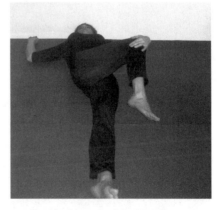

FIGURE 9-27 Outer Buttock (right): Lying on your back with your right knee bent up to your chest as in the stretch above (A), hold the outside of your right knee with your left hand on your outer knee. Pull your bent right knee across the left side of your body (B).

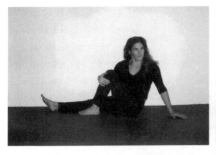
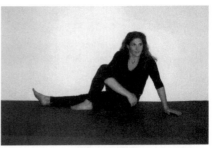

FIGURE 9-28 Seated Trunk Twist (right): Sitting with your left knee bent, with your right leg straight, twist your upper body to the left and hold your outer knee with your right hand (A). Increase rotation stretch by reaching back of your upper arm to outside of your knee (B). Further increase stretch by crossing your left knee over your right leg.

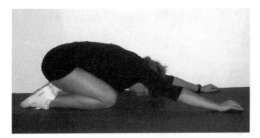

FIGURE 9-29 Lower Back Stretch: On your hands and knees, reach both arms as far out in front as possible at the same time stretching your buttocks back toward your feet.

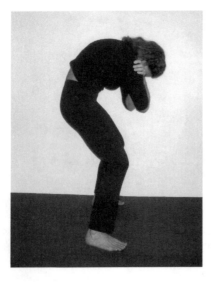

FIGURE 9-30 Upper Back Stretch: Standing with your knees slightly bent, feet shoulder width apart, cross your arms and hold your shoulders. Pull your shoulders down to round your back. This stretch can also be done while seated.

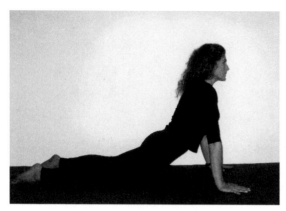

FIGURE 9-31 **Ab Stretch: Lying flat on your stomach, toes pointed behind you, push up with both arms to arch your back and stretch out your abdominals and front of your hips.**

Back pain syndromes are extremely common in active women due to both sports and other life activities. Sciatica is back pain that travels down the leg, due to a variety of causes. If your back pain lasts more than one week, is accompanied by leg weakness or numbness, or interferes with sleep, see a doctor as soon as possible for an evaluation. Most causes of back pain with or without sciatica are treatable with medications, mild rest, and appropriate strengthening and stretching exercises. These exercises should be continued indefinitely to maintain a strong core and prevent your pain from returning.

CHAPTER TEN

The Pelvis, Hip, and Thigh

Because the pelvis, hips, and thighs provide an essential weight-bearing area connecting the legs to the core, pain can develop here frequently, particularly in women. Causes of pain and injury can be confusing, as this area not only connects the spine and legs, but also surrounds internal organs of the reproductive, urinary, and digestive systems. Muscles and ligaments connect the spine to the pelvis, hips, thighs, and legs, sending pain signals from one area to another if they are irritated throughout their path. Hip and pelvic pain can also be closely related to back pain; therefore, if you have problems with one area, you might have problems with the other.

Repetitive motion activities such as running, cycling, swimming, skating, horseback riding, kickboxing, or aerobics can lead to overuse pain and injury. Common workout techniques such as lunging and squats, gym equipment such as stair climbers, or poor bike positioning can lead to hip pain. Having one leg slightly longer than another and running on banked roads can cause hip problems, as can hip and thigh alignment problems. Girls and women at various life stages including adolescence and pregnancy can also develop problems due to changes in ligament looseness. Pain syndromes can also be due to overuse or wear and tear, and sometimes also from underuse, or sitting or lying in one position for too long.

Functional Anatomy

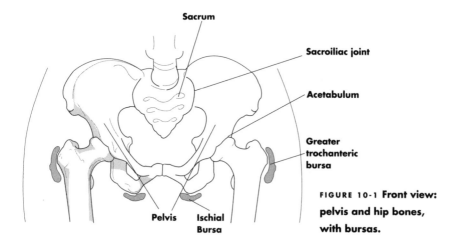

FIGURE 10-1 **Front view: pelvis and hip bones, with bursas.**

The hip joint connects the femur and pelvis as a ball and socket joint and allows movement in many directions. The socket of the pelvis is called the acetabulum. The pelvis is made up of three tightly connected pelvic bones, the sacrum and two iliac bones (one on each side). This makes up the cradle-shape connection between the torso and legs. The pelvic bone connections can loosen in pregnancy to allow the pelvis to expand for childbirth. There can also be a natural looseness at the sacroiliac joint. Occasionally, this loosening causes inflammation and pain.

Bursas are fluid-filled sacs around joints at areas of tendon attachment. In the hip, they are somewhat large. There are two bursas that cause the most problems in the hip and pelvis—the greater trochanteric bursa on the side of the hip and the ischial bursa at the "sit bones" (see figure 10-1). They are only noticed if they are inflamed; this is called bursitis.

The hips are anchored to the pelvis by ligaments, further strengthening the ball and socket joint. There are many layers of muscles that cover the hip and pelvis, allowing motion in six planes. The larger muscles cross more than one joint, such as the spine, pelvis, and hip, or pelvis, hip, and knee, to allow stable strength and motion in the hip and knee.

The hips, buttocks, and thighs are made up of the muscles that move the hips, knees, and upper legs. In general, "hip" muscles are considered your hip flexors and abductors. "Groin" muscles include your adductors and some hamstrings. "Thigh" muscles include your hamstring and quadriceps muscles. "Buttock" muscles are your gluteal muscles.

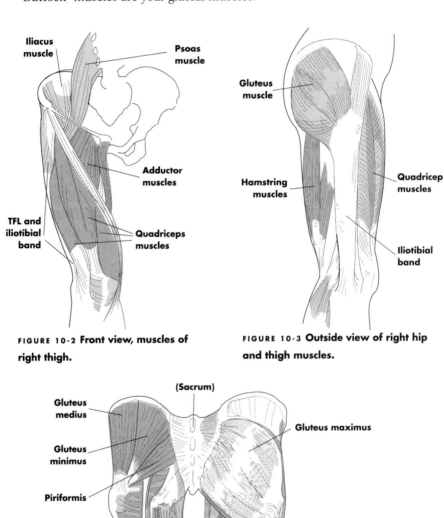

FIGURE 10-2 Front view, muscles of right thigh.

FIGURE 10-3 Outside view of right hip and thigh muscles.

FIGURE 10-4 Rear view: buttock muscles, deeper muscles illustrated on the left.

Understanding Hip Movement

DIRECTION	MEDICAL TERM	PRIMARY MUSCLES USED	EXAMPLE
Inward rotation	Internal rotation	Gluteus minimus, TFL	Turn knees in
Outward rotation	External rotation	Gluteus maximus, piriformis	Turn out knees
Forward movement	Flexion	Hip flexors (iliacus, psoas)	Climbing stairs
Backward movement	Extension	Gluteus muscles	Walking backward
Bring leg across body	Adduction	Adductor muscles	Crossing leg
Take leg away from body	Abduction	Gluteus minimus, medius, iliotibial band	Side kick

The pelvis also surrounds internal organs, including the uterus, ovaries, bladder, colon, vagina, and urethra. The pelvis's proximity to these internal organs and to the spine must be considered when evaluating causes of pain (see figure 10–5).

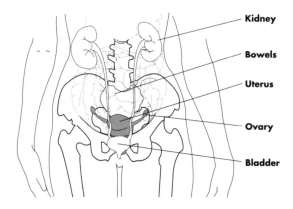

- Kidney
- Bowels
- Uterus
- Ovary
- Bladder

FIGURE 10-5 **Internal organs in pelvic region**

Pain and Injury Patterns

Pain and injury patterns are listed in decreasing order of frequency. Iliotibial band syndrome is listed first, as it is one of the most common problems causing hip and occasional knee pain in active women.

Iliotibial Band Syndrome

Iliotibial band (ITB) syndrome causes outer hip pain that can send aching or burning pain down the side of the thigh into the knee. ITB syndrome is a term used to describe inflammation of a band of muscle and tendon on the outside of the hip (see figure 10–3), that helps lift the leg out to the side, bend the knee slightly, and stabilize the pelvis when walking or standing. It is a very common injury in runners and also in athletic women who kick, lunge, and do martial arts. Not stretching, running on a banked surface, or a difference in leg length can predispose an athlete to ITB syndrome.

Iliotibial band syndrome can be relieved with a disciplined stretching and strengthening routine, icing, and anti-inflammatory medications. Stretching is one of the most important parts of treating and preventing ITB syndrome. Stretching should be incorporated into the regular exercise routine so ITB syndrome does not return.

Bursitis

Bursitis—inflammation and irritation of the bursa—causes an aching and stiff pain over the inflamed area, either over the side of the hip or at the "sit" bones. It is usually on one side but can occasionally be on both. The most common form is greater trochanteric bursitis, causing pain and tenderness over the side of the hip, which is usually felt when lying on that side, getting up from sitting, and walking. Bursitis over the ischium, or sit bones, often is associated with pain in the hamstrings. Runners, racewalkers, hikers, cyclists, and kickboxers can develop bursitis. It can also develop after sitting or sleeping in one position for a long period of time. Bursitis improves by taking pressure off that side (not lying or sitting on it as much), icing, stretching, and strengthening the muscles around it. Sometimes, a cortisone injection will help decrease the inflammation that causes pain.

Arthritis

Arthritis usually begins with symptoms of morning stiffness, progressing to pain with movement, limited internal rotation, stiffness after sitting, and weakness. Hip arthritis pain is often felt in the groin. Arthritis develops due to wear and tear, such as lifelong impact activities, and also due to genetic predisposition. For early hip arthritis, maintaining motion and strength with stretching and strengthening activities and avoiding impact activities is the best way to manage and lessen arthritis symptoms. If the arthritis is severe and disabling, a hip replacement can be done.

Sacroiliac Pain

Sacroiliac pain is usually one-sided low back pain between the buttock and back, causing very low back, pelvis, or buttock pain when twisting, turning in bed, or going up and down stairs or off a curb. Sacroiliac pain comes from an irritation of the sacroiliac joints, the connections between the triangle-shape bone at the base of the spine and the pelvis on each side. Although mostly stable, sacroiliac joints can become loose, irritated, and inflamed. Sacroiliac pain might become worse during menstruation, during growth spurts, and during and after pregnancy. Most pain is due to sacroilitis, or inflammation of the joint. Later in life, the joint sometimes fuses, causing sclerosis, a condition similar to arthritis causing stiffness and pain.

Joint pain in this area does respond to anti-inflammatory medications coupled with strengthening and stability exercises. If it is still problematic, cortisone injections can also reduce inflammation. Also, a sacroiliac belt worn low around the pelvis can give some relief (see figure 10–6). Because sacroiliac pain can be difficult to treat, chronic, and a great source of distress, there are many types of alternative medicine treatments designed to help the pain. Manipulation can be effective but should be done sparingly, as the joint can become irritated with too much manipulation.

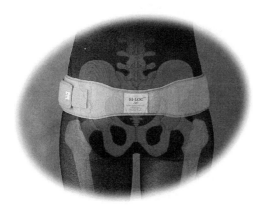

FIGURE 10-6 Sacroiliac belt, to be worn snug and low around the pelvis (photo courtesy of OPTP; see the resources at end of the book for purchase information).

Leg Length Discrepancy

Many people naturally have one leg longer than the other. Sometimes this can cause hip problems, especially in active athletic women. This can result in increased pressure on one side of the pelvis at the sacroiliac joint and can also lead to a tilted pelvis, which contributes to sacroiliac pain, back pain, bursitis, and tendinitis. To correct uneven leg length, a heel lift can be inserted under the insole of the shoe of the shorter leg, built into an orthotic, or added to the outside of the shoe. Usually, just half the leg length difference is corrected at first so the body can adjust to its new positioning.

Buttock Pain/Piriformis Syndrome

Buttock pain is very common in active women and can come from the back, pelvis, gluteal, or hamstring muscles. Deep buttock pain that is one-sided can be due to piriformis syndrome, spasm, irritation, or inflammation of the piriformis muscle, the deep muscle that outwardly rotates the hip (see figure 10–4). This pain can feel like sciatica and send burning or shooting pain down the back of the thigh. Because the piriformis muscle lies under the sciatic nerve, it can cause symptoms of sciatica. The muscle can become weak, making it painful to rotate the thigh out or abduct it when the thigh is at 90 degrees. This injury responds to anti-inflammatory medications, massage, strengthening, and aggressive stretching. Trigger point injections of cortisone can also help.

Hamstring Pain

Hamstring pulls and sprains are also common and often occur as an overuse syndrome without a noticeable injury. When severe, they can cause bruising and swelling and intense pain with walking and moving. Hamstring pain can be secondary to ischial bursitis, piriformis syndrome, and sciatica. Hamstring pulls and sprains respond to icing, stretching, strengthening, and rest from irritating activities.

Groin Pain

Inflammation of adductor, abdominal, and flexor muscle tendon attachment sites due to overuse can cause pain in the groin, lower back, and sacrum. These attachment inflammation sites usually improve with stretching and icing. Hip arthritis is another common cause of groin pain.

A groin pull is actually a strain or mini-tear of the inner thigh muscle. This injury is common in hockey players, horseback riders, and ice-skaters.

Field sports players can also develop groin pain from quick movements in a new or changed direction. Groin pulls respond to strengthening and stretching. Avoid painful activities until you are fully healed.

Snapping Hip Syndrome

Snapping hip syndrome is a condition in which athletes complain of a snapping, popping, or clicking sensation that occurs with hip movement. Occasionally, there is a sense of locking that releases after the snapping sound. This condition is caused by inflamed and occasionally scarred tendons rubbing across each other or even across the bone. Snapping hip syndrome is usually more annoying than serious and often does not even cause pain. Kickboxers, joggers, aerobic enthusiasts, and soccer players can develop this irritation. It usually responds to frequent stretching along with a gentle strengthening program and a decrease in irritating activity.

Hip Pointer

A hip pointer is pain over the top of the right front of the hip bone. It usually develops after a fall or impact directly to that area and can be associated with a bone bruise, which can take eight or more weeks to fully heal. Hip pointers are due to inflammation of the hip flexor muscle tendons and can cause pain with walking or kicking. Sometimes, abdominal muscle injuries can cause hip pointers. Often, field sports players suffer these injuries. Hip pointers respond to icing, anti-inflammatory medications, along with a gentle stretching.

Thigh Bruise

Medically known as a contusion, a large bruise to the thigh can occur with a severe muscle pull, fall, or injury to the thigh. These can take several weeks to heal and cause much pain and swelling. If there is also weakness or limited motion at the knee or hip, the injury should be evaluated by a doctor to make sure there are no muscle tears or the serious complication of bone growth within the bruised area.

Pinched Nerves

Pinched nerves tend to cause numbness or tingling sensations and are often associated with back pain, as nerves can be compressed or irritated on their way out of the spinal cord as they are heading into the pelvis and legs. If there is also weakness and disabling pain, see a doctor as soon as possible.

A numbness or burning over the side of the thigh and front of the hip is called lateral femoral cutaneous neuropathy. Also called merelgia parasthetica, it is due to a pinching of a sensory nerve as it enters the thigh through the groin. As long as there is no associated weakness, it is not serious.

Back Pain and Sciatica

Back, pelvic, and hip pain are very closely related and can cause similar pain conditions. There are some hip and pelvis problems that can cause sciaticalike sensations and buttock pain that shoots down the leg. In the pelvis, sciatica can also be due to muscles or tendons in the pelvis pressing on the sciatica nerve. This occurs in problems such as piriformis syndrome and ischial bursitis. Because of the complicated nature and many possible causes of sciatica, pain in the low back and buttock that radiates down the leg should be evaluated by a doctor. Most symptoms eventually resolve with conservative treatment.

Stress Fractures

Stress fractures can cause sharp or aching pain anywhere in the hip and pelvic region that is usually worse with impact activity. Stress fractures are the result of too much impact or weighted stress on one area of bone. Stress fractures should be considered if pain in the hip, low back, groin, or pelvis does not improve. In girls or women who have had other stress fractures, a history of eating disorders, have not had their period for four to six months or more, or are overtraining in a high-impact activity, stress fractures are more likely. Stress fractures only heal with proper rest. Unfortunately, rest can often be a challenge in highly motivated athletes.

Internal Causes of Pelvic Pain

Because the pelvis holds many important internal organs, pain can be due to gynecological, urinary, gastrointestinal, and deep muscle problems. Gynecological issues in this area include ovarian cysts, pain of menstruation, pelvic inflammatory diseases, and pregnancy. Urinary issues can include infections, bladder spasms, and occasionally kidney infections. Gastrointestinal issues include stomach cramping, irritable bowel syndrome, and constipation. Muscle causes of pain deep in the pelvis include tightness, spasms, or weakness in the muscles of the pelvic floor, deep hip, and deeper buttock muscles. Coccyx bruises, dislocations, and fractures can also cause pain deep inside the pelvis. Chronic pelvic pain can occur after abuse, trauma, or surgical procedures.

Pelvic pain often affects sex, urination, bowel function, and physical activities. Because possible internal causes are multiple and can mimic other back and pelvic pain problems, diagnosis and treatment of these causes of pelvic pain can be challenging. Follow-up with appropriate, sometimes multiple, specialists can be time-consuming, but is highly recommended to better resolve the cause of pain. A urogynecologist or pelvic pain specialist doctor or therapist can be very helpful for proper diagnosis and treatment of this often complex problem. (See the resources at end of the book for a recommended book on pelvic pain.)

Evaluation and Treatment

You should see a doctor if you have persistent pain at night, numbness, or tingling, or weakness; are limping; or the pain seems to be spreading or not improving over one week. Any fever, chills, numbness, pain while sleeping, unusual discharge or bleeding, or trouble voiding should be seen by a doctor as soon as possible.

Diagnosis and treatment is based on the history of the pain, presence of weakness, tenderness or restricted motion, potential nerve or internal organ involvement, and bone health. If the pain is deep and internal, a pelvic exam should be done. X-rays might be ordered to assess arthritis or bony problems. MRIs or bone scans will rule out a stress fracture. The doctor will likely prescribe medications for pain and inflammation, recommend rest from painful activities, and should prescribe stretching and strengthening exercises that do not cause pain.

Avoiding positions that make the pain more noticeable is also important to healing. Daily activities, including getting up from sitting, walking, sex, and turning in bed can also irritate the site of injury, and these activities should also be limited if they cause pain. Stretching, and icing should be done daily.

Massages are very helpful to help alleviate pain and release tightness in the lower back and over areas of dense muscle such as the buttock. Some massage therapists or other musculoskeletal professionals also stretch the muscles while massaging, which can further contribute to relieving symptoms.

There are many alternative disciplines of medicine that focus on relieving pain in this area. These include osteopathic manipulations, chiropractic release techniques, and acupuncture. These treatments can have variable benefits and should only be done in addition to stretching and strengthening. Stop alternative techniques of hip and pelvis pain treatment if there is no improvement in pain after one month of regular treatment; stop immediately if there is an increase in pain and consult with your doctor. Yoga is an excellent method of maintaining flexibility and strength in the hip, buttock, and pelvis.

Hip and Thigh Exercises

Exercises are described for the right leg (substitute with your left leg if that is the side that bothers you) and should be done on both sides if you have time. The motions should be done in a controlled motion by counting slowly to three for the up motion, holding for a slow count of three, and lowering for a slow count of three. Begin with a low weight or none at all. Perform one set of 10 repetitions of each exercise, then switch sides or rotate through the exercises before starting a second set of exercises. When the two sets of 10 repetitions feel easy, add an ankle weight of 1 to 2 pounds and increase by 1 pound every 2 weeks to a maximum of 10 pounds. You may also add a third set to increase the challenge.

Exercises that cause pain should be modified with lighter weights, smaller motions, and fewer repetitions. If there is still pain, stop the exercise and review the techniques with your doctor, therapist, or trainer educated in therapeutic exercises. If you are healing from an injury or pain, ice the uncomfortable area for about 10 minutes after exercise.

Strengthening and stretching exercises should be done regularly to prevent inflammation and pain due to weakness and tightness. For a female athlete without any specific hip or pelvic pain complaints, these exercises should be done two or three times a week. For those with pain or musculoskeletal issues in this area, the exercises should be done three to five days a week. As with any exercises, they should not cause pain but should feel like you are giving your muscles a good strength challenge.

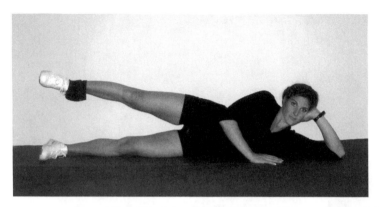

FIGURE 10-7 **Outer Thigh Lifts: Lying on your left side, lift your straight right leg up to 8 to 12 inches, hold for count of 3, then lower slowly.**
Gym version (more advanced): Use a standing cable with a strap around your right ankle, stand with the left side of your body toward the cable, and raise your right leg out to your side 8 to 12 inches, hold, and slowly release.

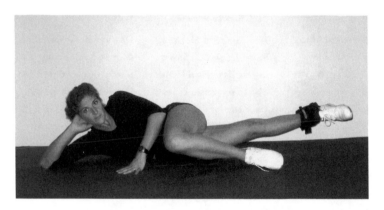

FIGURE 10-8 **Inner Thigh Lifts: Lying on your right side with your top left leg bent either in front or behind you, lift your straight right leg up 8 to 12 inches. Hold for count of three, then slowly lower.**
Gym version (more advanced): Use a standing cable with a strap around your right ankle, stand with the right side of your body toward the cable and cross your right leg over your left 12 inches, hold, and slowly release.

Standing Hip and Pelvic Stability

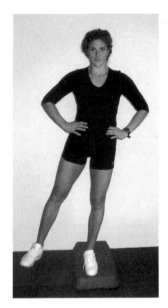 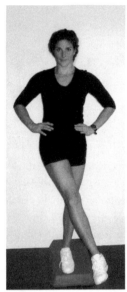 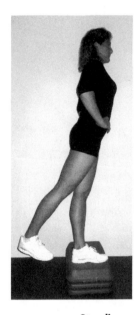

FIGURE 10-9 Standing Leg Raise: Standing with good posture (stomach in so your abdominal muscles are tight, pelvis straight, not tilted) on the right side of a step (or on floor), lift your straight right leg out to your side slowly, hold for slow count of three, and slowly return to center. Make sure you are not tilting your body to the left side (watch in mirror). Switch sides.

FIGURE 10-10 Standing Inner Thigh Lift: Standing as described in the above exercise, cross your straight right leg over your left. Hold for a slow count of three and slowly return to center. Make sure you are not tilting your body to the left side (watch in mirror). Switch sides.

FIGURE 10-11 Standing Glut Strengthening: As above, lift straight right leg out to back slowly, hold slow count of 3 and slowly return to center. Switch sides.

Advanced Hip Exercises

Advanced standing hip and pelvis stability exercises (10-9 through 10-11): Use a 3 to 10 pound ankle weight on your lifted leg.

More Advanced: Stand on a balance board while doing exercise.

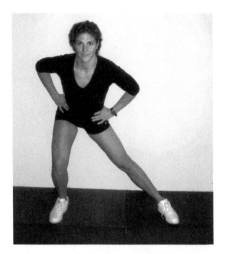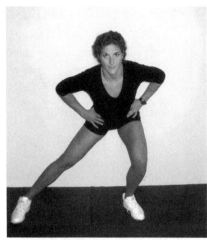

FIGURE 10-12 **Side Lunges: Standing, lunge your right leg out, bending your right knee to land (A). Push off your right leg back to standing center. Repeat 10 times and switch sides (B).**

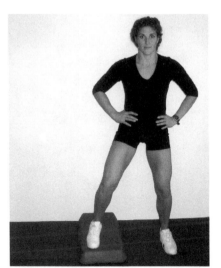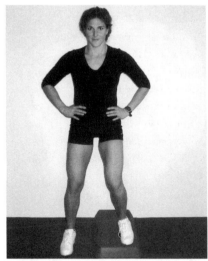

FIGURE 10-13 **Two-Step Step-Overs: Standing with a step on your right, step onto step (A) with your right leg, bring your left leg onto the step, and step down to right side on your right leg, bringing your left leg off the step (B). Reverse direction.**

Advanced Plyometric Hip Exercises

Plyometric exercises are explosive exercises involving jumping with a controlled, soft, silent landing to protect the joint and improve landing balance and technique.

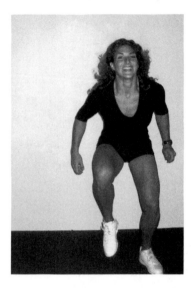

FIGURE 10-14 Side-to-Side Hops: Hop side to side, landing softly. (May hop over blocks, cones, or taped lines on the floor.) Advanced: Perform these on one leg.

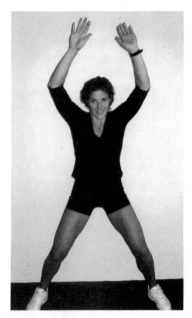

FIGURE 10-15 Jumping Jacks: Perform jumping jacks, landing softly.

Pelvic Stabilization Exercises

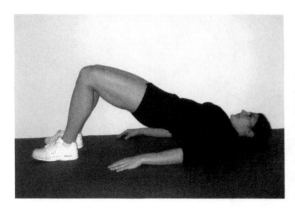

FIGURE 10-16 **Bridge: On your back with your knees bent and shoulder width apart, lift your pelvis and hips up, keeping your lower stomach sucked in tight. Hold for slow count of three and slowly lower.**

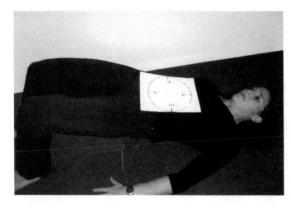

FIGURE 10-17 **Pelvic Clock: Imagine a clock face on your lower abdomen and pelvis. Raise your hips to bridge position and tilt your pelvis to 12, hold for 3 seconds, tilt to 3, hold 3 seconds, tilt to 6, hold 3 seconds, and tilt to 9, holding 3 seconds. Lower hips; start next circle in reverse direction so the progression is counterclockwise (12, 9, 6, 3).**

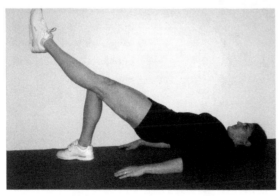

FIGURE 10-18 **Bridge with One Leg Up: Perform bridge exercise with one leg straight, keeping your leg up for full set of 10. Lower leg and switch sides.**

Advanced

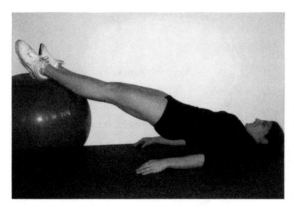

FIGURE 10-19 **Bridge with Legs on Ball: With both legs on a large stability ball, lift your hips and pelvis up, holding for three count.**

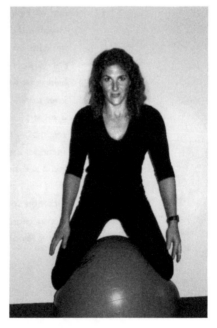

FIGURE 10-20 **Stability Ball Balance: Squeeze your thighs and tighten your abs and hips to be upright while kneeling on large stability ball. Try to hold for 10 seconds, and work up to 20.**

Hip and Thigh Stretches

Hold each for a slow count of five. Repeat five times. Stretches that are one-sided describe right-side hip stretching.

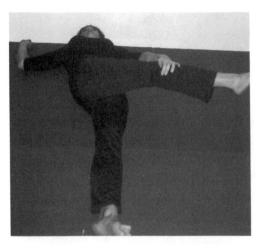

FIGURE 10-21 Outer Thigh Stretch (Iliotibial Band): Lying on your back with both legs straight, raise your right leg up, then across your body to the left, pulling your right leg down with your left hand on your outer right calf or with a strap around your right foot. Stretch intensity increases the higher you lift your right leg before bringing it across.

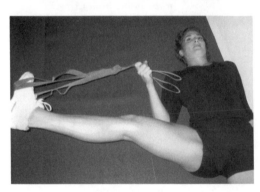

FIGURE 10-22 Inner Thigh Stretch (Adductor): Lying on your back with both legs straight, raise your right leg up, then out to the right side to open your legs, holding with your right arm on your right calf or with a strap around your right foot. Stretch intensity increases the wider your right leg opens to the side.

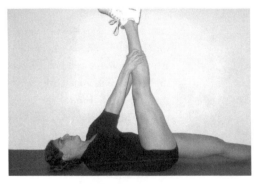

FIGURE 10-23 Hamstring Stretch: Lying on your back with your left knee bent and your right knee straight, lift your right leg up, holding on to your calf or with a strap. Pull in toward your body, keeping your right knee straight.

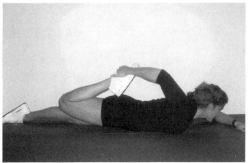

FIGURE 10-24 **Hip Flexor Stretch:** Lying on your stomach, reach back with your right arm to top of your right ankle. Pull your foot back toward your buttocks, lifting your knee off the floor. (This stretch can also be done standing, allowing your knee to go behind the plane of your body.)

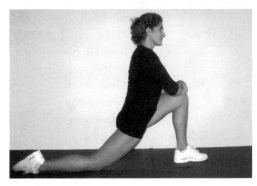

FIGURE 10-25 **Advanced Hip Flexor Stretch:** Standing in lunge position with your right leg back and toes pointed, bend your left knee forward to feel the stretch through the front of your right hip.

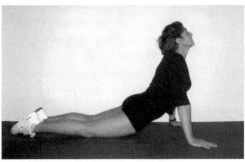

FIGURE 10-26 **Both Legs Hip Flexor Stretch:** Lying on your stomach, with your toes pointed down, press up with your elbows straight.

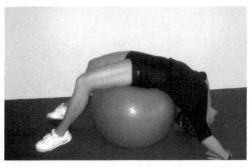

FIGURE 10-27 **Hip Flexor Stretch on Ball:** Lying on your back with a large exercise ball under your mid back, arch your back to feel the full stretch through the front of your hips and thighs, reaching your arms and legs to the ground.

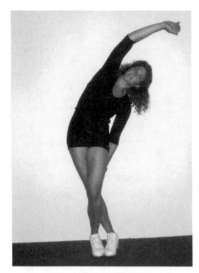

FIGURE 10-28 Outer Thigh Stretch (Iliotibial Band): Standing, cross your right leg behind your left. Reach your arms up and over to the left.

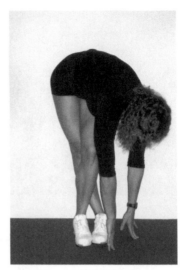

FIGURE 10-29 Outer Thigh and Hamstring Stretch: Standing as above, your right leg behind your left, bend over to the left side, reaching for the floor.

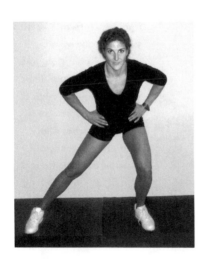

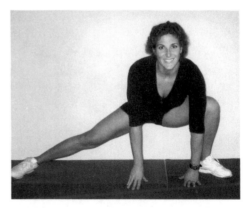

FIGURE 10-30 Inner Thigh Stretch: Standing with your feet wide apart, facing forward, lean in lunge from to the left with your right knee bent, left knee straight, toes facing forward. Hold when stretch in your right inner thigh and groin is felt (A). Advanced stretch: Bring your hands to the floor (B).

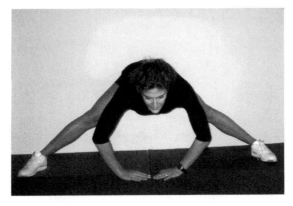

FIGURE 10-31 **Both Legs Inner Thigh Stretch:** For both legs, bend forward from your hips with your legs straight and wide apart, feet forward or pointed out slightly.

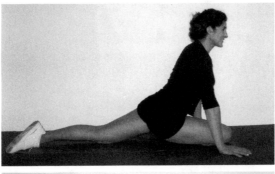

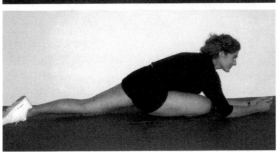

FIGURE 10-32 **Advanced: Pigeon Stretch:** From lunge position, with your right foot forward, cross your right foot forward toward your left, allowing the outside of your right knee to come to the mat, then your left front of thigh to come down onto mat (A). More advanced: Allow your arms to reach out forward onto the floor (B).

Pelvis, hip, and thigh pain is very common in women and tends to linger. It can also be difficult to identify and treat. Consult with a doctor to ensure that there is no internal or gynecological problem and to rule out back problems For true hip, pelvic, and thigh pain, treatment involves avoiding painful activities and pursuing active strengthening, stretching, and stabilization exercises, including those that challenge balance and pelvic stability.

CHAPTER ELEVEN

The Knee

Knees take a lot of stress throughout the day, particularly with stairs, bending, kneeling, and carrying. In sports, impact, twisting, jumping, squatting, and lunging activities can lead to joint wear and tear. Knees can be more susceptible to problems due to the amount and type of activities, history of injuries, joint alignment, and genetics. Athletic activities including basketball, volleyball, soccer, skiing, martial arts, rowing, and dance tend to cause an increased risk of knee problems. Recent changes in activity type or amount can also cause knee pain.

Knee pain and injury is very common, especially to girls and women. These problems can be very limiting, as the pain often becomes worse with exercise or athletic activity. As with other joints, pain on one side leads to favoring that side, causing the muscles to become weak, increasing the risk of more serious injuries in the future. For active women, it is important to learn how to strengthen and protect these valuable joints and identify any potential problems early so that both fitness and life activities can continue without limits.

Functional Anatomy

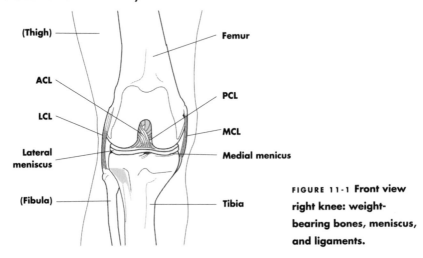

FIGURE 11-1 **Front view right knee: weight-bearing bones, meniscus, and ligaments.**

The femur (thigh) and tibia (leg) bones serve as the strong foundation of the joint and allow your bodyweight to be supported in standing and movement. The knee functions as a hinge joint between the femur and tibia, allowing bending. The other two bones around the knee joint are the patella (kneecap), a small bone that functions as a lever and point of attachment for the tendons of the quadriceps muscles. The patella and femur form the patellofemoral joint, a common site of pain in women.

The ligaments are very important to stabilize the knee and keep the joint moving in the right direction while preventing the bones from sliding forward, backward, or sideways over each other. The major ligaments of the knee are the anterior cruciate ligament (ACL), the posterior cruciate ligament (PCL), the medial collateral ligament (MCL), and the lateral collateral ligament (LCL) (see figure 11-1). The ligament injury that can cause the most problems in female athletes is the ACL, as it is the main stabilizer of forward motion of the thigh bone.

The bones are cushioned by cartilage and the medial and lateral meniscus. Tendons attach the muscles to bone and are named for the muscles they attach. Where tendons pass over the bones, there are bursas, fluid-filled sacs that cushion and allow tendons to move smoothly across, also named for the area they are in (see figure 11-2).

The muscles surrounding the knee joint allow movement of the joint and provide strength and stability to the ligaments. They attach to the bone

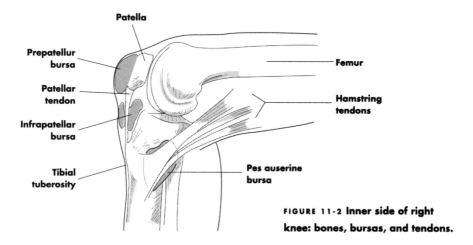

Patella

Prepatellur
bursa

Patellar
tendon

Infrapatellar
bursa

Tibial
tuberosity

Femur

Hamstring
tendons

Pes auserine
bursa

**FIGURE 11-2 Inner side of right
knee: bones, bursas, and tendons.**

via tendons. Some of these muscles also cross the hip joint, working to control the entire lower leg (see figure 11-3). The muscles that control the knee include the quadriceps, a group of four muscles that make up the front of the thigh and straighten the knee, and the hamstrings, a group of four muscles that make up the back of the thigh and bend the knee. The muscle that plays an important role in preventing knee pain is the medial quadriceps muscle, also known as the VMO. The hamstrings play an important role in stabilizing the ACL. The adductors on the inside of the joint and abductors on the outside also provide side-to-side stability. Because the thigh muscles control both the hip and knee, the hip can sometimes be involved with knee problems.

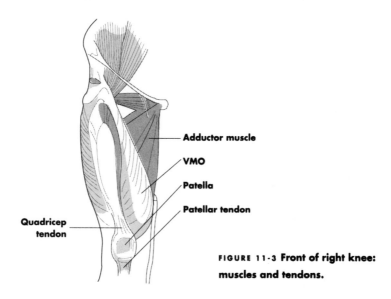

Adductor muscle

VMO

Patella

Patellar tendon

Quadricep
tendon

**FIGURE 11-3 Front of right knee:
muscles and tendons.**

Pain and Injury Patterns

Pain and injury patterns are listed in descending order of frequently. Patellofemoral pain is the most common type of knee pain in active women and is often a component of other pain and injury syndromes.

Patellofemoral Pain

Patellofemoral pain is the number one reason for knee pain in women, causing aching stiff, creaking, and crackly sounding knees that are sore in the front or underneath the kneecap. Although it can cause mild swelling, patellofemoral pain usually develops without injury. Pain is worse when climbing stairs, squatting, or sitting for long periods of time.

Patellofemoral pain, also known as "chondromalacia patella," is caused by an irritation between the patella and the front end of the femur. This irritation occurs due to muscle weakness, overuse, or alignment problems. Patellofemoral pain is more common in girls and women due to angled alignment of the femur to tibia, resulting in a joint that angles or kneecaps that tilt or are loose. This alignment is measured by a Q angle; one that is 17 degrees or more is often associated with patellofemoral pain (see figure 11-4). Having a greater Q angle indicates a greater likelihood that the patella will press against the femur during bending and straightening due to poor tracking in

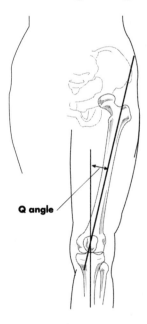

Q angle

FIGURE 11-4: The Q angle is measured as the angle formed between the line that crosses the anterior pelvic bone (ASIS) and the patella, and a vertical line crossing the patella and tibial tuberosity.

the groove of the top of the knee. This causes grinding and popping noises, along with inflammation and pain.

Patellofemoral pain has also been called "runner's knee," as it often occurs in runners who do not do any quadricep-strengthening exercises. It becomes more noticeable running up and especially down hills. It can also be common in cyclists, from riding up hills or after a sudden increase in distance. Fitness class enthusiasts can also develop patellofemoral pain due to repeated stair climbing, squats, or lunges. This also commonly occurs due to weaker muscles when returning to sports after a period of inactivity due to an injury or an overly busy schedule.

Patellofemoral pain improves with icing and anti-inflammatories and decreasing irritating activities including hills, stairs, squats, and lunges. Strengthening and stretching the surrounding muscles is key to preventing the pain from returning and allowing you to go back to pain-free athletic activity. Surgery (to "realign" your knee) is not recommended, as it usually causes more problems in the long run.

Corrective braces, straps, or taping to attempt to improve alignment, tracking, and tilt of the patella can sometimes be helpful, although these techniques are tolerated differently in each person. Orthotics that support the arches in flat feet can also help correct joint alignment from below.

Patellofemoral pain tends to return, especially if you take a break from athletic activities and start again or if you are injured. To prevent its return, make strengthening and stretching exercises a regular part of your workout program. Avoid repeated squatting or lunging. Refer to the exercises at the end of the chapter for both maintenance and prevention of patellofemoral pain.

Symptoms of Patellofemoral Pain

Cracking, popping noises during bending

Pain going up or down stairs

Pain after sitting for a long time

Pain with squats, lunges, kneeling

Pain running up or down hills

Bursitis

Bursitis causes stiffness, swelling, and pain due to inflammation of the bursa. The inflamed bursa is often tender and warm and might also feel boggy or even numb due to the swelling. Bursitis occurs mostly due to overuse, such as overtraining or a sudden increase in distance or force, but can also be secondary to injury or a fall directly on the knee. Bursitis can also be associated with tendinitis, as one irritates the other during movement. Bursitis responds to icing, stretching, and moderate rest. Anti-inflammatories can help with the swelling. If the bursas are swollen and painful, they might occasionally need to be drained by a doctor using a needle. An injection of cortisone can also help. If there is a lot of fluid and you are not able to bend your knee or walk on it normally, see a sports medicine doctor as soon as possible so it does not result in muscle weakness or tendon irritation.

Tendinitis

Tendinitis causes symptoms similar to bursitis with stiffness and achy pain especially when first moving the knee joint in the morning or after sitting for a long time. The most common type of tendinitis, patellar tendinitis, is also known as jumper's knee. This is an overuse injury that is painful below the kneecap and bothersome with running or jumping. It can occur on both sides due to inherent weakness and tightness of the patellar tendon. It responds to rest from painful activities, ice and anti-inflammatories, and stretching and strengthening of the quadriceps muscles.

Arthritis

Arthritis of the knee joint causes stiffness, swelling, pain, and weakness. Osteorthritis is the most common type of arthritis, due to wear and tear. It is also hereditary. Osteorthritis usually occurs later in life, over the age of 45, and seems to be more common in people who were very athletic in running and jumping activities. It is also more common in people who are heavier and those who were power lifters or bodybuilders. Osteorthritis can also occur after an injury. Unfortunately, arthritis cannot be reversed or "cured," although there are many treatments now available to make it less painful and preserve the joint motion and function.

Arthritis causes a loss of the protective cartilage of the knee, and on x-ray, there is narrowing of the normal joint space. The bones tend to rub together, causing the symptoms of swelling, stiffness, creaking, and pain. In severe cases, there can be swelling and loss of motion. It is usually recommended that high-impact activities be avoided as much as possible to prevent the arthritis from getting worse. Osteoarthritis is managed with regular strengthening exercises, stretching to maintain motion, and medications to decrease swelling and pain. Glucosamine chondroitin is a supplement that can sometimes reduce the symptoms and slow progression of osteoarthritis.

Medical treatments include steroid injections into the knee joint to decrease inflammation and pain, or a series of cartilage-lining injections (called synvisc, suparts, and hyalgan). These provide symptomatic relief. The most aggressive, definitive treatment of osteoarthritis is joint replacement. Total joint replacement is a surgery that requires several months of therapy and recovery and is usually done as late as possible in life, as the replaced joints might need to be revised. A uni-knee is partial joint replacement, a less-invasive surgery with shorter recovery time. Both types of joint replacement prohibit running and jumping activities to prevent loosening of the artificial joint.

Methods to Treat Symptoms of Osteoarthritis (In Increasing Order of Severity of Symptoms)

Ice or heat

Exercise and stretching

Decreasing high-impact activities

Wearing well-cushioned shoes

Glucosamine chrondroitin supplements

Anti-inflammatory medications

Physical therapy

Joint injections with steroids or cartilage medicines

Knee replacement surgery

Meniscus Tear

A meniscus tear is a common injury that can occur in almost any sport, usually due to a fall or twisting motion. A meniscus tear causes sharp pain with twisting or impact. There can also be pain at rest, when crossing the legs, or turning in bed. There can be swelling, popping, and locking sensations. If it is a small, a meniscus tear can heal with strengthening exercises and by avoiding painful activities. If pain is limiting motion and activity, arthroscopic surgery, through small incisions on the sides of the knee, is recommended. For athletes, recovery from this surgery is usually quick. Therapeutic exercises are recommended to maximize healing as quickly as possible. With proper rehabilitation the athlete might be able to return to sports in six to eight weeks.

ACL Injury

ACL injuries occur due to collision or bad landings involving twisting or being off balance. A pop is usually heard, and there is sharp pain. Swelling develops within a few hours after injury. Most athletes who tear their ACL end up in emergency rooms because pain and swelling makes walking and bending difficult. X-rays in the emergency room are usually normal, because there is no injury to the bone. Usually, the emergency room will give you an immobilizer to keep your knee straight and suggest that you see an orthopedic surgeon, as ACL injuries often require surgical repair. Over the next week, the swelling and pain usually improves, and it is important to try to bend and straighten the knee without weight while you are sitting or lying down. You should try to stay off it as much as possible until you are evaluated by the orthopedist or sports medicine doctor. If you are diagnosed with an ACL tear, you may walk on it without the immobilizer as soon as swelling and pain have decreased.

Because the ACL is an important knee stabilizer and because injury is usually associated with a meniscus tear, surgery is usually necessary to return you to full function. Recovery from surgery can be grueling, as stiffness and swelling can cause pain, and full healing can sometimes take three to six months.

There are some athletes who choose not to have surgery and who recover with aggressive strengthening of the hamstring and knee muscles. These women must be diligent about strength training three to five times a week. Also, athletes who do a lot of activities requiring jumping and landing, including basketball and volleyball, dance, or downhill skiing, usually are not able to do these activities as well without surgery.

ACL injuries occur more commonly in female athletes and can be prevented with strength and technique training. This training focuses on correcting the weaknesses that have been found to contribute to ACL injuries, because weak muscles are not able to protect the joint or contribute to proper body mechanics. Hamstring strength is very important to ACL stability, as the hamstrings protect the ACL. Correcting alignment, improving balance, and strengthening other areas of weakness due to ankle sprain or hip or back pain is an essential part of preventing and recovering from ACL injuries. Being aerobically conditioned is also an invaluable way to prevent ACL tears, as fatigue can also cause injuries. Making sure shoes fit well and playing surfaces are not bumpy or slippery also reduces all injuries.

Risk Factors for ACL Injuries	
Hamstring muscle weakness	Landing off center
Poor balance	Irregular playing surface
Ankle weakness	Slippery playing surface
Landing too far forward	Collision
Landing with a twisting motion	Previous history of knee injury

Other Ligament Injuries

The MCL and LCL can be sprained and torn, causing pain and sometimes swelling on the inside or outside of the knee joint. This can be bothersome in twisting or side-to-side motions and can cause a sense of looseness at the joint. PCL injuries similarly cause a sense of instability in the backward direction. These ligaments tend to heal on their own, and their weakness can be supported by strengthening the surrounding muscles. Rarely do these injuries require surgery.

Osgood-Schlatters

Bone growth and development in girls and young women can cause irritation of the tibial tuberosity, the bony area at the top of the tibia where the patellar tendon attaches. Known as Osgood-Schlatters, it causes pain similar to patellar tendinitis with the addition of swelling and tenderness over the top of the tibia. Osgood-Schlatters improves with icing, stretching, and avoiding painful impact activities. Over the age of 20, the pain of Osgood-Schlatters usually disappears, although some athletes develop a residual bump over the top of the tibia.

Fractures

Fractures due to injury can occur to the patella, tibia, and occasionally the femur. Fractures usually require surgery and eight weeks of rest with crutches. Physical therapy is always recommended after fracture to ensure normal motion and strength. Osteoarthritis can sometimes develop later in life at the site of an old fracture.

Evaluation and Treatment

Evaluation

See a sports medicine doctor, orthopedist, or a rehabilitation specialist if your knee pain lasts more than one week, interferes with sleep or activity, and especially if there is swelling, a feeling of buckling, or you are limping. The doctor will ask you about your pain, including if you have had this in the past, if there was an injury, or if there was a recent change in activity or intensity of training. The examination will measure your strength, motion, and determine if there is swelling, ligament looseness, or joint dysfunction. X-rays might be done to evaluate the bone and joint space. If your pain has not responded to treatment or you have unusual symptoms, an MRI might be ordered to visualize the soft tissue structures, particularly the menisci, cartilage, and ligaments.

Knee Symptoms You Should See a Doctor For

Pain lasting longer than one week

Swelling

Buckling

Locking

Pain that keeps you from sleeping

Limping

Limited motion

Treatment usually involves ice and resting from any activity that causes pain. As soon as you are allowed, start gentle motion to preserve the normal bend and straightening of the knee. If surgery is recommended to repair a torn ligament or meniscus, exercises and physical therapy afterward is crucial to the success of surgery, and preventing any other problems. Occasionally, pain syndromes such as patellofemoral pain and bursitis can develop on the other knee as it takes more stress. Maintaining strengthening exercises on both sides is crucial to preventing further problems.

You might be given an immobilizer or brace immediately after injury. Ask the doctor specifically how long you must wear it and if you are allowed to remove it to bend your knee. Try not to wrap or brace your knee yourself without the approval of your doctor, as this can restrict motion and lead to further weakness and long-term stiffness of the joint. Some doctors recommend braces for patellofemoral pain; however, these tend to irritate more than relieve symptoms due to tight and improper fit. If there is a tender area due to bursitis or tendinitis that the brace is rubbing on, it can actually make you feel worse. If you have a stable knee and the brace seems to be irritating you, do not wear it. Unless it is a hard, custom-fitted brace with a hinged or locked joint, as sometimes used after ACL injury, it will not prevent further injury.

Some athletes like braces because they feel more secure. The feeling is one of gentle support to the muscles, not to the actual joint. This can be helpful if there is swelling, or within the first few weeks of injury, when soft braces can sometimes make sleeping and walking more comfortable. It is not recommended to wear the brace for much longer, however. Straps perform a similar function. It is believed that they help support movement of the kneecap or take tension off the tendons. They are not essential to knee recovery, and like braces, can sometimes cause more pain by irritating tender areas. If you feel more comfortable with a strap or a brace, only wear them for a short time and be aware that you might develop an unnecessary dependence on them.

PERFORMANCE TIP **Ice is your knee's best medicine.**

Knee pain indicates inflammation, which responds to ice and anti-inflammatory medications. Cortisone injections also decrease inflammation but are only used in certain knee conditions, as they can weaken tendons if used repetitively. Because of this risk to tendons, cortisone injections should not be repeated more than twice. Icing is always helpful to knee problems and should be done for 10 minutes at the end of each day, after strengthening exercise and athletic activities, and when sore. Wrapping a cold gel pack in an Ace wrap snuggly around your knee while keeping it elevated can reduce swelling dramatically. Muscle rubs and pain-relieving creams can also help decrease soreness. A cryocuff is a device providing ice and compression that speeds healing after surgery or injury. (See the resources at back of the book for purchasing information.)

Physical therapy is helpful to recover from knee injuries and pain that has been limiting sports or activity. Therapists have special training in techniques to reduce inflammation and pain and increase strength and motion. If you are getting physical therapy, you should continue until you have all your motion and at least 90 percent of your normal strength back. Therapists and athletic trainers can also give you specific exercises and training to help you return to your sport. Your therapist should also give you exercises to do on your own to increase the speed of your recovery.

If your pain is mild to moderate and you have most of your full motion, you can do your own therapy by performing the exercises below followed by stretching and 10 minutes of icing. You will make significant progress by doing these low-resistance exercises every day; if you are recovering from an injury, this is recommended over high-resistance exercises every other day. You should see your doctor at least one more time for follow-up; return sooner if your pain gets worse. If your pain does not improve within two to four weeks, go back to your doctor to reevaluate your diagnosis and treatment.

Exercises and Stretches

Exercises are very important to strengthen the muscles that support the joint. Strong muscles allow proper tracking and take stress off ligaments and cartilage. Stretches maintain motion in the joint and flexibility in the tendons to prevent them from becoming stiff and strained. Exercises can be done at home with ankle weights and using body resistance, or on gym equipment.

If you choose to use exercise machines to strength train, exercise one knee at a time to build up equal strength on each side (most equipment is designed to do both knees together). Make sure the motion does not involve extreme bending or too heavy weight, which can strain the joint. Increase weight and number of repetitions slowly over several weeks.

Squats and lunges should be avoided by anyone with knee problems or pain, as they put excessive, unnecessary strain on knee joints. If you have healthy knees, squats and lunges still must be done with caution, if done at all. If you feel you *must* squat or lunge, do not squat deeper than 90 degrees and keep your knee centered over your foot. Do not increase the strain on your knee with added weight. There are many other exercises that strengthen buttocks and thighs that are recommended instead of squats and lunges, including biking, low steps (less than nine inches), extension leg lifts, and stairs. Aerobic activity with low stress to the knee joint also includes swimming (avoid the breaststroke kick), elliptical trainer, and walking (if tolerated).

PERFORMANCE TIP **Avoid squats and lunges if you have any knee problems.**

Exercises

Try the exercises first without weights. If this is too easy, use an ankle weight starting with one to two pounds. Gradually increase the weight by one pound each week as long as you do not have pain with the exercise, until you reach 10 pounds. Try to do these exercises three to five days a week. If you are also doing other exercise or sports, do the knee exercises after your workout.

Remember to do all movements slowly. You should be able to comfortably do two sets of 10 repetitions without pain or soreness in the joint. If you have pain with an exercise, try reducing the amount of bend, weight resistance, and repetitions. If the exercise is still painful, do not do it; try it again with a lower weight in one or two weeks when your muscles are stronger.

Exercises become more advanced in the order they are described; if you feel sore after the first two exercises, do only those exercises for the first week and gradually add a new exercise as you become stronger.

It is always a good idea to do both legs, as problems on one side often also occur on the other. Remember to ice your knee for at least 10 minutes after exercises, especially if you are sore. (If you do not have time for this, ice sometime later that day.)

Hold each exercise at the end of the motion for a slow count of three, counting slowly to three as you move up and release. Repeat each exercise 10 times per set; do at least two sets per day, rotating through exercises or switching sides to allow the muscles to rest between sets. When two sets of 10 exercises become easy, increase the amount of repetitions per set to 15 or add a third set. Exercises are described for the right knee; it is recommended to focus on the side that is painful, but try to do exercises on both sides if you have the time.

Quadricep Strengthening and Patellofemoral Exercises

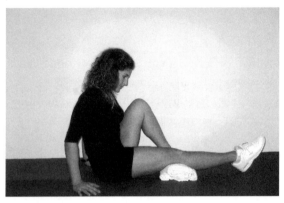

FIGURE 11-5 **Quadricep Tighteners: Sitting with a rolled towel (or pillow) under your extended knee, press your knee down into the towel to fully straighten your knee and tighten the muscles. Hold for a slow count of five. Release.**

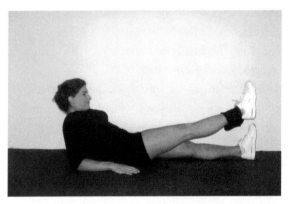

FIGURE 11-6 **Straight Leg Raises: Half sitting or lying flat with your right leg straight out in front and your left knee bent for stability, slowly lift your right leg up about 8 to 12 inches. Hold for a slow count of three, then lower for a slow count of three. Gym version: Use a standing cable machine, with the cable attached to your right ankle. Stand on your left leg with your back toward cable machine, tighten your muscles, and lift your straight leg forward. Slowly release.**

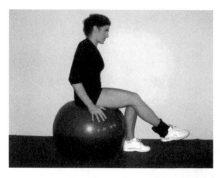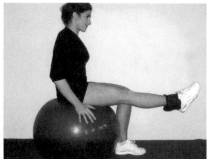

FIGURE 11-7 **Leg Extensions: Sitting, start with your right leg out in front, bent to about 60 degrees (A). Straighten your right knee to lift your foot for a slow count of three, hold straight with tight muscles for slow count of three (B), then lower for slow count of three.**
Gym version: Single Leg Extensions on Leg Extension Machine: First, set machine to very low weight (5 to 10 pounds). Raise machine with both legs so your feet are in front of you underneath the leg bar. Lower one leg and perform the exercise one leg at a time, lowering only to the half-bent position (shown in A above).

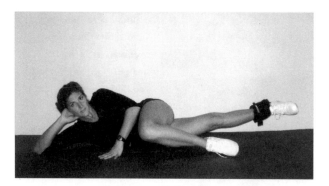

FIGURE 11-8 **Inner Thigh Lift: Lying on your right side with your top knee bent in front or behind you (whichever is more comfortable), straighten and tighten your right knee while lifting your inner thigh to the ceiling 8 to 12 inches for a slow count of 3. Hold for a count of three, then lower for a slow count of three.**
Gym version: Use standing cable attached to your right ankle, stand on your left leg with your right side toward cable; cross your right leg in front of your left.

Hamstring and Quadricep Exercises

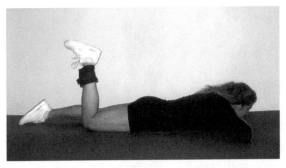

FIGURE 11-9 **Knee Curls: Standing or lying on your stomach, bend your right knee behind you. Hold for a slow count of three, then lower.**
Gym version: Hamstring Curl Machine: Do one leg at a time with very low weight, not bending knee past 90 degrees.

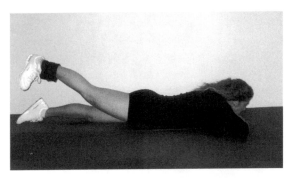

FIGURE 11-10 **Rear Leg Extensions: On your stomach, raise your straight right leg behind you, lifting while keeping your knee straight.**

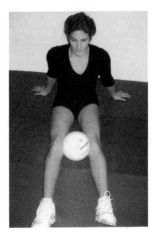

FIGURE 11-11 **Adductor Squeeze: Sitting with your legs straight out in front, squeeze a volleyball, basketball, or small exercise ball between your thighs. Hold for slow count of five.**

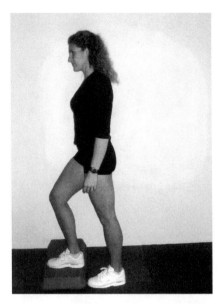 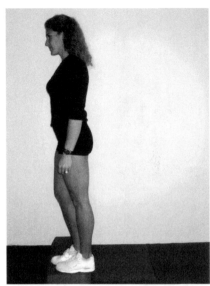

FIGURE 11-12 **Step-Ups: Standing behind a low stair, step, or telephone book shorter than nine inches high, place your right foot on the step (A). Put all your weight on your right leg and straighten to step up with your left foot (B). Leaving your right foot on the step, slowly step down onto your left leg to starting position.**

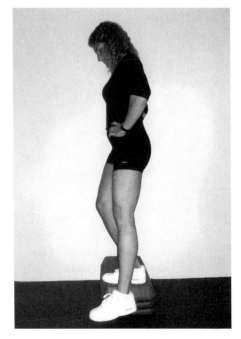

FIGURE 11-13 **Side Step-Ups: With a step to your right place your right foot sideways on the step. Step up onto your right foot, bringing your left foot up. Keep your right foot on the step and place your left leg back down on the floor to starting position.**

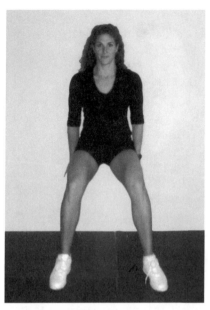 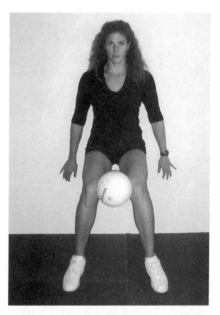

FIGURE 11-14 **Wall Seats: Standing with** your back against the wall and your feet about 18 inches away from the wall, slowly slide your back down the wall with both knees bending to a few inches above a full sitting position. Hold for a count of 10, making sure you are putting your weight evenly on both legs, not avoiding the painful knee. If this is uncomfortable, turn your toes out slightly and do not slide down as far.

FIGURE 11-15 **Advanced Wall Seat: Per-**form wall seat as above, holding a basketball, medicine ball, or large pillow. In sitting position, place the ball between your thighs and squeeze together for 10 to 20 seconds. Hold the ball with your hands to slide back up the wall.

Stretches

Stretches should be held for a slow count of five and repeated five times per stretch. They should be done after strengthening exercise or sports activity and can also be incorporated into your athletic warm-up. Stretches are described for the right leg but should also be done on the left.

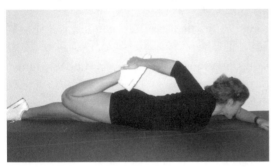

FIGURE 11-16 **Hamstring Stretch/Runner's Lunge: Standing, reach your left foot forward onto a step, chair, or cube. Keeping your right knee straight, shift your weight onto your bent left leg. Hold for a slow count of five. (Can also be done on the floor.)**

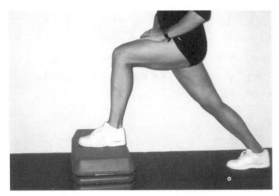

FIGURE 11-17 **Quadricep Stretch: On your stomach, bend your right knee behind you and reach back to pull your foot toward your rear. Hold for a slow count of five. (Can also be done standing.)**

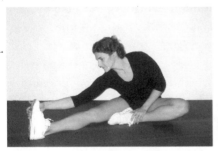
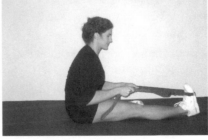

FIGURE 11-18 **Seated Hamstring Stretch: Sitting, straighten your right knee out in front of you with your left knee bent and turned out, and lean forward to reach for your toes (A). This exercise may also be done with strap around your foot to enhance the stretch and allow your back to remain straight (B).**

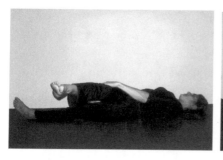 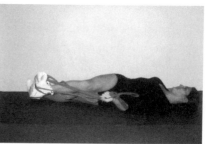

FIGURE 11-19 Outer Hamstring Stretch: On your back, cross your straight right leg over your left and pull across to your left side with your left hand (A), or use a stretch strap for more effective stretch (B).

Exercises to Prevent ACL Injuries

To prevent serious knee injuries, particularly ACL injuries, you should work on balance and agility. This will prevent off-center landings. Using a balance board fine-tunes your nerves and muscles to keep you upright during activity. Balance exercises are crucial for preventing knee instability or imbalance. One-legged activities such as one-legged squats, hops, and raising on your toe and heel on one leg with your eyes closed will allow you to develop skillful athletic balance.

Hopping activities and jumping rope on one leg helps increase agility, balance, and strength. Practice jumping and landing with your body weight over the center of your feet, knees bent, not leaning forward. Jumping and hopping activities should focus on a soft landing (that makes as little noise as possible) to decrease impact on your knee joints. Plyometric exercises are best for injury prevention and reducing stress on your joints. Plyometrics involve explosive jumps with soft, quiet landings, strengthening your muscles and reducing the impact and force of landing. The more practice you have in jumping and landing, the less likely you are to fall or injure yourself or your knee joint.

Cutting maneuvers such as running around cones, side-stepping around a gym, and jumping over low obstacles improves agility and balance. You should try to keep each step light and quiet to reduce impact and stress on joints.

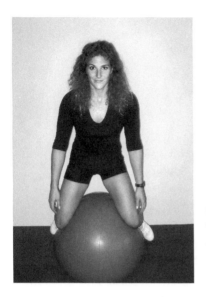

FIGURE 11-20 **Balanced Hamstring Strength:** Try to kneel on a large stability ball without touching your feet to the floor. Squeeze your knees into ball to hold yourself upright. Try to hold for 10 seconds and increase to 20.

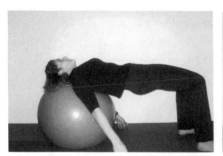

FIGURE 11-21 **Hamstring Strength Using Ball: On your back, with your torso parallel to the floor and with your upper back on a large stability ball with your knees bent less than 90 degrees and your feet shoulder width apart (A), pull with your legs to roll the ball forward, lowering your torso close to floor (B). Slowly push the ball back, rolling your torso back up parallel to the floor.**

Advanced

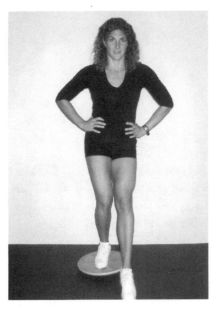

FIGURE 11-22 Balance Board Mini-Squats:
With your right foot on a balance board,
slowly bend your knee about six inches
for a mini-squat on one leg, maintaining
a straight spine and hips with good bal-
ance, lightly touching your left toe to the
ground. Straighten your knee to starting
position.

Plyometric Hops

Land softly and quietly with each activity. Perform each exercise 10 times, alternating directions or legs after each set. As you become more advanced, you may hop over cones, ladders, or taped markers spaced farther apart and increase the repetitions, trying not to "double hop" (land twice).

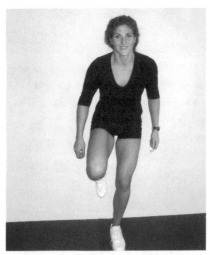

FIGURE 11-23 One-legged hop.

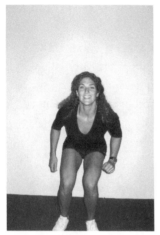
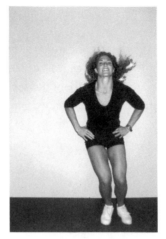

FIGURE 11-24 **A, B,** **Side-to-side hops.**

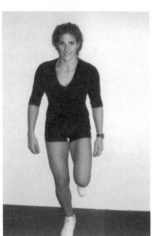
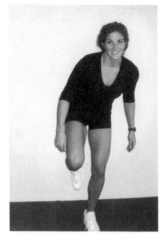

FIGURE 11-25 **A, B,** **Side-to-side hops on one leg.**

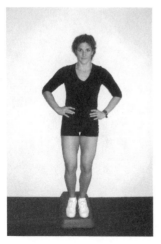
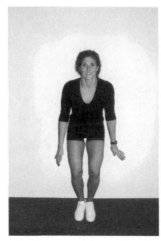

FIGURE 11-26 **A, B,** **Side-to-side hops on and off step. Also perform hops forward and backward on and off step.**

Knee pain and injury syndromes are extremely common among active women. Some require surgery. With aggressive and appropriate strengthening exercises, practice in jumping and landing technique, and balance exercise, the severity of and number of injuries and pain syndromes can be reduced.

CHAPTER TWELVE

The Leg, Ankle, and Foot

In women, the lower legs, ankles, and feet take a lot of abuse. When injured, they tend to be a challenge to heal, because rest is difficult due to the necessary activity of walking. During athletic activities, feet are challenged to hold you upright in many directions and speeds of travel. Feet strike the ground first, absorbing all your body's shock and holding you up. Leg, ankle, and foot pain and injury can lead to strange walking patterns, resulting in pain at the knee or hip.

Legs, ankles, and feet can suffer from repetitive stress injuries, including ligament and tendon strains and stress fractures. Dance, running, kicking, and field and court sports are notorious for causing lower limb problems. Ankle sprains are the most common sports injury overall, and although they might seem minor, they can cause future problems to other joints if not correctly healed and rehabilitated. Shoes also play a large role in leg and foot pain, especially if they are too pointed, flat, hard, large, or small. There are many factors contributing to lower leg, ankle, and foot problems. Keeping these areas strong and pain-free will prevent many other activity and sports injuries.

Functional Anatomy

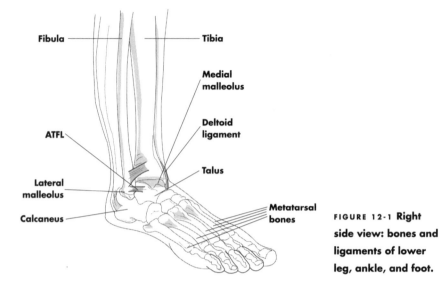

Fibula

Tibia

Medial malleolus

Deltoid ligament

ATFL

Talus

Lateral malleolus

Calcaneus

Metatarsal bones

FIGURE 12-1 **Right side view: bones and ligaments of lower leg, ankle, and foot.**

The ankle joint is made up of four bones, the tibia, fibula, talus, and calcaneus (see figure 12-1). These are connected by ligaments named for the bones they attach to. The most commonly injured ligament is the ATFL (anterior talofibular ligament), on the outside of the ankle; the deltoid ligament performs a similar supporting role on the inside of the ankle joint in front of the medial malleolus. There are also supportive ligaments: the spring ligament and the plantar fascia ligament, at the base of the foot that support the arch and lessen the stress of impact.

The ankle and foot movements are controlled by muscles in the lower leg. The largest and strongest muscles required for push off in walking and jumping are the calf muscles in the back of the leg, the gastrocnemious and soleus (see figure 12-2). These control the downward motion of the foot (toe point). Muscles in the front of the leg control the upward movement of the foot, including the anterior tibialis and peroneus. The muscles are attached by tendons; the Achilles tendon is the largest tendon and is the attachment of the calf muscles. Other major tendons that serve supportive roles are the anterior tibialis and peroneus tendons. Calcaneal bursas are the fluid-filled sacs that help the tendons glide smoothly over the bony sites of attachment (see figure 12-3).

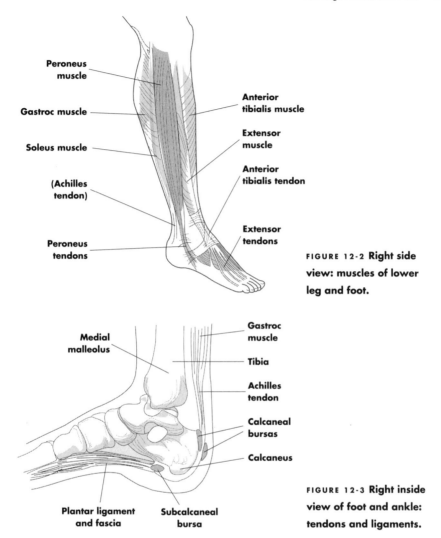

FIGURE 12-2 Right side view: muscles of lower leg and foot.

FIGURE 12-3 Right inside view of foot and ankle: tendons and ligaments.

Pain and Injury Patterns

Pain and injuries are listed in descending order of frequency. Ankle sprains, the most common overall sports injury, are often part of or contribute to other pain and injury patterns.

Ankle Sprain

Ankle sprains are the number one sports injury. They occur commonly in field sports, aerobic activities, dance, and hiking during a twisting injury, trip, or fall when the ankle gives way. Sprains can be painful, causing difficulty with each step. Swelling often occurs within a few hours, and there might be a large area of bruising.

The most common ankle injury is a sprain called an inversion injury, or ATFL sprain. This occurs when the foot turns in under you and puts stress on the outside of the ankle. Often, once this happens, the ankle remains loose in this direction and is prone to repeated ankle sprains. After each sprain, the ankle joint becomes unstable, contributing to other ligament injuries in the foot or knee, or risk of fracture due to the weak base of support. A severe ankle sprain might require the use of crutches for a few days or longer if there is also a fracture. Usually, a soft cast or walking boot is recommended for the first one to three weeks after injury to limit twisting motions and reinjury.

A severe ankle sprain might limit activity for several weeks, but for most people, walking can begin normally again in a day or two and sports activities can be resumed within the month. Bracing can be used if your ankle feels wobbly, but don't get dependent on them—they can prevent your muscles from being as strong as they should. If you are still healing from a sprain and must play sports, wear a supportive sports ankle brace or air cast during play to prevent reinjury.

Also be careful of what you do with your feet when you are sitting. Often, girls sit with their feet turned in or curled under, the exact position of stretch that mimics a sprain. Try to avoid this as much as possible, because your goal is to tighten those ligaments, not stretch them. Activities that help prevent further ankle sprains include balance exercises. Shoes are also important in preventing ankle sprains—if you are hiking uneven terrain or doing aerobics or kickboxing, running shoes are not recommended, as they have no lateral support.

Avoiding Ankle Sprains

Try to run on even terrain.

Avoid hiking through leaves or slippery terrain.

Wear well-fitting shoes, and lace them properly.

Do exercises for balance and lower leg strength.

Walk slower if you are feeling tired.

Do not run in the dark on ground you cannot see.

Do not sit with your feet turned in.

Shin Splints

Shin splints are a generic term for pain and tenderness in the front of the lower leg. The pain can be aching or burning and usually develops during exercise. Shin splints are usually painful with running or jumping and occasionally even with walking. They are an overuse injury that can arise due to a sudden increase in mileage, type of training, or wearing different or worn-out shoes.

Shin splints can be caused by a variety of medical diagnoses, including tendinitis of the anterior tibialis muscle tendons, inflammation of the soft tissue that surrounds the bone, and stress fractures. Often, the surface of the bone is inflamed; this is called anterior tibial stress syndrome. A more serious but less frequent cause of shin splints is compartment syndrome, where the muscles get inflamed within their soft tissue structure. This might require surgery. Stress fractures also cause shin splints and require strict rest for proper healing.

Shin splints that do not get better with ice or rest after a week should be evaluated by a sports medicine doctor. Mild to moderate shin splints (not due to compartment syndrome or stress fractures) can improve with cushioned orthotics, changing to a newer pair of well-cushioned shoes, changing running surface, or cross-training. If you have pain in the shins, stretch, strengthen, and ice them regularly. Shin splints are often a sign that you are training too much, have increased your mileage too quickly, or your shoes have lost their support and conditioning.

Plantar Fasciitis

Plantar fasciitis is heel pain that is felt when getting out of bed in the morning, getting up from sitting a long time, or after standing for a long period. It is an inflammation of the plantar fascia, a thick, strong band of tissue on the bottom of the foot that supports your arch. This is more common in people with flat feet who wear flat shoes or do not wear arch supports, as their plantar fascia is under more stress. Although it does not lead to serious problems, it can cause frustrating, activity-limiting pain that tends to return. Plantar fasciitis is the source of the pain of heel spurs.

Treating plantar fasciitis requires daily stretching, strengthening, and icing after standing and at the end of the day. Anti-inflammatory medications also help speed healing. Cushioned gel heel cups are often recommended to treat the pain of plantar fasciitis; however, these should only be worn for the initial period of severe pain. For more effective, long-term treatment, full-foot, cushioned orthotics with a well-supported arch are recommended.

Custom-made orthotics are costly and rarely covered by insurance. A cheaper, sometimes as-effective treatment are sports or cushioned arch supports available in sporting good stores and drugstores. These tend to wear out faster and might need to be replaced every six months. You will know if an orthotic or arch support is effective, as you will feel virtually no pain when your feet are in them. If you have plantar fasciitis, you should wear shoes with orthotics or arch supports at all times, even at home. Walking barefoot, especially on surfaces like hard tile floors, pavement, or sand, can cause a return of symptoms.

Ultrasound and ultrasonic treatments, done by a therapist or foot specialist, can contribute to healing. Wearing night splints to keep the heel cord stretched can also be very effective. In severe cases of plantar fasciitis, corticosteroid injections are used. Heel injections are painful and are used sparingly, as they can lead to rupture of the plantar fascia.

Once you have healed from plantar fasciitis, you should continue stretches and toe curl exercises and wear arch supports on a regular basis to prevent the pain from coming back. Also, avoid wearing shoes with flat insoles without good arch supports. Low-heeled, well-cushioned shoes will also support the plantar fascia and prevent repeat inflammation.

Tips to Prevent Plantar Fasciitis

Try not to walk barefoot.

Do not wear wet sneakers, as they lose their cushioning.

Wear shoes with well-supported arches.

Do not wear flat shoes unless they have a supportive arch.

Wear well-cushioned shoes.

Stretch your heels and calf muscles daily.

Curl your toes and stretch them several times throughout the day.

Achilles Tendinitis

Achilles tendinitis is a soreness and stiffness that occurs when the heel strikes the ground, when going down stairs, or when landing on your heels. It is an overuse injury but can often be due to a new or different pair of shoes that are not well cushioned or that make the heel strike the ground differently. Achilles tendinitis responds best to icing, stretching the heel and calf muscles, and wearing well-cushioned shoes. You can decrease pressure and tension on the Achilles tendon, allowing it to heal faster, by wearing cushioned or gel heel cups in all shoes. Dress shoes with a (low) heel are easier on the Achilles tendon than flat shoes.

Calf Pain

Pain in the back of the calf can be due to a twisting injury or to overuse. The most common cause is a gastrocnemius sprain, and sometimes a tear of the calf muscle can occur ("tennis leg"). If not treated, a calf injury can lead to a muscle tear, or Achilles tendinitis. Calf pain usually is more bothersome with stairs, getting out of bed, or getting up from sitting for a long time. It often causes stiffness and sometimes swelling. Calf pain that includes swelling, redness, warmth, numbness, or fever can be a sign of a more serious medical problem and should be seen by a doctor within the day. If you have these symptoms, rest and keep the leg still and elevated until your doctor evaluates you.

Most calf pain goes away on its own but can return if stretching is not done regularly. To heal quickly, move your ankle in circles as much as possible, ice as often as possible, and gently stretch out your calf muscles frequently with calf and heel stretches.

Tendinitis

There are various forms of tendinitis that can occur in the foot and ankle. Tendinitis can have similar symptoms as an ankle sprain or shin splints, but tends to cause stiffness when getting out of bed or after sitting for a long time. Pain occurs with motion, and bracing or ankle wraps are sometimes recommended to prevent any aggravating motion. There is usually weakness because pain has blocked the muscles. Tendinitis of the peroneus tendons is often due to rotation of the foot outward with each step. Tibialis tendinitis can cause pain that feels similar to shin splints. The three best things you can do for tendinitis are stretching, exercise, and applying ice.

Bunions

Bunions are a great source of pain and are a frequent reason for surgery in women. Bunions appear as a bump with redness and swelling over the outside of the big toe. When severe, a bunion causes widening of the front of the foot, chronic callus or blisters, and misaligned and often crossed toes. Infections can also occur, which makes this condition even more painful. Although most bunions are hereditary, they are also caused by tight-fitting shoes and walking with more weight on the inside of the foot.

Once the toes have started to turn in, surgery is often the only way to correct it. Therefore, it is very important to address bunions early on and prevent them as much as possible. Prevention includes wearing shoes with plenty of room in the front, supporting the inside arch with orthotics to prevent the weight from being mostly on the toes, and doing toe strengthening and stretching exercises. Avoiding high heels, especially those with pointed toes, is crucial.

Strategies to Prevent Bunions

Wear shoes with wide toe areas.

Avoid pointy shoes.

Avoid high heels.

Never wear shoes that are too small.

Wear shoes with arch supports.

Keep your toes flexible and strong with toe curl exercises.

If you have bunions that have bothered you for more than six months, are painful with walking and activity, and do not respond to any of the above treatments, ask your doctor to refer you to a physical therapist for pain relieving, stretching, and strengthening techniques. Custom-made orthotics might also be very helpful. Surgical foot specialists that you might need to consult include podiatrists and orthopedic surgeons. You may require surgical correction if you continue to have pain or are having frequent infections.

Neuroma

A neuroma causes pain between the toe spaces, noticed when landing or stepping down, usually in tight-fitting or closed shoes. The pain is often shooting, zinging, or burning. A neuroma is a painful nerve cluster that develops from too much pressure between metatarsal bones in the forefoot. The causes include tight shoes or laces and sudden increase in impact and weight-bearing activities. Neuromas occasionally can occur from wearing shoes that are not well cushioned and from activities involving impact (such as aerobics, dance, and running). Treatment is based upon the severity of the pain—for mild pain that has been present only for a few days or weeks, wearing wider shoes and looser laces can be curative. Toe pads to space out toes or support them from underneath can also relieve the pain. These tend to be more effective when they are part of a custom-made orthotic, which can be designed to take pressure off the front of the foot. Corticosteroid injections can also provide a cure. Physical therapy, including strengthening the toes, stretching the foot and heel, and using methods to decrease inflammation, can help relieve pressure on the nerve. Finally, if these conservative measures do not work, a surgeon can do a minor procedure to remove the nerve bundle.

Numbness

Numbness is caused by a pinched nerve, most commonly in the foot or toes, due to tightness or pressure of shoes. Occasionally, this can be due to back problems, so see your doctor if you also have back pain or foot weakness. An injury to the foot, ankle, or toe can also cause numbness, which often recovers over several months, as most pinched nerves do with pressure relief. Try taking 100 mg a day of vitamin B_6 (or a B complex with B_6) to help nourish the nerves.

Stress Fracture

Stress fractures are hairline fractures caused by too much stress on a healthy bone or average stress on a weak bone. They usually cause pain with walking or weight bearing but can also cause an ache when resting. Stress fractures most often occur in the metatarsals, tibia, fibula, and occasionally the calcaneus. Dancers, runners, and aerobic or fitness enthusiasts tend to suffer the most stress fractures. Stress fractures can occur out of the blue and are not related to a fall or injury. They can occur with a sudden increase or change in activity or training schedule, change in playing surface or running terrain, or if shoes have lost their cushioning.

Stress fractures usually take six to eight weeks to heal, after which time you can gradually begin impact activity. While healing from stress fracture, the best exercise activities include swimming or underwater running while wearing a floatation vest. You might be able to ride a stationary bike using more pressure on the noninjured side, but check with your doctor before taking on this activity. You should otherwise try to keep your legs strong with lower body exercises either by working out at the gym or using ankle weights at home. If you have a lot of pain and limited motion, you might need a referral for physical therapy. Usually, stress fractures heal by avoiding impact activities, but they can progress to full fractures if they are not rested properly. Having had two or more stress fractures without injury is a sign you can be at risk for thin bones (see chapter 5, "Bone Health and Osteoporosis").

Athlete's Foot

Athlete's foot—a common condition due to foot fungus—causes itchy, scaly, sometimes red, peeling, and cracked skin around the bottom and sides of feet. This is also a very common condition due to foot fungus. Nails can also be affected, appearing scaly, yellow, and ingrown. The fungus that causes athlete's foot grows in warm, moist environments, and can be worse if you wear nonbreathable shoes, do not dry your feet thoroughly, and tend to have sweaty feet.

If you have a mild case of itching, you can try over-the-counter powders, sprays, and lotions that should help cure your athlete's foot. Taking off your shoes as much as possible and wearing breathable shoes or sandals helps prevent and treat the problem. If your athlete's foot does not improve within one week of treatment, make an appointment with a dermatologist to treat it more effectively. If you have open sores, darkened skin or nails, or ingrown toenails, make an appointment as soon as possible.

Nail Problems

Field sport players, kickers, dancers, skaters, skiers, and runners tend to develop nail problems from injury. Nails can develop ridges, change color, develop bleeding underneath, and can become ingrown. These conditions are all due to abnormal pressure on the nail area and should be avoided by making sure shoes fit properly. Sometimes, these problems are unavoidable and must be managed as best as possible with protective taping, padding, and icing banged toes after injuries to decrease swelling.

Nail fungus can cause scaly, thick, discolored nails and usually requires medications. Frostbite also causes nail discoloration and pain. Keeping your toenails as short as possible also decreases stress on the nail. As much as possible avoid any pressure on the injured toe by wearing roomy, protective shoes.

Plantar's Wart

A hard, darkened nodule on the bottom of the foot is described as a plantar's wart. These are caused by a virus, usually obtained from walking barefoot in public places. Plantar's warts are not always painful, and they are fairly easy to cure by scraping or cutting the thick wart and applying salicylic acid (such as Compound W) or medicated wart pads. A wart will usually go away in about two weeks with daily scraping and application of medication. If it does not, a dermatologist or podiatrist can remove them with a freezing application, laser, or surgery. If the wart becomes painful, a cushioned shoe insert can help, along with the medicated wart pad to further relieve pressure. Pain that limits walking or activities should be evaluated by a doctor.

Evaluation and Treatment

If you injure your foot or ankle, rest, elevate, and ice the injured area for 15 to 20 minutes as soon as possible. Wrap it snug with an ice wrap and try to keep it elevated as much as possible over the next 24 hours, icing three or four times a day. If you feel you cannot walk on it, see a doctor immediately. If you can walk on it but are still having pain one week later, see a doctor.

The doctor will evaluate your joint for looseness, check your strength, and feel for any areas of tenderness or pain. X-rays might be taken to make sure there is no fracture. If you are placed in an ankle brace, gel or air cast, or walking boot, ask your doctor how often you can remove the device to allow yourself to maintain your motion and work on strength. The sooner you can begin motion and strength exercises, the sooner you will be able to return to normal activity. You should continue icing the injured area at the end of each day and whenever sore to control inflammation, especially if there is swelling. For pain, anti-inflammatory medications can be helpful.

You should begin strengthening and balance exercises as soon as your doctor allows it and as soon as you can do them without pain. If you have a lot of swelling, pain, or weakness, ask your doctor for a referral to a physical therapist. A complete strength and balance rehabilitation program will allow you to recover faster and prevent reinjury.

If orthotics are recommended, break them in slowly by wearing them for only a few hours at a time the first week and increasing a few hours each week thereafter. If they seem to irritate you, take them back for adjustments.

Athletic Footwear Tips to Prevent Injury

Wear comfortable, well-fitting shoes.

Do not lace shoes too tight.

Make sure shoes have an arch support, or use an orthotic.

Replace athletic shoes every 250 to 400 miles, or after 40 to 60 hours of playing time.

Wear a shoe appropriate for the activity.

Socks should be breathable without bunching or wrinkles.

Once shoes become saturated with water, they can lose their cushioning and should be replaced.

Exercises and Stretches

The exercises described in this chapter are helpful for all lower leg and ankle problems. Ankle sprains, both first time and repeat, can be avoided with proper exercises. Once you can easily do all the exercises listed, maintain your strength and stability with challenging balance activities at least three times a week. Advanced balance activities include balance board exercises, yoga, and jumping rope on one leg. Balance exercises are beneficial to all athletes.

Ankle exercises are listed in increasing order of difficulty. Progress through the exercises slowly if there is pain, starting with the first two exercises the first week, then adding one exercise each week thereafter. Try to do at least two sets of 10 repetitions for each exercise, increasing to 15 repetitions per set, then adding a third set. If you are doing the exercises to prevent injury and have no pain, focus on the balance exercises, heel stretches, and toe strengthening exercises.

If you are sore after exercise, apply ice for 10 to 15 minutes. If the soreness continues to the next day, take that day off from exercises and start again the following day with less intensity. Ice should always be applied if there is swelling.

Ankle-Strengthening Exercises

The first three exercises begin with the foot flat on the ground or in the air. Keep the movements slow and try to create as large a motion as possible without causing pain. Motion will improve as your ankle heals. If you have trouble limiting motion to just your ankle, cross your right knee over your left to stabilize the knee and hip joints.

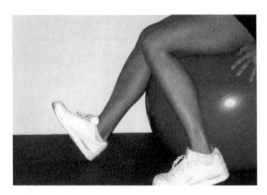

FIGURE 12-4 Ankle Pumps: Sitting, starting with your foot flat on the ground, lift up your toes and front of foot as high as you can. Hold for three, then lower.

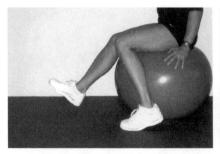 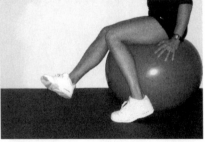

FIGURE 12-5 Ankle Rotations: Rotate your ankle clockwise in large circle slowly 10 times (A) then counterclockwise slowly 10 times (B).

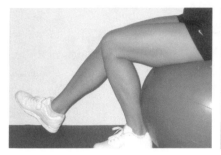 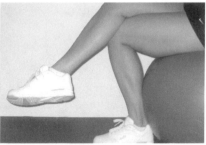

FIGURE 12-6 The Alphabet: Pretend you are holding a piece of chalk between your toes and have to draw giant capital letters on a blackboard beneath you (A). Draw out each letter slowly, making the movements as big as possible (B). Try to make it to M, and continue the second half of the alphabet later in the day.

Balance and Strengthening Exercises

If you need to, hold on to a wall, counter, or chair back for balance, gradually increasing your balance so you do not need any support.

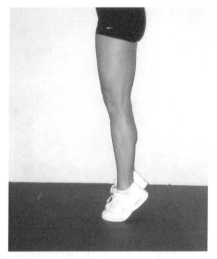 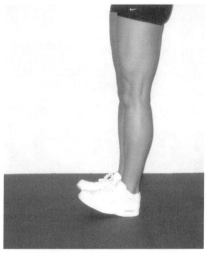

FIGURE 12-7 Heel Raises: Standing, lift your heels to rock into your toes.

FIGURE 12-8 Toe Raises: Standing, lift your toes to rock onto your heels.

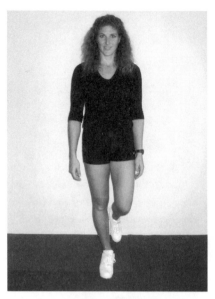

FIGURE 12-9 **Single Leg Balancing: Stand on your right leg for 20 seconds. Advanced: Balance on one leg with your eyes closed.**

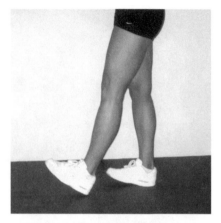

FIGURE 12-10 **Heel Walk: Standing on both legs, lift the front of your feet and toes to walk 20 steps on your heels.**

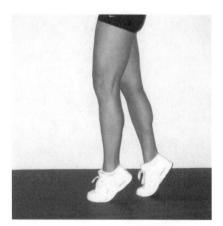

FIGURE 12-11 **Toe Walk: Standing on both legs, raise your heels to stand as high as you can on your toes and walk 20 steps.**

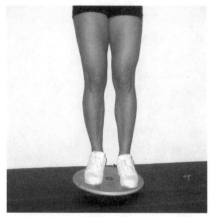

FIGURE 12-12 **Balance Board: Stand on a balance board and rock side to side, then front to back. Can be done as an easier exercise by standing on a couch cushion.**

Advanced Exercises

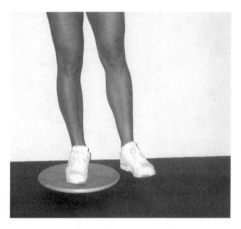

FIGURE 12-13 **Advanced Balance Board: Stand on one leg on a balance board, rocking back and forth and side to side.**

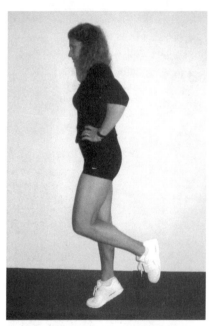

FIGURE 12-14 **Single Leg Heel Raise:** Stand on your right leg and raise your heel 10 times.

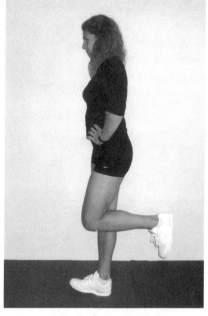

FIGURE 12-15 **Single Leg Toe Raise:** Stand on your right leg and raise your toes and the front of your foot 10 times.

Very Advanced

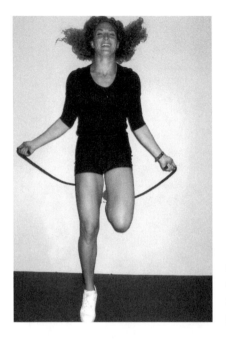

FIGURE 12-16 **Jump Rope: Jump rope doing 10 hops on both legs, 5 on the right, and 5 on the left. Repeat 10 times. (Can also be done without a rope.)**

Foot and Toe Exercises

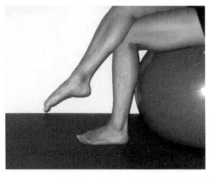 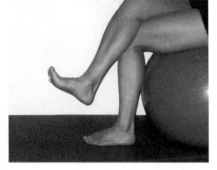

FIGURE 12-17 **Toe Curls and Spreads: Curl all your toes as if you were making a tight fist with your foot (A). Hold for three, then spread your toes as much as possible (B) and hold for three, returning to curls.**

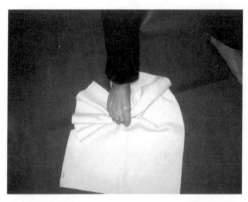

FIGURE 12-18 **Towel Scrunch: Barefoot, grab the closest end of a towel with your toes and pull it toward you, scrunching it with your toes. Continue until you have scrunched the entire towel toward you.**

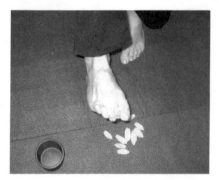 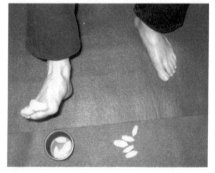

FIGURE 12-19 **Item Pick-Up: Pick up each of 10 shells (A), pens, marbles, or other small items with your toes and release them into a container (B).**

Stretches for the Lower Leg

Hold each stretch for a slow count of five. Repeat each stretch five times and try to do at least twice a day.

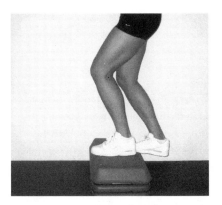 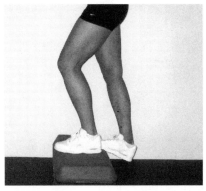

FIGURE 12-20 **Heel Stretch (right): Standing on a step, curb, or large telephone book, tilt your right heel off the back of the step so only the ball of your foot is on the step. Slowly lean into that heel, putting most of your weight on your right leg. You will feel a stretch in your heel and calf. Perform the stretch holding your heel down with your right knee bent (A) and straight (B).**

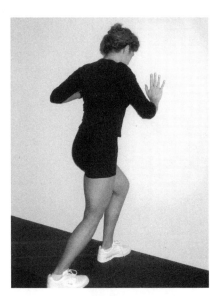 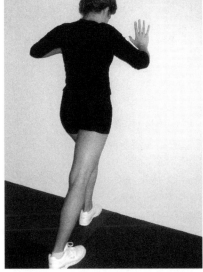

FIGURE 12-21 **Calf Stretch (right): Stand three to four feet from a wall. With your right leg farther behind you than your left and both knees bent (the front knee will be bent more than the back), lean into your back leg (A). Repeat with straight right knee (B).**

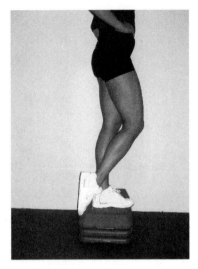

FIGURE 12-22 **Shin Stretch: Stand with your left foot in the middle of a step, your right foot off the step and your toes behind the edge of the step, point the toes of your right foot down and pull the top of your right foot into the step to increase the toe down motion.**

Leg, ankle, and foot pain and problems are common in active women. Due to improper shoe wear and fit, overuse, and alignment, pain can become chronic. Correcting shoe and alignment problems, improving strength and balance, and avoiding overuse will help keep your lower body healthy and pain-free. Balance and strengthening exercises should be done on a regular basis to prevent flare-ups or reinjury.

PART III

The Fitness System: Maximizing Athletic and Workout Performance

CHAPTER THIRTEEN

Exercise Problems and Injuries

Athletic and fitness activities challenge your body and mind to push to a higher level of performance. If your body is not conditioned properly, if equipment or conditions are not what they should be, or if pain or weaknesses are ignored, both short-term and long-term problems can develop. Short-term problems include discomfort, severe pain, and swelling. Long-term problems including chronic injuries, weakness, pain, and difficulty with nonsports activities. These problems can lead to feeling depressed, confused, overchallenged, discouraged, and frustrated, making athletic activity less enjoyable.

Grueling training is required to be in the peak physical condition required of a competitive athlete. Part of this training is teaching your mind to ignore your body's signal warnings such as fatigue and pain. As these body signals are ignored, you can become overtrained, actually decreasing effective conditioning. Overtraining can affect your physical body, mind, hormones, blood systems, and chemical balance. It can cause mental stress and extreme fatigue, leading to poor performance, illness, and injuries.

Pain

Pain has many consequences and can affect more than just the body area that is painful or injured. Pain can lead to weakness, poor posture, and difficulty walking or playing sports, with inefficient modifications to avoid discomfort. Pain that lasts for several days or weeks can limit activities and sleep and cause depression. Medications taken to treat pain might cause digestive problems, or, if painkillers are taken, addiction. Frequent doctor visits take time, and expenses can add up. This cycle can be very frustrating! Therefore, avoiding pain is the best goal.

How Pain in One Joint Can Affect an Athlete's Body and Mind

It is very common for young girls and women to have knee pain, especially during adolescence when the body is changing and growing. This knee pain is most often due to patellofemoral pain, an irritation of the kneecap and front of the knee joint. The knee pain can seem quite limiting, causing pain when going up or down stairs or hills, running, biking, and even sitting for long periods of time. There might also be swelling, stiffness, and clicking noises. To avoid pain, the young athlete might stop doing stairs, running, or biking, and even limit walking. This decrease in activity and movement leads to weakness, not only in the knee muscles, but throughout the leg from the ankle to the hip. This weakness will persist if it is not corrected, often even after the knee pain is improved, leading to future problems such as ankle sprains or hip problems.

Unfortunately, doctors' and health professionals' advice is not always appropriate for an athlete, as most doctors recommend the same overly conservative treatments for everyone. Some doctors treat patellofemoral pain by advising young women not to play sports or go to the gym and instructing them to wear a bulky brace (which interferes with most activities and is often uncomfortable). If a young woman follows this faulty advice, she might never play her sport again because she feels it causes too much pain and frustration.

In this example, pain has changed the young woman's entire outlook on sports activity because she has pain with activity and was advised not to do the sport. Unfortunately, this scenario is common. However, the correct treatment of joint or muscle pain is to do selective activities and rest, which means rest only from activities that cause pain. This includes sports activities that do not cause pain, while avoiding other painful activities, such as stairs. It might also mean her switching to another conditioning athletic activity, such as cycling, until the pain is resolved.

Another important factor for treating pain is maintaining motion and strength. Every joint can be strengthened in some way without causing pain; it might take a physical therapist or athletic trainer to show you how.

Medications for pain should be well tolerated without uncomfortable digestive complaints, moodiness, sleepiness, or other unwelcome side effects. There are countless pain relievers on the market; your doctor should try to find the right one for you. You can also try topical pain-relieving ointments, patches, or creams, which can work quite well, or heat or ice packs either, instead of, or in addition to, medications.

Also, bracing is not always helpful, especially if it causes more pain. In fact, most braces for all pain syndromes are just designed to make symptoms better. Braces are not a substitute for strengthening exercises. If the brace irritates you, do not use it! In the case of patellofemoral pain, a brace is not necessary; it often just feels bulky and uncomfortable.

The bottom line is, treating pain should be individualized for you. Sometimes, if there is an important tournament, you might be allowed to play through the pain if it will not cause you any long-term problems. Find a doctor who will tailor your healing program to you; if you cannot, work more closely with an understanding and insightful physical therapist or athletic trainer. They can help guide your treatment and will better understand your limits and expectations, facilitating a faster recovery and a stronger return to athletic activities.

The following questions can help your sports health care provider determine the best treatment for your cause of pain:

When did it start?

When does it happen?

What makes it worse?

What makes it better?

How do you describe it?

Pain: Your Body's Warning System

Pain is your body's warning that something is not right. Cause, type, and description of pain provides a clue to the underlying problem. Important clues include when the pain started, when it occurs, what makes it worse, what makes it better, and how it is described. For example, pain is most often described with the following words:

- *Sharp, stabbing*—Usually indicates a tear or severe sprain of muscle tendons or ligaments, pinching of scar tissue or nerve, or bone fracture.

- *Dull, aching*—usually indicates a swollen, inflamed joint; overworked or strained muscle; or bone pain.

- *Stiffness*—usually indicates joints, tendons, ligaments, and muscles that can cause stiffness when they are overworked and inflamed, then rested for a while.

- *Knawing, burning, shooting*—usually indicates nerve irritation or severe muscle damage.

Pain Signals That You Should See a Doctor For

Sharp, knifelike pain that interferes with function

Pain that keeps you up at night

Pain that requires pain relievers every four hours in order to feel comfortable

Pain accompanied by swelling, fever, or a large amount of bleeding or bruising

Pain accompanied by numbness or weakness

Not all pain is a sign of a serious problem. Most active and athletic woman have pain from time to time; if it lasts less than half hour or is mild enough not to interfere with activities, it is usually not serious. Sometimes the body is just trying to figure out what it needs to do to meet your challenges and heals itself quickly.

To help your body heal on its own, you can take anti-inflammatories available without a prescription such as ibuprofen/Advil/Motrin, naprosyn/Aleve, or ketoprofen/Orudis. You can also try pain-relieving muscle rubs, creams, and patches. Applying ice packs is recommended over hot packs for any new pain, as heat can increase swelling. If the pain keeps you from sleeping, walking, or performing daily activities, or is not getting better, see a doctor.

Widely Available Pain-Relieving Methods

Aspirin-like products (ibuprofen/Advil or naprosyn/Aleve)

Non-aspirin pain relievers (acetomenophen/Tylenol)

Pain-relieving muscle rubs, creams, and patches

Ice packs

Heating pads

Muscle Cramp

Muscle cramps are a common exercise problem, experienced by nearly everyone who exercises. Fortunately, they are not usually serious. They can take various forms but occur mostly as the following types: in the calf, foot, or toe during exercise or stretching; in the calf at night while resting or sleeping; or in the side of the trunk or abdominal area as a side stitch during running.

Types of Muscle Cramps

TYPE	COMMON LOCATIONS
During exercise or stretching	Leg/foot/toe
Night cramp or charley horse	Calf
Side stitch	Chest wall/breathing muscles

Muscle cramps are primarily an annoyance. They do not pose any health threats, do not lead to injury, and do not limit sports or activities. The worst that happens is an athlete loses her momentum from the pain of the cramp, which can result in poor performance. Cramps are usually a result of a combination of factors, including the following:

- *Low potassium*—Potassium is an electrolyte the body needs for muscle firing (including the heart muscle) and chemical balance. Potassium is lost in sweat and urine and needs to be replenished if exercise lasts longer than an hour. Good natural sources of potassium are bananas, oranges and orange juice, kiwis, strawberries, and tomatoes. During events, potassium is usually supplemented in sports drinks and gels.

- *Low sodium*—Sodium is an electrolyte also required by the muscles to contract. It regulates body fluids, as water within the body follows sodium into the cells (that is why after eating a salty snack or meal, your hands or feet will often become bloated or swollen). Low sodium develops with loss of fluids through exercise in heat, contributing to potentially serious problems of dehydration. Sodium is in salt and salty foods and can be replenished during sports with sports drinks.

- *Overexertion*—If the muscle is overworked, it cannot meet your demands to perform and can go into spasm. Overexertion is a very common reason for cramping and is a common cause of calf cramps in marathon runners. It is more likely to occur with improper conditioning, at extremes of temperature, and with dehydration.

- *Poor conditioning*—Poor conditioning is a very common reason for cramping. As with overexertion, the muscle firing system is overworked and gives out, causing muscles to fire improperly and eventually shut down temporarily.

- *Overheating*—Overheating can also cause light-headedness, weakness, and nausea and lead to heatstroke, muscle breakdown, and hyperthermia, a medical condition that can be life-threatening. Overheating can be prevented by avoiding exercise during hot times of the day, not exercising in gyms that are not air-conditioned properly, and dressing in light, breathable clothing. Drinking cool fluids also helps control body temperature. Avoiding overheating is essential to exercising during pregnancy.

- *Dehydration*—Not drinking enough fluids is a significant cause of cramps. Without enough fluids, the blood thickens, decreasing the amount of nutrient and waste exchange in the muscle cells. This is usually also associated with low sodium and potassium. These are replenished most effectively with a sports drink, which will restore both electrolytes and fluids needed to prevent cramping muscles (see chapter 14, "Exercise Fuel").

- *Improper rest*—Improper rest leads to overexertion and injuries. Rest is needed for muscles to heal, clear lactic acid, and refuel glycogen, sodium, and potassium. Muscles can develop slight tears if they are overworked and require rest to repair themselves. If they are not rested and repaired, they are more likely to weaken and not fire properly.

- *Low calcium or magnesium*—Because these minerals are involved with muscle firing, low levels can contribute to cramping. If you are not already taking a calcium supplement and a multivitamin that contains magnesium, take 600 mg calcium and 100 mg magnesium at night to treat cramping.

Although the pain of a cramp can be sharp and severe, it usually resolves within minutes. Resting or slowing down the pace is usually required for the cramp to stop; if the cramp does not resolve after 10 minutes, this might be a sign of an injury. Most often you can return to the sports activity within minutes of the cramp; some athletes even walk or run through them by slowing their pace. There can often be increased muscle soreness in the cramped area the evening or day after exercise.

Treating and preventing muscle cramps is important for more comfortable future workouts. Massage, heat, Epsom salt baths, and pain-relieving muscle rubs can relieve soreness, restore blood flow, and encourage waste-nutrient exchange. Stretching is important to return motion to the area. Because cramps often occur when muscles are not conditioned or in an injured or overused area, they might occur repeatedly until the muscle area is strengthened and reconditioned.

To prevent cramps during exertion, make a potassium- and sodium-rich food or drink part of your pre-workout routine. Have sports drinks available during the workout, especially if it is hot or the workout lasts longer than 30 minutes. Make sure you are taking at least 1,200 mg calcium and that your multivitamin contains magnesium.

Treatment Methods for Muscle Cramps

Increase potassium (orange juice, bananas) in your diet.

Increase sodium (salt) in your diet.

Drink sports drinks while exercising.

Do not get dehydrated.

Stretch before and after exercise.

Do not overdo your strength program.

Double your calcium intake.

Take a magnesium tablet.

Soak in Epsom salt baths (1 to 2 cup bath salts in warm tub; soak for 15 to 30 minutes).

Night Cramps

Night cramps, also known as charley horses, feel similar to muscle cramps that happen during exercise and stretching but occur during rest. Usually due to the same combination of factors as muscle cramps in general, they can also result from fatigue that occurred during the day. They seem to occur more often in people who are not as active, those beginning a new sports or workout program, and women who are pregnant. They are relieved with stretching, massage, and proper conditioning. Potassium, magnesium, and calcium should be part of the diet. Night cramps can also be alleviated by drinking tonic water and stretching before bedtime. For persistent night cramps, your doctor might prescribe a muscle relaxer.

Abdominal Pain

Side Stitches

Side stitches are a feeling of sharp tightness and pain on one side of your chest wall or abdomen that occur while quickly walking, running, or sprinting. Side stitches can be very painful. Many runners stop due to the severe pain and feel they cannot stand up straight for fear of increased pain. Side stitches can also make breathing feel difficult.

Side stitches are usually the result of a cramp in the breathing muscles. Most often, they are brought on by fatigue or spasm, usually occurring if you are out of shape, training too hard, or not properly rested. They can be due to inefficient blood flow to the breathing muscles, especially with heavy breathing. They can also be caused by eating a large meal, drinking too much fluid, or starting your run too fast.

If a side stitch occurs, you can try to run or walk through it. If it continues, try to slow down, raise your arms overhead, or even sit or lie down if you cannot "walk it off." Breathe shallow, through pursed lips, and slow your breathing rate to allow your breathing muscles to rest. You can also try gently massaging the painful area. If the pain does not go away after 5 to 10 minutes, travels into your arm or back, continues to get worse, or is accompanied by a feeling of doom, call for emergency medical care to rule out any problems with your heart.

Side stitches usually go away the more you train. Strengthening your abdominal muscles, along with stretching your arms overhead and doing slow, trunk rotations and side stretches with deep breathing daily can help prevent side stitches. You can also try treatments used for cramps, increasing potassium, sodium, calcium, and magnesium; getting more rest; and drinking more fluids.

Strategies to Relieve a Side Stitch

Slow down to a walk.

Take shallow breaths.

Raise your arms overhead.

Lie down on your back.

Gently massage the painful area.

Runner's Trots

Runner's trots is a term for diarrhea that occurs during a run, caused by many factors, most of which can be controlled. Runners trots are painful because the bowels are cramping and pressing on the surrounding nerves and muscles. Runner's trots can be a symptom of irritable bowel syndrome, colitis, or hernia, so if the cramping and diarrhea do not resolve with the strategies mentioned here, see your doctor or a gastroenterologist.

Nervousness can cause runner's trots and pre-event diarrhea. If this happens to you, plan around it. Schedule bathroom time into your pre-event planning, and bring toilet paper in case you need it. If your bowels are sensitive, you should avoid caffeine and foods that tend to cause loose stools—certain fruits, salads, prunes, melons, milk products, orange juice, chocolate, sugary, spicy, and fatty or greasy foods—12 hours before your activity. You will likely be comfortable eating bananas, energy bars, and low-fiber bread or cereal products. Also, be very careful to avoid irritating foods or drinks the night before your event.

Foods to Avoid to Prevent Runner's Trots

Fatty foods

Dairy products

Caffeine

Fresh fruits

Sugary foods

Spicy foods

Fatty/greasy foods

If you tend to develop runner's trots, wait two to three hours after eating before you exercise. Avoid caffeine, dairy products, and fatty foods at least three hours before running. Drinking large amounts of fluid can sometimes be the cause of runner's trots; during exercise and before exercise, sipping small amounts is preferred to filling your stomach with fluid. Experiment during practice to learn the best ways to avoid runner's trots.

Breathing Problems

Difficulty catching your breath is common under both physical and emotional stress. The most common cause of this in athletes is exercise-induced asthma, causing wheezing, chest pain or heaviness, and feeling unable to breathe. Coughing can also be a problem, especially after completing the exercise. The most common trigger for breathing problems is working out in the cold; others include dehydration, anxiety, stress, environmental allergies, pollens, molds, pollution, smoke, dry air, and heavily chlorinated or chemically treated pools. Colds or respiratory infections can make you more likely to experience an exercise-induced asthma attack. Attacks usually end within 20 to 30 minutes after exercise, although coughing and hoarseness can last for a few hours.

Asthma is a spasm of the muscles in the small airways of the lungs caused by an airway irritant, usually one of the factors mentioned above. These spasms result in wheezing, coughing, and shortness of breath both during and after exercise. Asthma can be a problem in young girls and is more common in athletes with environmental allergies. Athletes with asthma should be aware of the warning signs and symptoms. Having doctor-diagnosed asthma not related to exercise makes exercise-induced asthma attacks more likely and also more dangerous. Although it is rare that exercise-induced asthma is life-threatening in healthy athletes, athletes who already have asthma as a diagnosis must be careful to avoid exercise-induced asthma, as it can lead to a full-blown asthma attack requiring emergency medical care. Fortunately, many young girls grow out of severe attacks of both asthma and allergies.

Warning Signs of an Impending Asthma Attack

Chest pain or heaviness

Shortness of breath

Wheezing

Feeling unable to breathe or catch your breath

Coughing

Anxiousness

Severe episodes of asthma causing life-threatening respiratory distress can occur but are preventable with medications, including an inhaler used before and, if needed, during and after exercise. Athletes, coaches, and trainers should be aware of warning signs such as trouble catching your breath or breathing, wheezing and coughing, and chest pain and heaviness.

To date, there are no known long-term consequences of exercise-induced asthma as long as it is treated. If you have any symptoms, speak with your doctor. You might be sent for tests to evaluate if you have asthma, which will likely be normal. Still, ask your doctor for a (ventolin) inhaler. You might have to convince your doctor to give you one, as there is no specific test for exercise-induced asthma, but symptoms such as wheezing during exercise and coughing after exercise lead to the diagnosis. Exercise-induced asthma is very common and can occur in nearly one out of three exercising women. Sports medicine doctors are more accustomed to treating this.

Triggers of Exercise-Induced Asthma	
Cold air	Stress/anxiety
Allergies	Pool chemicals
Pollen/molds	Colds or respiratory infection
Pollution	Dehydration
Smoke	Humidity

Headaches

Headaches are a common problem in all women. They can be due to many causes and can occasionally be due to a serious condition such a change in blood supply to the brain or a tumor. Most headaches, however, are not serious. If the pain is excruciating or associated with any numbness, vision problems, nausea, or weakness, go to an emergency room and call your doctor on the way.

Tension Headaches

Tension headaches tend to occur at times of stress and feel like a pressure in one area of the head. Often this is a true aching, mostly dull, but occasionally sharp headache with or without a throbbing sensation. Tension headaches respond to relaxation techniques and stress management, massaging the forehead or temples, and rest. Aspirin and aspirinlike products are usually very effective for these headaches. Caffeine can also help.

Exertion Headaches

Exertion headaches, also known as weight lifter's headaches, can be of different levels of intensity. These headaches occur during or immediately after exertion. At their worst, they can feel similar to migraines. They can get worse with coughing or abdominal pressure. Although it is not yet clear what causes these types of headaches, they are usually not serious and respond to aspirin medications.

Sinus Headaches

Sinus headaches cause a feeling of fullness, pressure, and forehead and face pain that gets worse if you are bent over with or without nose stuffiness. These can occur in outdoor exercisers with allergies, in an indoor environment with poor air quality, and often in swimmers or divers exposed to airway irritants in the pool chemicals. Sinus headaches improve with decongestant medications, nasal sprays, and aspirin or nonaspirin pain relievers. Antihistamines can help prevent them if environmental allergies are a problem. Using a saline nasal mist frequently is a natural way of relieving and preventing sinus pain and pressure.

Migraines

Migraines are severe headaches that are often accompanied by eye pain, nausea or vomiting, and generally not feeling well. They can last from several hours to a few days. Because these headaches can affect balance or prevent you from eating or drinking enough, intense exercise should be avoided during a migraine, although mild exercise might lessen the intensity of pain. Migraines can be related to hormonal cycles and occur more frequently in women during the menstrual years. If you have them or suspect you might have them, see your doctor or a neurologist. There are various lifestyle modifications and medications to prevent and treat migraines.

Footballer's Headache

Footballer's headache, pain that results after striking the head with a ball as in soccer or in a fall or collision, can be felt as different intensities of headache. If the injury has occurred a few times, the headaches can return without injury. The pain can be anything from a dull to a strong, severe ache or feel similar to a migraine. If this headache lasts for more than a few hours, has other symptoms besides pain in the head, and started after a blow to the head that also caused dizziness or passing out, you should see your doctor to make sure you do not have a concussion.

Breast Soreness

Breasts can become sore from being stretched during impact activities such as running, aerobics, and court or field sports; become bruised from impact with fast-moving equipment in front of the chest such as golf, rowing, and kayaking; or from impact or collision in contact sports. The breasts are supported by the pectoralis muscles that lie underneath and by the ligaments above and within them. These ligaments can become stretched and cause breast soreness after unsupported jumping activities. Although this is not a medical problem, the loosening of ligaments can lead to "saggy" breasts. Nipple tenderness and even bleeding can occur if the nipple rubs against loose clothing such as running without a bra. This problem can be easily prevented by putting Band-Aids or a lubricant (such as Vaseline) over the nipples and wearing a well-fitting athletic bra that does not rub. To date, there is no evidence that any of these complications can lead to serious medical problems such as trouble breastfeeding or increased risk of cancer.

Athletic bras are very helpful in preventing exercise-related breast problems. They take the pressure off the ligaments, skin, and muscles and keep the breasts protected. These bras are now available in all sizes, shapes, and fabrics. Find the one that is comfortable and provides the most support, especially if you are a runner or field sport player (see the resources at end of the book for purchase information). In contact or ball sports, chest guards can also be worn.

Skin Problems

Rashes

Allergic rashes, the most common of which is poison ivy, can be troublesome for outdoor exercisers. Poison ivy is present in the summer and fall and causes an itchy, red rash that can ooze yellow liquid after a few days. Although the rash does not spread from person to person, the contagious resin from the plant can remain infectious on clothes, furniture, or pets for an indefinite time. Thus, poison ivy can develop or return long after being outside if you have had skin contact with the resin. The resin can be rinsed and washed off; therefore, it is wise to wash any skin, clothing, and pets that might have come into contact with poison ivy.

Poison ivy and many types of rashes will feel less irritating with the use of nonprescription creams and lotions. If your case is severe and covers more than a small area of your body, see a dermatologist for stronger medicine. Although not everyone is allergic to poison ivy, it is quite possible to develop an allergy later in life. Poison oak is very similar to poison ivy and is treated similarly. For other types of rashes that last more than a few days, see a dermatologist for identification and treatment. Whenever there is a question of an allergy or severe skin itching, take 50 mg diphenhydramine HCI (Benadryl). This will make you sleepy but should decrease the itch and reduce the intensity of the allergic reaction.

Chafing

Chafing, raw, reddened skin from friction, commonly occurs between the thighs in runners or cyclists, at sites of equipment rubbing, and around the neck and under the arms in athletes who wear wet suits. Chafing can be prevented by using petroleum jelly (Vaseline), sports lube, or nonstick cooking spray between your skin and the clothing, equipment, or area of friction before you do the activity. Because these rashes can be very painful and irritating and affect sports performance as you try to avoid the movement that causes chafing, anticipate possible friction areas and use lubrication.

Sunburns

Sunburns should be prevented by wearing sunscreen or clothing and a hat or visor. Severe sunburns can cause illness, dehydration, and swelling. Skin cancer is related to frequently unprotected, sunburned skin.

Yeast and Fungal Infections

Itchiness and bumpy redness is often due to a yeast or fungal infection. These types of rashes can occur in the groin, underneath the breasts, or between the toes. Creams and powders available without a prescription can be very effective. Vulvar and vaginal itching suggests a yeast infection; often, this can be treated by keeping the area dry and using nonprescription creams. Changing out of wet clothing or workout gear as soon as possible after exercise will make these infections less likely. Wearing breathable, fast-drying shorts and workout pants are recommended (avoid cotton or wool). If you have itchiness or a rash that does not improve, see your doctor for diagnosis and stronger treatment.

Numbness

Numbness is a sign that nerve functioning is disrupted. Most numbness is due to temporary causes, including nerve crushing and stretching due to pressure or injury. It is common for active women to develop numbness in their feet or toes. This feeling is usually caused by shoes that are too tight, or toes banging into the front of your shoes or exercise equipment, causing a crush injury to the nerve. Mostly, numbness in the feet is resolved by wearing wider shoes or lacing less tightly. Other reasons for foot and toe numbness can be due to weak ankles or falling arches. Thigh numbess might occur while sitting or wearing tight pants or a tight belt. When pressure is relieved from the nerve, the numbness usually resolves after a month or two. If the numbness persists, a doctor or podiatrist can help you determine how to avoid permanent injury due to repeated damaging nerve pressure.

Just as common as numbness in the feet is numbness in the fingers and hands. This, too, is caused usually by pressure on the nerves as they go through the wrist or are stretched across the elbow. (Carpal tunnel syndrome is the most common, although not usually a problem in active women.) Bikers tend to get numbness of their fingers from leaning on the handlebars; gel-padded handlebar wrap and biking gloves along with redistributing hand weight throughout the ride prevents this from becoming a permanent problem. Occasionally, athletes feel their hands fall asleep or get tingly while running. This is usually due to stretching the nerves from repetitive swinging or hanging and is not serious as long as it stops at the end of the run. This can also occur in the thighs or legs. Numbness during exertional activity can also be a sign of fatigue or dehydration.

Field or court players can also experience numbness and pain after a contact injury. Called burners or stingers (see chapter 6, "The Neck"), when they occur in the arms, these are due to a neck injury. Although they can suggest a serious neck injury, they usually are not, but the athlete should be taken out of play and evaluated by a doctor.

It is normal to wake up occasionally with a numb hand, arm, or leg after having slept on it in an unusual position. Sometimes wearing a watch to bed can cause a numb hand. As long as your feeling comes back over the next 5 to 15 minutes and you regain full function, there is no need for alarm or even to see a doctor—your nerve signals were disturbed by positional pressure on the nerve or blood supply.

Numbness alone is usually not a reason to rush to a doctor or emergency room. Complete loss of sensation along with pain and weakness should be treated as an emergency, however, as it can be a sign that the nerve might be permanently injured (from a spinal cord or head injury, for example). Rarely does the combination of numbness, pain, and weakness occur without injury, but these problems should always be evaluated by a doctor as soon as possible.

The best way to protect your nerves is pay attention to these signals. If you are getting repeated episodes of numbness in an area, change your position, loosen restricting clothing, or get proper-fitting equipment to alleviate pressure on the nerves. If the situation continues every time you do the activity and is accompanied by weakness or pain, see a doctor.

Fatigue

Fatigue can feel like a weakness in one body area, overall body weakness, not feeling rested in the morning, falling asleep in places you are not supposed to (seminars or classes, sitting, eating), and feeling your muscles give way. Fatigue can be dangerous if ignored, because it can lead to falls, injuries, and illness. Fatigue in one area of the body is usually due to injury or overuse. Feeling weak and sore is very common among active athletic women after a hard workout, race, game, or training session. This should be treated with rest—one day off completely, then a very light workout the following days until the area feels strong again.

If there is no apparent reason for the weakness, and if there is pain in the neck or back, there could be a problem with the motor (or movement) nerve signal. If you do not recover from this fatigue in a day or two or it is getting worse, definitely see a doctor. Weakness can also result in an area that has had pain—for instance, after a fracture or sprain. Muscles lose their strength after just five days of rest, so weakness after an injury is normal. A strength program is recommended to reverse the weakness.

Often, weakness is not noticed because the opposite side compensates. An athlete with a long-standing knee problem and pain, for example, might not notice the weakness on one side because she habitually favors it by standing, pushing off, and squatting more on the good leg.

PERFORMANCE TIP **When strength training, do each side individually for at least half of your exercises to make sure that you are balanced on both sides. (For example, use dumbells for bicep curls instead of a bar or arm curl machine with both arms together.)**

General fatigue can be due to poor sleep, not consuming enough calories, stress, chronic overtraining, underlying illness, or pregnancy. It can also cause mental fatigue, which interferes not only with your activity, but with other aspects of your life as well. It can make you irritable, moody, and distracted and can disrupt your balance and coordination; it can even cause tremors. If you are an elite athlete, this is a real problem. Battling fatigue is the reason why relaxation techniques, sleep, and sports psychology is an important aspect of every athlete's life. Mental performance is a large percentage of overall performance.

Signs of Fatigue

Headaches	Trouble sleeping
Muscle pain	Trouble staying awake
Weakness	Trouble concentrating
Tremors or twitching	Poor memory
Poor endurance	Poor coordination
Loss of appetite	Balance problems

Although it might be tempting, avoid products that are sold to promote energy. Most of these products are dangerous because they can cause life-threatening dehydration, accelerated heart rate, high blood pressure, and irregular or skipped heartbeats. Particularly avoid energy products that also promote weight loss (see chapters 3, "Nutritional Health," and 14, "Exercise Fuel"). Safer, quick-energy fixes include a small snack or a short nap. Other brief energy perks include peppermint gum or candy, deep breathing, laughter, and fresh, cold air. Caffeine is effective but can have side effects such as addiction, dehydration, stomach upset, and diarrhea.

Healthy Ways to Increase Energy

Peppermint

A small snack

A nap

Deep breathing

Fresh, cold air

Caffeine (watch for dehydration and other side effects)

Incontinence

Leaking urine during sports activities occurs in up to 30 percent of active women. It occurs when the stress of lifting, jumping, twisting, or coughing puts pressure on weakened bladder muscles. Common causes include childbirth, hormone dysfunctions, nerve disorders, urinary tract infections, too much caffeine, or an overly full bladder.

The best exercise to train these muscles to become stronger is Kegel exercises, an easy exercise where you contract the muscles that hold your urine. If you are struggling with incontinence, try to do this exercise, holding for a count of ten, ten to twenty times, three to five times a day. Kegels can be done anywhere and no one will know you are doing them! Physical therapy specialists in women's health issues can also be helpful with incontinence by using techniques such as muscle stimulation and biofeedback for muscle training and strengthening.

Injuries

In an ideal world, you would never get injured, always get stronger, and continue to improve with each season. Because that is not realistic, it is important to learn how to recover faster and get back to athletic and fitness activities sooner. Regardless of the severity or nature of the injury, there are some basic principles that can help you manage and prevent problems with injuries.

Medications

The prescribed medications used to relieve pain when you are injured are either painkillers or anti-inflammatories. (Additional types of medicines prescribed include muscle relaxers or sleeping pills, which are used more often for treatment of back, neck, or chronic pain.) Do not mix prescription medications with nonprescription medications unless you have reviewed this with your doctor or pharmacist. Taking several types of nonprescription medications is not recommended. Also, do not compare number of milligrams of different pain medications or anti-inflammatories, as this has nothing to do with effectiveness and is like comparing apples to oranges. For example, the common medication ibuprofen at 400 mg, is about as effective as Vioxx at 12.5 mg.

Pain Killers

Pain killers are strong medications that usually have sedating side effects such as making you feel relaxed or sleepy. It is recommended that you do not drive or operate machinery while taking these drugs. If taken regularly for a few weeks, painkillers can also be addictive and hard to stop once the pain is gone. They also tend to cause upset stomach, nausea, or vomiting. The most common painkillers used are Tylenol with codeine (Tylenol 3), hydrocodone (Vicodin) and oxycodone (Percocet). It is best to avoid these medications as much as possible and use them only in cases of severe pain. Do not use them as a sleeping pill; if you do, they can become addictive. Instead, ask your doctor to prescribe a safer sleeping pill to take.

Nonsteroidal Anti-Inflammatories

Nonsteroidal anti-inflammatories are the medications most commonly prescribed for pain and inflammation. There are more than 50 types of these drugs, the most common of which is aspirin. They are available in many forms both with and without a prescription. Anti-inflammatories can have side effects that are more likely to occur if the drug is taken every day for more than a few months. The most common side effects are stomach irritation, reflux, and ulcers. More serious side effects are increased blood pressure and kidney problems. Because of potentially dangerous side effects, three new "Cox 2 Inhibitor" anti-inflammatories have been developed over the past few years with the brand names Celebrex, Vioxx, and Bextra. Until these Cox 2 inhibitors were developed, all anti-inflammatories were both Cox 1 and Cox 2 inhibitors, affecting more sites in the body than just those that control pain and inflammation. Because Cox 2 inhibitors are more specific to blocking the sites of pain and inflammation, these new-generation anti-inflammatories have less side effects overall and less risk of stomach ulceration.

Although the safety of anti-inflammatory medications is fairly high, there are some risks. In certain people, anti-inflammatory medications can affect the heart and blood vessels by raising blood pressure. (Those that have a reputation for this in particular are Vioxx, Ibuprofen (Advil), and Diclofenac.) It should be noted that people with multiple medical problems, severe high blood pressure, kidney problems, liver disease, or ulcers or people who are taking medications such as wararin (Coumadin) or steroids (Pred-nisone), usually cannot take anti-inflammatories. It should also be noted that problems can occur if you are taking two types of anti-inflammatories at once; this is easy to do because there are many types of both prescription and non-prescription pain medications. Avoid mixing medications by letting your doctor or pharmacist know all the medications—prescription and nonpre-scription—you have been taking.

Nonsteroidal anti-inflammatories are excellent medications for relieving pain and inflammation. The bottom line is, some are more effective than others for certain people. If you have had success with an anti-inflammatory in the past, let your doctor know which it was so you can take it again; likewise, if you have had problems in the past, let your doctor know that as well to avoid these and try something new.

Having a variety of treatment options is to your benefit. The greater number of treatment options available today allows you to have a better chance of pain and inflammation relief with the least side effects. This allows quicker healing, more comfort and compliance with exercise and therapy programs, better sleep and work, and quicker return to normal activities—the best results for both doctors and patients. If you still have pain, speak to your doctor. Be prepared to discuss when and how often your pain occurs. If you are already taking medications, know what kind, how much, and how often, as this is a good measure of how uncomfortable you are. Having pain that keeps you up at night or does not let you focus on daily activities is not normal. Speak to your doctor and discuss pain management techniques if you have such pain.

Common Nonsteroidal Anti-Inflammatories

BRAND NAME	GENERIC NAME
Bayer, Ecotrin, Emperin	Aspirin*
Advil, Nuprin, Motrin	Ibuprofen**
Aleve, Naprosyn	Naproxen**
Orudis, Oruvail	Ketoprofen**
Indocin	Indomethacin
Voltaren, Arthrotec, Cataflam	Diclofenac
Relafen	Nabumetone
Lodine	Etodolac
Mobic	Meloxicam
Celebrex	Celecoxib***
Vioxx	Rofecoxib***
Bextra	Valdecoxib***

*No prescription needed
**Available at lowest doses without a prescription
***Cox 2 inhibitors

Staying Fit While Your Injury Heals

Depending on your injury, you can keep your heart and lungs fit with alternative activities to maintain aerobic conditioning such as biking, swimming, cycling, and using a UBE (upper body ergometer). If you are using crutches or limping, these are both more strenuous aerobic activities than walking (and require more calories).

If you have a lower body injury, you can circuit-train in the gym, raising your heart rate by doing upper body exercises at high repetitions with low weights and little rest in between sets. Keep your recovery goals in sight with inspirational pictures, images, and phrases. Work out every other day if you feel tired, and remember that healing from injury takes energy so make sure you are eating well and taking a vitamin plus calcium.

Preserve Flexibility

If you are in a cast, sling, or brace, you must stretch a few times a day to prevent your surrounding joints from becoming tight and stiff. For example, if you have an ankle fracture and must be in a cast without bearing weight on it, your hip and knee might remain in a bent position as you walk with crutches and sit most of the time. Toes also become tight, stiff, and perhaps even swollen if you do not wiggle them. Hip and back tightness can lead to poor posture; prevent this by lying on your stomach several times a day to straighten it out, putting your leg up to straighten the knee and do a hamstring stretch, and stretching your leg out straight as often as possible (see figures 13-1 through 13-6 at the end of the chapter).

For other injured joints, refer to the following charts to increase and maintain flexibility. Move each joint through the full motions described 10 times in the morning and 10 times in the evening. For any movement limitations in your noninjured joints, see a physical therapist or athletic trainer for assistance on regaining that motion. This might take regular, aggressive stretching but is essential to full recovery from injury.

When Injured, Maintain Strength and Flexibility in the Surrounding Joints

INJURED JOINT	SURROUNDING JOINTS TO KEEP FLEXIBLE
Shoulder	elbow, wrist, fingers, neck
Elbow	shoulder, wrist, fingers
Wrist	fingers, elbow, shoulder
Hip	back, knee, ankle, toes
Knee	hip, ankle, toes
Ankle	toes, knee, hip

Maintaining Full Active Range of Motion in Each Joint

JOINT	MAINTAIN MOTION
Shoulder	Reach arms behind head, reach behind back, reach straight overhead, reach across front to opposite shoulder.
Elbow	Bend to touch tops of shoulders, straighten arm fully, rotate palms up and down.
Wrist	Bend wrist up and back, rotate in full circle, turn palms up and down.
Hip	Lying on back, knees bent, pull knees into chest, then rotate hips in circles; on stomach, push chest up to arch front of hip.
Knee	Sitting, bend to reach foot to buttocks, straighten fully by pressing back of knee into floor or mat.
Ankle	Circle foot around; toe tap up and point toes all the way down; tilt side of foot up and down.

Strengthening

Try to do strengthening exercises three days a week in the surrounding joints and on all joints on the noninjured side. For lower body injuries, do balance exercises if possible. Research shows that strengthening the noninjured side can help the injured side heal faster and prevent it from becoming as weak as it would otherwise.

Keep Your Spirits Up!

It is easy to feel sad and blue after an injury. While injured, you are not able to participate in the activity you love, and you are also having trouble with other day-to-day activities, such as walking, going to the bathroom, or driving. Remember that this is only temporary, and by keeping your spirits up, you will heal faster. The mind has very strong power over the body, particularly when it is healing. Do what you can to make yourself feel better: spend time with friends, read lighthearted books, watch funny TV shows. Laughter is truly the best medicine, and being in a good mood will allow you to be happier and more effective at everything you do.

Remember that you will get better. There are many athletes who feel that they became better at their sport after an injury taught them to strengthen new muscles, improve their balance, fine-tune their technique, improve mental toughness, or took better care to eat and rest more properly. Every experience is what you make of it. Every mistake or injury has the potential to be an opportunity to improve.

Keep Your Mind "in the Game"

Every day for about 10 minutes, imagine yourself playing your sport. Close your eyes and "see" yourself playing in a game or doing your exercise routine. Try to imagine all the senses that go along with it—smell, sounds, feelings of exhilaration, muscles burning. . . . Envision yourself playing your best and feeling *great*. This is called mental imagery and is used by many elite and professional athletes to keep themselves mentally and neurologically fine-tuned to their game.

Consider Other Types of Activities

Often, an injury leads to learning a new sport or activity. A runner who has repeated tendinitis might take up swimming or biking. A skier who has repeated knee problems might take up snowboarding. Trying new activities to increase workout variety can be beneficial to overall health and wellness. From each new activity, you can make new friends, develop new muscles, and keep yourself young with the thrill of a new challenge.

Improve Your Nutrition

If you are not already taking a multivitamin, now is the time to start. A good multivitamin contains the essential vitamins and minerals your body needs while it is healing. If you have any tingling or feelings of numbness, as can happen after injury, take an additional B complex daily, especially one containing 100 mg vitamins B_6 and 100 mcg B_{12}. (If you cannot stand the smell of vitamins, try brand-name vitamins and avoid those that are "natural," as these tend to have strange aftertastes and smells. You can also try taking vitamins with a delicious drink or with a spoonful of ice cream to help them go down easier.) Also, make sure you are eating at least three servings of protein and eating four servings of dairy products (or taking 1,200 mg calcium) a day for your bones and muscles to heal optimally.

Returning to Your Sport

If you are allowed to return to your sports activity, remember to do so *gradually*. Also remember that the biggest cause of reinjuries and poor healing is doing too much, too soon. You must cut back to less than one-fourth the amount you were doing before the injury and increase no more than 10 percent each week.

When you are healed enough to return to your sport, remember two phrases and start with one-fourth the distance, weight, or repetitions you were doing before you got hurt:

Start low, go slow.

Avoid too much, too soon.

Recommended Postural Exercises and Stretches While Healing from Leg Injury

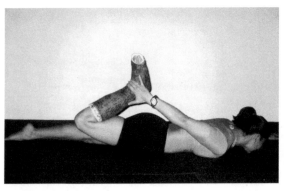

FIGURE 13-1 **Hip Flexor Stretch: On your stomach, reach back and pull one calf in while bending your knee and lifting your knee off the mat. Hold for count of five, release, and repeat five times.**

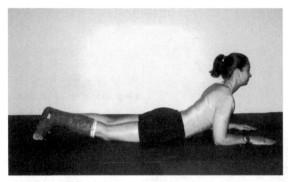

FIGURE 13-2 **Hip and Back Stretch:** On your stomach, arch your back to lift your upper body off the mat, placing your bent elbows on the mat, gently pressing your upper body up with your forearms. (May advance this stretch by straightening arms.)

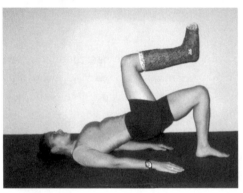

FIGURE 13-3 **Advanced Back and Abdominal Strengthening:** On your back, starting in bridge position (see figure 9-9), leave your left leg on the mat, lift your right (injured) leg in the air with your knee bent, and perform a bridge by lifting your hips and pelvis up. Hold for slow count of three. Keep your right knee up, lower pelvis, and repeat 10 times.

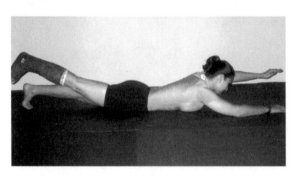

FIGURE 13-4 **Upper and Lower Back Strengthening:** On your stomach, perform swimmer by lifting your left straight arm and right straight leg, and hold for three. Switch sides and repeat 20 times.

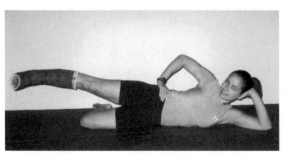

FIGURE 13-5 **Abductor Strengthening:** Lying on your side, lift your straight top leg six to eight inches toward the ceiling. Hold for slow count of three, then slowly lower. Repeat 10 times.

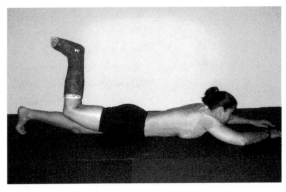

FIGURE 13-6 **Glut Strengthening: Lying on your stomach, bend your right knee and lift your knee up toward the ceiling. Hold for slow count of three. Slowly lower and repeat 10 times.**

Being active has many rewards. As with all rewarding things, there are some risks and occasional problems. Most are minor and easy to overcome. Addressing the problem and taking care of it as soon as possible is the best way to keep it from becoming a long-term issue. Knowing when to stop and when to see a specialist or doctor is the most important aspect. Face the problem as a challenge and meet it appropriately. Do not get discouraged for too long. Appreciate the experience your healing provides. Soon you will be healed and stronger than ever!

CHAPTER FOURTEEN

Exercise Fuel

Food is fuel. Just like the right gas fuel in your car makes it run smoother and more efficiently, the right food fuel in your body will make you run longer and more comfortably. Getting the right amount and type of exercise fuel can be a challenge, and there are overwhelming and confusing amounts of food products and advice on what is best for performance. The goal is to fuel your body with the healthiest, most nourishing energy and fluid supply appropriate for your athletic activity and caloric needs.

Maximizing nutrition throughout your training and exercise, not just the week before an event, will result in the best physical and mental performance. Performing better while training allows for better overall conditioning. Each practice or training session is a chance to improve performance. In effect, with each meal, as with each workout session, you are improving your level of fitness. Finding the optimum type and amount of exercise fuel specific to your body and activity can be a challenge and will take some practice. A working knowledge of the benefits (and risks) of sports nutrition is very important.

Hunger, Thirst, Cravings

Most nutritionists and health-care professionals will tell you to listen to your body signals—hunger and thirst are signals that your body needs food or fluids. Sometimes the signals get confused; for example a craving for sweets could actually mean you are thirsty. Sometimes boredom leads to "hunger" or an acidic stomach can make you feel "hungry." But mostly, hunger means you need food.

In athletes, salt cravings might mean you need sodium; red meat cravings might mean your body needs iron; ice cream or cheese cravings might mean you need calcium; french fry or dessert cravings might mean you need more calories, carbohydrates, and fat.

Thirst is one of the most important cravings. Being thirsty actually means you are already a little dehydrated, as thirst is a catch-up body signal. If you feel thirsty, your body almost always needs water. (There are very few false thirst signals, other than medicines such as antidepressants or antihistamines that dry out your mouth and make you feel thirsty.) Because athletes and active people rarely take time to drink enough fluids, thirst should always be honored.

The Importance of Fluids

The body is mostly water and needs plenty to function. Water is essential for all organ system functions, especially muscles. Not having enough fluids puts you at a risk of dehydration, a state in which your body does not have enough water. To protect the vital organs such as your brain, lungs, and heart, when you are dehydrated the water first is taken from the bloodstream and muscles. This causes poor, slow function and makes your body work harder to do all movements. You feel fatigued and can develop weakness, slowness, muscle cramping, and even nausea and confusion. Your heart rate increases, requiring your body to work harder, and you also feel that you are working harder than you actually are. With dehydration, muscle firing takes longer, so your muscles work less efficiently. You are unable to maintain your body temperature as well and can be subject to frostbite and heat stroke at extreme temperatures (both can be very serious). Your blood actually thickens without enough water in the body and does not work as well to supply oxygen to the muscles and take away waste products such as lactic acid (one reason for muscle cramping).

During competition, dehydration is a serious risk, as it will decrease your performance and can even risk your health. If you are severely dehydrated, your body will shut down, which can result in long-term kidney failure and bodily damage. Also, if you are dizzy or light-headed from too little fluids, your coordination can be affected, resulting not only in poor athletic skills and performance but falls, which lead to further injury.

Temperature and Dehydration

The environment plays a large role in body fluid losses. Dehydration negatively affects performance in extremes of temperatures. In the cold, dehydration stunts circulation, putting you at greater risk for frostbite. Heat is the most dangerous temperature variable, especially when it is over 90 degrees Fahrenheit. At this temperature, the risk of heat exhaustion is increased and can occur even before you feel thirsty. Heat exhaustion can lead to heat stroke, as indicated by symptoms such as flushed skin, chills, stomach cramping, goosebumps, vomiting, dizziness, headache, confusion, irritability, and eventual fainting, breathing difficulties, and convulsions. Heat exhaustion takes a serious, sometimes permanent toll on your heart, kidneys, and muscles. Humidity complicates the effects of high temperatures by preventing sweat from cooling the body.

High Temperature and Dehydration = a Dangerous Combination	
SIGNS OF HEAT EXHAUSTION	**SIGNS OF HEAT STROKE**
Flushed skin, goosebumps	Vomiting
Confusion	Muscle spasms
Headache	Convulsions
Nausea	Tremors
Weakness, tremors	Loss of consciousness

Dehydration is measured and researched in percent body water lost. This easily translates into bodyweight before and after exercise, as each pound equals about two cups of fluids. (One pound is 1 percent of a 100-pound woman; 1.4 pounds is 1 percent of a 140-pound woman.) Heat exhaustion can occur with only a 1.5 percent decrease in body water; this can occur before thirst even kicks in! After this, for each 1 percent of your bodyweight that you lose of fluid, your body temperature rises a small amount. If there is a great amount of dehydration, up to 7 percent of body fluid loss, sweating decreases, causing a further rise in body temperature. Performance decreases if you lose just 2 percent of your body fluids associated with decreased blood volume. (If you weigh 140 pounds, that would mean when you have lost 2.8 pounds in sweat.) This is easy to do in one hour of exercise, particularly if it is hot.

Percent Body Fluid Loss and Its Effects

PERCENT LOSS	EFFECTS
1	Each percent over 1.5 percent causes a slight body temperature rise.
1.5	You feel thirsty and have a greater risk of heat exhaustion.
2	Performance begins to decrease, blood volume shrinks.
7	Sweating decreases or stops.

Fluid Recommendations

It is important to take the time to drink enough healthy fluids such as water, flavored waters, vegetable and fruit juice, caffeine-free drinks, and sports drinks throughout the day. Drinks containing alcohol or caffeine do not increase your body fluid supply, as both these ingredients are diuretics (causing water loss through urination). Therefore, although you might feel you are quenching your thirst with a beer or cola, you are not increasing your body fluids. If you do drink these beverages, alternate with water or seltzer so you will increase your body fluids.

Good Sources of Fluids

Water	Caffeine-free drinks
Flavored water	Sports drinks
Juice	

Alcohol should be avoided before and during exercise due to its slowing effects on the brain and nerves. Alcohol also slows muscle firing, reflexes, and reaction time and impairs balance. In cold weather, alcohol decreases circulation in the arms and legs, increasing risk of frostbite. Most important, alcohol impairs judgment, making sports and activities dangerous.

Drinks That Do Not Increase Body Water

(If you must drink these, drink an extra glass of water for each serving.)

Alcohol	Tea
Coffee	Caffeinated sodas

Reasons Never to Drink Alcohol Before or During Exercise

Impairs judgment	Increase risk of overheating
Decreases coordination	Slows brain function
Increases injury risk	Slows reflexes
Causes dehydration	Decreases circulation
Increases risk of frostbite	

Symptoms of Dehydration

Light-headedness	Muscle cramping
Nausea	Goosebumps
Vomiting	Not urinating in more than three hours
Sluggishness	Confusion
Tiredness	Muscle twitching

Body fluid regulation also depends on the amount of sodium and potassium in the bloodstream. These are important electrolytes that are lost through sweat and urine. If it is very hot or the exercise lasts longer than one hour, you need to drink a sports drink or electrolyte solution to replenish sodium and potassium. Otherwise, your body will go into an electrolyte imbalance called hyponatremia (low sodium). Symptoms include weakness, fatigue, and slowness. At extreme low levels of sodium, the heart and muscle functions can be impaired. In its most dangerous case, hyponatremia causes seizures and can be life-threatening. For this reason athletes are advised to eat salted foods without restrictions.

What are the best fluid recommendations? Drink throughout the day and before exercise. If it is hot or if you are exercising for more than an hour, you must drink ½ to 1 cup (4 to 8 ounces) of fluid every 15 to 20 minutes of exercise; if the temperature is over 75 degrees Fahrenheit, try to drink 1 cup. If the exercise lasts longer than one hour, you need to drink a sports drink with 6 to 8 percent carbohydrates to maximize how much water the body absorbs. This sports drink should also contain sodium and potassium. The amount of electrolytes you consume should be higher if the exercise lasts longer than two hours. Electrolytes are also found in some food bars, gels, or higher electrolyte solutions (read labels).

After the exercise, try to drink another two cups of fluid as soon as possible. To learn how much your body needs after activity, weigh yourself naked before and after exercise; for each pound lost, drink two cups of healthy fluids. You can also estimate your body's fluid status by paying attention to your urine color and amount. Plentiful, light-yellow urine is a sign you are drinking enough; small amounts of dark-yellow or brown urine is a sign you need to drink more.

Fluid Replacement Recommended During Exercise of Various Lengths*

<1 hr: 8 to 16 ounce water (or sports drink, if desired)

1 to 2 hr: 32 ounce fluid, at least half from sports drink or electrolyte solution

>2 hr: minimum of 16 ounce sports drink per hour plus extra sodium and potassium

*In temperatures above 90 degrees, add 8 to 16 ounce sports drink per hour.

PERFORMANCE TIP Sports drinks are recommended to replenish carbohydrates and electrolytes if exercising for more than one hour, especially in hot temperatures.

PERFORMANCE TIP Drink two cups of fluid for every pound lost during exercise.

Sports Drinks and Their Nutrient Content

SPORTSDRINK	CARBOHYDRATE	SODIUM	POTASSIUM	DRINK CALORIES
Gatorade	19g / 6 percent	55 mg	30 mg	70
Powerade	14g / 5 percent	110 mg	30 mg	50
Powerade	7g / 2 percent	55 mg	30 mg	25

Drinks containing other additives such as vitamins or oxygen have no effect on performance or nutrition. Vitamins in drinks other than juices are usually a very low percent and are not necessary during exercise. The oxygen in oxygenated waters gets released in the stomach and is not absorbed in the blood or lungs, where the body can use it. Other additives such as energizers or stimulants are not recommended due to potential health and dehydration risks.

Oxygenated waters do not have any effect on body oxygen content.

Fueling for Exercise

The best, most efficient fuel for exercise are carbohydrates. They are easily and quickly broken down into glucose, your body's direct source of fuel. Therefore, carbohydrates are the best foods to eat immediately before and during performance, as they are the most easily broken down for immediate energy. Carbohydrates are chains of sugar molecules such as fructose, sucrose, lactose, and glucose. The length of these chains identifies the carbohydrates as either simple or complex. Simple carbohydrates are short sugar chains easily digested; complex carbohydrates are longer chains such as starches and fibers that take slightly longer to digest.

The glycemic index can be used to measure how quickly your bloodstream will receive the glucose contained in a certain food. The glycemic index is based on a scale of 0 to 100. High glycemic index foods, such as sugar, honey, and exercise gels, reach the bloodstream within minutes. (Sugar has a glycemic index of 100.) Low glycemic index foods can take one to three hours to reach the bloodstream as glucose, and the glucose is released slowly in small amounts.

You can use the glycemic index to determine what is best for you before and during exercise. Two hours before competition, low glycemic index foods are recommended, as they will provide a slow, long-lasting source of glucose. Thirty minutes to one hour before, medium glycemic index foods are recommended. Immediately before and during exercise, high glycemic index foods are recommended to quickly replenish glucose supplies. Before and during exercise, avoid high-protein and high-fat bars or foods, as they are not efficient quick sources of energy. Protein breakdown also requires water, which your body needs to exercise. Carbohydrates are to you like gasoline is for your car; eating protein and fats are like getting your car fuel from coal—they need several processing steps before becoming directly usable energy.

Of course, an important feature of this recommendation is that your body is able to tolerate the food without developing gas, bloating, or an urge to go to the bathroom. Most people cannot tolerate a heavy meal immediately before exercise, so try to eat a meal at least two hours before. If you are exercising or competing early in the morning, have a small, high-carbohydrate, low-fiber, medium glycemic index meal 30 to 60 minutes before the event, followed by a high glycemic index snack immediately before. You should also have small, low-fiber (high glycemic index) carbohydrate snacks available during endurance events that last longer than an hour to replenish blood glucose. The American College of Sports Medicine recommends consuming 30 to 60 grams of carbohydrates during each hour of exercise after the first hour. Foods such as dairy products, fresh juices, and fatty foods are not recommended, as they might cause diarrhea if eaten before or during exercise.

Carbo Loading

For endurance and aerobic events lasting one hour or longer, maximizing your body's glycogen stores during the days before competition is the best way to maximize the amount of energy you will have available during the event. Study after study has shown better performance in endurance events after carbo loading—increasing the amount of energy your body has stored in the liver and muscles.

The technique is to make sure you are eating a diet made up of at least 60 percent carbohydrates the three weeks through sixth day before your event. Beginning on the third day before the event, your diet should be mostly carbohydrates to increase diet content of carbohydrates to 80 percent. This can make you feel a little bulkier, as the extra stored carbohydrates cause your body to hold on to more water, but you will need it (and lose it) during the event. Balance the rest of your diet with higher amounts of protein than fat. Also, make sure you are taking a multivitamin and continue taking your calcium supplements.

Recipe for Carbo Loading

Three weeks to six days before event	60 percent carbohydrates
Six to four days before event	70 percent carbohydrates
Three to one day before event	80 percent carbohydrates
Meal before event	100 percent carbohydrates

Carbohydrates can have various effects on your bowels. High-carbohydrate diets are tolerated differently from person to person; while some women might feel comfortable, others can feel bloated, gassy, become constipated, or have loose stools. Bland carbohydrates such as pasta, rice, bananas, apples without skin, and bread usually will not cause as much stomach upset and are the kinds of foods usually well tolerated the night before an event. If you still have difficulty tolerating such a high-carbohydrate diet, adding just two extra servings of carbohydrate-rich foods a day can help.

Fueling During Performance

Fueling for Activity

Energy sources should be tailored to your activity type and duration. If you are doing a sprint event, you do not need to worry about replenishing fuel stores, as your body has enough; simply make sure your digestive system is comfortable by avoiding high-fat or heavy foods. In moderate-distance events, your body uses glycogen stores; these can be maximized by carbo loading as described above. You might want to eat a 100 to 200 calorie carbohydrate snack if the activity lasts slightly longer than one hour to give yourself an energy boost, but this is not essential, and the carbohydrates in a sports drink can provide this extra fuel. In events lasting two hours or longer, you must take in 30 to 60 grams (120 to 240 calories) of high glycemic index carbohydrates per hour, or your body will begin to break down fatty acids (and possibly muscle protein) to obtain fuel. This is not ideal, as this conversion also takes energy and extra water. Therefore, providing your body with enough quick glucose sources throughout the exercise event is the best way to keep your body running smoothly. In longer-endurance events lasting more than three hours, you should eat whatever you can. If foods are not tolerable during exercise, you can obtain calories through a combination of carbohydrates in sports drinks and in easily digested energy gel, paste, or Gu.

Activity-Specific Energy Sources Recommended During Event

Sprint events (fewer than four minutes)	No need to refuel
Short events (fewer than one hour)	No need to refuel
Moderate-endurance events (one to two hours)	120 to 240 calories of high GI carbohydrates helpful, not necessary
Endurance events (two to three + hours)	120 to 240 calories high GI carbohydrates per hour
Ultra-endurance events (more than three hours)	at least 120 to 240 calories high GI carbohydrates per hour along with any additional carbohydrate sources you can tolerate

Fueling After Exercise

Researches have now discovered a window of opportunity in which your muscles and liver are more receptive to replenishing glycogen stores. This occurs within the first hour after exercise and, to a lesser extent, for the next several hours. It is highly recommended by sports nutritionists that you take advantage of this opportunity and eat 200 to 300 calories of carbohydrates within the first hour after exercise, followed by the same amount each hour for the next few hours if you have completed a hard workout or endurance event. Consuming carbs in this way will decrease the amount of fatigue you might feel over the next few days and make your next workout easier. Recent studies suggest that eating protein immediately after exercise will help your body more quickly repair torn or stressed muscle tissue and similarly speed recovery. Therefore, add 100 calories of protein to the 200 to 300 carbohydrate calories within the first hour after exercise. A sandwich, milk shake, or energy bar would make excellent post-workout snacks.

Energy Bars

The original sports food bar, the Power Bar was designed to refuel an athlete during an event. It is an excellent source of ready-to-use carbohydrates in an easily digestible form; bikers and triathletes find them a favorite as they stick to their bikes and can be peeled off in pieces during a race or long workout. Newer bars on the market contain more protein and some fat. These function better as small meal replacements or for recovery after exercise. High-protein bars are less-effective sources of energy during exercise.

Bars made especially for women are smaller, thus lower in calories. They also contain some nutrients that benefit women especially—soy protein (thought to prevent breast cancer), calcium, iron, and folate. They can be more expensive, however, so beware. If you are taking your recommended multivitamin and calcium supplement, you do not need these special bars. If you like to use energy bars as snacks or during athletic activities, make sure you read the labels to find out which bar is best for your needs.

Not only are meal replacement and energy bars expensive, but they don't necessarily taste as good as they promise, and some can cause gas. You should experiment with what tastes best to you and does not cause other side effects. Exercise fuel does not need to be in the form of a sports bar. A recent research study actually compared the performance of athletes who ate white bread, Snickers, or a sports bar before and during exercise. They all performed the same! For fuel immediately before and during exercise, the common essential ingredient is carbohydrates.

It is wise to consider what you are using these bars for. If you do not need the extra protein or vitamins, especially if you eat a well-balanced diet and take a multivitamin, you can save money and enjoy a tastier snack by eating high-carbohydrate treats such as Fig Newtons or chocolate (moderate glycemic index), Rice Krispie treats or Pop Tarts (higher glycemic index). Like energy bars, experiment with these fuel sources in practice to make sure they do not cause uncomfortable side effects.

FOOD	CAL.	PROTEIN (G)	FAT (G)	CARBS (G)	CA (MG)	B (%)	FE (%)	FOLATE (%)	GI*
Power Bar	230	10	2.5	45	300	100	35	100	M (56)
Cliff Bar	240	10	4	43	250	15	30	0	M
Luna Bar	180	10	4.5	27	350	100	35	100	M
Oasis Bar	180	9	3.5	26	350	35	35	35	M
Pria Bar	110	5	3	16	300	30	20	60	M
Balance Bar	190	14	6	22	100	25	20	20	L/M
MetRx Bar	310	34	8	25	500	50	40	100	L/M
Fig Newton	180	2	0	44	40	NA	8	NA	M
Rice Kr Treat	160	1	3.5	30	0	15	4	10	H (90)
Snickers	280	4	14	35	40	NA	2	NA	M (55)
Pop Tart	200	2.5	10	37	1	10	10	10	H
SlimFast	220	10	3	40	400	40	15	30	M

* GI = glycemic index, if not specifically available; L is low, M is medium, H is high, and NA is not available.

Energy Gels or Pastes

Energy gels are high glycemic index, simple carbohydrate sources, and excellent fuel supplies for athletes during a long workout or a race. They taste good, do not require chewing, and provide instant energy. They are made of maltodextrin, a long glucose chain that quickly breaks down as soon as it is digested. Each packet usually contains 25 grams (100 calories) of high GI carbohydrates. Gels and pastes come in many flavors and thicknesses; brand names are Gu, CliffShot, and Power Gel. They are often fortified with vitamins or minerals, but these are not necessary during competition. They also are available with caffeine, the amount found in about a half cup of coffee ("double caffeine" equals 1 cup of coffee). Be careful that you are not using products designed for recovery during an event, as these have too high a percentage of protein to be an efficient fuel source. Before using these fuel sources in an event, try them in training, as the sugary taste or unusual texture or flavor might make them unpleasant.

Energy Drinks

There are many different types of energy drinks that provide a liquid source of quick carbohydrates. It is not recommended to use drinks that contain "metabolic enhancers," proteins, or a complex concoction of chemicals during an event. If the event is more than an hour, all you really need is a good source of carbohydrates, sodium, and potassium. (For exercise lasting less than one hour, water is fine.) The basic sports drinks do provide some carbohydrates, and if they are consumed regularly—8 ounces for every 15 minutes—these carbohydrates can be enough in medium-endurance events. Sometimes, a large load of liquid carbohydrates can result in having to go to the bathroom or diarrhea. Again, it is very important to test these products before you participate in your race, hike, or event.

Supplements

Creatine

Creatine is a legal supplement that has been shown to increase performance in short bursts of intense activity, such as sprinting and power lifting. It also decreases fatigue and improves strength and power. Creatine causes weight gain and muscles to bulk up and get bigger. Creatine is naturally found in fish and meats and is available as the supplement creatine monohydrate.

Creatine naturally functions as part of the energy cycle in the body, and by supplementing creatine, this energy cycle might work more efficiently. Creatine also allows muscles to absorb glycogen faster, increasing muscle fuel supply. Because of this glycogen increase, creatine produces weight gain and increases muscle bulk.

Creatine has not been around long enough to know what the full spectrum of long-term health effects might be. There is some question about its safety; it has recently been made illegal in France, where it has been found to be related to cancer. High blood levels of creatine suggest kidney problems, the most serious risk due to high doses of creatine taken for an extended time. Taking creatine can cause muscle cramping and dehydration, both of which further stress the kidneys. Creatine can also predispose compartment syndrome, a serious and very painful lower leg condition in which the muscles expand beyond their soft tissue compartments.

Creatine is not recommended for long periods of time at high doses (no more than 30 mg daily over no more than 7 days). At a low dose, such as 5 mg, creatine may be safe, but even at this low dose, it is still not recommended to take creatine for longer than 3 months. Because of kidney risks, it should never be taken by diabetics or people with kidney compromise. Due to both known and unknown health risks, it should never be taken during pregnancy or by children or adolescents. Creatine has no effect during exercise, as it does not reach the muscle energy cycle quickly.

Ribose

Ribose is a sugar found naturally in foods and in the body that is thought to increase the efficiency of the energy-producing cycles in the body. Similar to creatine, it is a direct ingredient of the cell's energy cycle and is thought to increase strength by improving supplies of energy to the muscles. The research has not yet provided enough specific evidence of this; because it is a sugar, however, the body can use it as basic carbohydrates for direct energy. Although ribose supplies quick energy as a sugar carbohydrate with no health risks, the expense might not be worth the questionable benefit. Also, large amounts can cause bloating and diarrhea.

Caffeine

Caffeine, a naturally occurring chemical found in plants, is the only legal, inexpensive, proven performance enhancer without risks of serious health consequences. Caffeine has stimulating effects to both nerve and muscle tissue, making it easier for nerves and muscles to fire. Caffeine also has effects at the cell level to speed up the production of energy and allow fatty acids (stored muscle energy) to be burned more easily. With more easily accessible energy, and nerves and muscles that fire more quickly, the body can work longer, harder, and with increased endurance.

Caffeine also has numerous effects on the brain, including decreasing your sensation of exercise intensity, and stimulating the pleasure receptors in the brain, allowing you to feel better and work harder for longer. Caffeine improves brain reaction time and memory retention and blocks sleep receptors. It also constricts blood vessels to reduce headaches.

Performance-Enhancing Effects of Caffeine

Less feeling of discomfort	Quicker nerve and muscle firing
Greater enjoyment	Quicker burn of fatty acids
Less sense of fatigue	Improved alertness
Greater attention to tasks	Faster reaction times

Caffeine reaches maximum effect within 30 to 60 minutes after intake. It has a half-life of about six hours, which means that six hours later, half the amount you drank is still in your system! This is why afternoon coffee can interfere with sleep. In athletes, where sleep is important to performance, caffeine products should not be consumed within at least six hours before bed.

Caffeine can have some harmful effects; it raises blood pressure a few points, can contribute to heart palpitations, and can mildly reduce levels of iron and calcium absorption. Caffeine can become harmful to athletes because it is a diuretic, leading to greater risk of dehydration if not enough fluids are consumed. Caffeine is addictive to your body and mind; withdrawal can cause headaches, depression, and constipation. Your body also can become dependent on caffeine and might require a little more each day to provide the same effects. These effects are all short term and reversible by decreasing amounts of caffeine consumed. If done gradually, this should not cause problems.

Caffeine at extremely high doses has been made illegal by the U.S. Olympic committee. The illegal amount is the equivalent of 10 cups of coffee, well above the 2- to 3-cup equivalent (200 to 300 mg) amounts of caffeine needed to provide performance-enhancing benefits. At extremely high doses—equivalent to 40 cups or more or 50 caffeine pills (5 to 10g) at once—life-threatening seizures and heart arrhythmias can result and lead to death. Caffeine is not metabolized well by children and should not be consumed by girls under age 16. While planning to become pregnant or during pregnancy, total caffeine should be limited to less than 200 mg a day (2 small cups of coffee or 4 small servings of tea or cola), as more than 200 mg per day can contribute to miscarriage and low birth weight infants.

Caffeine Precautions

Limit amount if you have high blood pressure.

Have less than 200 mg daily if you are planning to become or are pregnant.

Drink extra fluids if you are working out or competing.

The more caffeine you have, the more likely you will become addicted.

Do not consume caffeine if you are under 16 years old.

Cut down on caffeine if you regularly have trouble sleeping.

Caffeine is not recommended if you have heart palpitations or arrhythmias.

Under no circumstances should you have more than 1 g a day (10 cups of coffee).

Just like any substance or drug, some people tolerate caffeine better than others; it can also be metabolized quicker in some people than others. Therefore, caffeine is something you should definitely try in practice first. The most common problems associated with caffeine before or during exercise are having to urinate or move your bowels, as caffeine is a diuretic (a substance causing fluid loss) and a laxative (causing bowel movement). If not taken with enough water, dehydration can be a risk. Also, stomach irritation and regurgitation from the increased stomach acidity due to coffee can occur. All these side effects pose problems during an athletic activity. Caffeine can cause some people to be anxious and jittery, and should be avoided by those involved in precision sports, which can become a problem for athletes.

Uncomfortable Side Effects of Caffeine

Stomach cramps	Indigestion
Diarrhea	Irritability
Frequent urination	Tremors
Acidic stomach	Poor sleep

If you can tolerate caffeine, the benefits are increased endurance, concentration, and quicker reaction time. Caffeine can be obtained in pills, coffee, tea, soda, and specified energy gels and bars, waters or other drinks, and candy. There are legal limits for caffeine content in various countries. In the

United States, there is a limit of 6 mg of caffeine per liquid ounce and a limit of 200 mg per pill.

The amount of caffeine in a drink or food varies the most in brewed teas and coffees, depending on the strength and brewing time. A breakdown of caffeine content is seen in the following chart.

Average Caffeine Content of Various Products (milligrams)					
COFFEE (8 OZ.)	TEA (8 OZ.)	SODA (12 OZ.)	PRODUCT (1 SERV)	CHOCOLATE (1 OZ)	PILLS (1 TABLET)
Brewed/ drip 110 to 135	brewed 50	Diet Coke 47	Red Bull 130	milk 6	Vivarin, no Doz Max 200
Espresso 90	green 30	Dr Pepper 42	Guarana 250	dark 20	No Doz (reg) 100
Instant 95	bottled 20	Mountain Dew 55	PowerGel 25 to 50	chips 10	Anacin 32
Starbucks 200	instant 20	Pepsi 37 Coke 35	Gu gel 20	syrup (2 T) 5	Dexatrim 200
Frappucino (12 oz.) 130		Jolt 70	coffee ice cream 20	hot chocolate 5	Excedrin 75
Venti Starbucks 500		Coke 35 Sunkist 45	Cliff ice bar 50	baking (unsw) 25	Midol 32

If caffeine is something you would like to try to help performance, the equivalent of two to three brewed cups before an event or a workout is usually all you will need to get the full performance-enhancing effects, although many athletes feel an effect with less. You can also try caffeinated gels, gums, waters, or energy bars, which might not irritate your stomach and digestive system as much as coffee. (Often, they do not contain as much caffeine.) Make sure you take caffeine with at least equal amounts of water to avoid dehydration. Like any food or drink you plan to take before a race, make sure you try it out in practice first!

Amino Acids and Protein Supplements

These supplements are highly popular in gyms and among people trying to lose weight; protein supplements are also used as meal replacements. Some studies suggests increased muscle bulk with extra protein, but extra protein is simply used by the body just as any other nutritional substance would be: for calories and fuel. Any proteins that are not burned as calories will turn into fat, no matter how much exercise is done.

Overloading proteins can be hazardous to your body as it tries to break down the proteins. The kidneys, in particular, can suffer damage with a diet too rich in protein. The fact is, most Americans are already eating enough protein. Heavy weight and endurance training does require more than the RDI of .8 g/kg/d, but this can easily be obtained with a healthy diet. There is no scientific proof that specific amino acids help with performance or bodybuilding. Often, protein supplements are just overpriced calories!

Illegal Substances

Unfortunately, in the quest of athletes, performers, and bodybuilders for extreme physique and performance, illegal substance use can be common. These substances are illegal for many reasons, the most important of which is that they have serious and long-term negative effects on health.

Steroids

Steroids come in many forms and, unfortunately, are very easy to find, even though they are illegal. Common types of steroids include andro (androstenedione), testosterone, and "natural" alternatives to steroids. Precursors or metabolites of steroids are also available. Steroids can be taken in both pill and injectable forms. Do not be fooled by a pill, thinking it is not as dangerous as an injection. Regardless of the form, steroids have the same unhealthy effects; muscles will bulk up and become stronger, but the body also will change in very negative ways, many of them permanent. The risks are much greater than their benefit.

Side Effects of Steroids

Deepening of voice (not reversible)

Severe mood swings

Depression

Aggressive behavior (" 'roid rage")

Hair growth on the body

Loss of hair on the head

Widening of shoulders

Decreased breast size

Loss of your period

Loss of your ability to have (healthy) children

Osteoporosis

Liver failure (life-threatening)

Cancer

These drugs pose *serious harm* to the female body, especially because steroids are technically all anabolic (muscle building), androgenic (masculinizing) steroids. There are no steroids that are muscle building without the mostly irreversible masculinizing effects. Steroids are dangerous, expensive, and illegal.

Growth Hormones

Growth hormones, such as human growth hormone (HGH), also pose serious health risks and can cause liver failure and cancer. Many bodybuilders have died prematurely because they used these substances throughout their careers. Unfortunately, these hormones are found in many substances labeled for improved performance and can be bought at vitamin shops, at health food stores, and over the Internet. Your health can quickly deteriorate when taking these drugs and not only take you out of competition, but also kill you. Liver failure can happen literally overnight and be so severe as to require a liver transplant.

Erythropoietin

Erythropoietin is a medical drug used to build up blood cells in patients who do not have enough, such as in cancer patients undergoing cell destroying chemotherapy. It is a banned substance by the U.S. Olympic committee. Not only is taking erythropoietin cheating, it is dangerous, as it can thicken the blood and cause high blood pressure, resulting in a stroke, heart failure, and accelerated dehydration.

Metabolic Enhancers

Matabolic enhancers—including amphetamine, ephedrine, ephedra, ma huang, and xenedrine—are all mild forms of speed that raise blood pressure, and cause nervousness, heart dysfunction, seizures, heart stroke, and potentially death. They are also addictive. These metabolic enhancers have dangerous effects on performance. They are found in pills, teas, food products, diet pills, and dietary supplements.

In athletes, these products are particularly not recommended. None of these have passed the strict guidelines posed by the Food and Drug Administration (FDA), because supplements are not regulated by the FDA and manufacturers are not required to report specific benefits or risks. The dangers associated with taking these products cannot be stressed enough.

––––––––

With the right nutrition, performance can be improved. This includes not only eating the right foods, but also drinking enough fluids. Eat a well-balanced diet and take a multivitamin daily. Always bring snacks and water if you are exercising more than one hour. In the heat, you need water within 15 minutes of beginning a workout. If you are exercising over an hour, you should have a sports drink and try to drink 1 cup every 20 minutes. This is the equivalent of one large water bottle per hour of working out. The best food during exercise contains all or mostly carbohydrates. You need to refuel every hour at least, depending on the exertion. When training, try to eat and drink 20 to 30 minutes after exercise; this will best refuel your muscles for your next workout. Stay away from illegal performance enhancers. They are dangerous, expensive, and often ineffective. If you need a lift and can stomach it, try caffeine.

CHAPTER FIFTEEN

Pregnancy Fitness

Athletic activity is a regular part of many expectant mothers' lives. During pregnancy, exercise provides multiple benefits to body and mind: the enjoyment of the activity, better fitness and health, weight management, stress management, improved mood, and body benefits, including improved strength and decreased pain. Exercise can make labor easier, decrease back pain, and make child care less tiring. Although there are some important changes you must make to protect your child, with modifications, most types of exercise can be continued throughout pregnancy.

As with all aspects of pregnancy, there are many factors of which you need to be aware, especially if this is your first pregnancy. Remember, pregnancy is the beginning of a new stage of your life. You are responsible not just for yourself, but also for a wonderful child. This child's well-being and health depend on you. Using your skills in health management with exercise and fitness will preserve the health of both you and your baby.

Basic Guidelines

Once you suspect or know you are pregnant, you must start to listen to your body signals while exercising. Pay close attention to the four "F" fitness factors: *fahrenheit, fluids, food,* and *fatigue.* Ignoring these factors can cause problems with the development of your baby and the health of your pregnancy.

Fahrenheit

This refers to exercising in extreme temperatures. It is very important that you do not get overheated or feel hot while exercising. Your core body temperature actually rises while you exercise in extreme heat (over 80 degrees Fahrenheit). Problems with the neurological development of your baby can occur when your temperature goes up. For this reason, saunas, hot baths, and Jacuzzis are prohibited during pregnancy. This is particularly important during the first trimester. High temperatures also accelerate dehydration, another health risk during pregnancy.

Fluids

To avoid dehydration, a cause of early labor, make sure you are drinking plenty of fluids—about two cups a day more than before. During exercise, always have water or a sports drink available. You should sip at least every 10 minutes, and drink 1 cup for every 20 minutes of exercise. Your blood volume increases significantly with pregnancy and requires more fluids to maintain it.

Food

Because pregnancy is a higher state of metabolism and you burn sugars quicker than normal, you must provide your growing baby and yourself with enough fuel at all times. Before exercising, make sure you have eaten within the past two hours, and have a snack within the half hour after. If you are exercising for longer than one hour, it is recommended that you take a break and have a carbohydrate snack at least every half-hour during activity.

Fatigue

Because your baby's development depends solely on your body, it is much easier to feel fatigued during exercise. Do not push yourself through this. Stop when you feel tired, and especially if you are light-headed or short of breath. You might only be able to do one-third or one-half the exercise you did when you were not pregnant; some days, especially if you are active all day, you might not have energy to exercise at all. Rest if you are tired, and do not push your exercise to extremes. On these days, instead of a hard workout, consider a 20-minute walk, a gentle yoga class, or easy cycling. Sometimes, what you might really need is a nap.

The Four "F" Fitness Factors to Consider While Exercising During Pregnancy

FACTOR	WHAT TO CONSIDER	DETAIL
Fahrenheit	Avoid high temperatures.	You should *never* exercise or even relax in heat or temperatures above 90 degrees. Saunas, hot baths, and Jacuzzis are prohibited.
Fluids	Drink plenty!	You should never let yourself feel thirsty to prevent dehydration.
Food	Food is your fuel and is used up more quickly in pregnancy.	During pregnancy, you use up your body fuel stores faster; a carbohydrate snack should be eaten within a half hour of exercise and during exercise longer than one hour.
Fatigue	Rest is essential to your developing baby.	Fatigue is your body telling you that you need rest. Listen to your body and modify (or skip) your workout when you feel you need rest.

It is very important to discuss your athletic and workout activities, as well as your work and home schedule, with your doctor. Unless you have a chronic illness or problems with past pregnancies, you will probably be advised that it is safe to exercise in moderation. When asked for specifics, most physicians follow the very conservative and strict American College of Obstetric and Gynecology Exercise Guidelines.

Standard American College of Obstetric and Gynecology Exercise Guidelines

A 10- to 15-minute warm-up

An aerobic portion lasting no more than 20 to 30 minutes of easy to moderate intensity

A nonimpact activity (no jumping or running)

Careful heart rate monitoring to make sure heart rate does not go above 150 maximum, 145 if you are between the ages of 30 and 40, and 140 if you are over age 40

A gradual cooldown over a 5-minute period, followed by 5 to 10 minutes of gentle stretching to prevent blood from pooling in the legs and to maintain flexibility

---

These guidelines are designed to reduce health risks in all women. Athletic women who start at a much higher fitness level can usually tolerate more activity than these guidelines recommend, and no specific research has shown that impact activities are dangerous in healthy pregnancies. There are many accounts of women who jog for exercise throughout their pregnancies. Although this is not recommended for everyone and certainly very few doctors will admit that it is okay, there are also no specific studies to prove that it poses harm to the developing baby.

Still, moderation is an excellent adjective for all things in pregnancy; nothing, especially not exercise, should be done to excess. If you are a high-level athlete or exerciser who routinely does more than one hour a day of exercise, one hour a day should now be your maximum. Remember, even elite professional and competitive athletes can stay well trained with less activity during pregnancy because pregnancy is a constant "training state," stressing the body to physical limits in similar ways that exercise does. If you feel you are someone who is "addicted" to exercise and are not comfortable limiting yourself to one hour a day, you should see a counselor or therapist to determine why. Your mental health is just as important to the baby's health as your physical health is.

Basic Guidelines for Exercise in Pregnancy

Rest if you feel tired.

Avoid feeling hot.

Do not let yourself get thirsty.

Slow down if you feel short of breath.

Do not work out for more than 45 minutes at a time.

Have a snack immediately if you are working out for one hour.

Be flexible with your workout goals and cut back if you do not feel comfortable.

Skip your workout if you are nauseous, overly tired, or feel weak.

How Your Body Adapts

Your body changes to nurture the health of both you and your growing baby. The priority is to optimize blood flow and its supply of oxygen, fluid supply, nutrients, and temperature control to your baby. Just as your organs function to do this for you, they work at their maximum to do this for your baby.

Your heart rate increases to handle the larger volume of blood it pushes throughout the body in order to reach the fetus. Heart rate increases as the pregnancy goes on. By the third trimester, your heart rate can actually increase 10 to 15 beats per minute to accommodate the baby. This is demonstrated by an increase in pulse rate both at rest and while exercising.

Your blood increases in many ways: number of cells, volume (overall amount of fluid), and size of vessels. This allows it to more efficiently transport oxygen and nutrients to both mother and baby. Blood can also become slightly thicker, as it is carrying more nutrients and cells. This requires drinking increased amount of fluids to maintain proper blood flow.

Breathing can sometimes seem like work in pregnancy. Your breathing rate increases to supply oxygen to your baby and also to accommodate for your higher metabolism. Your body also becomes more sensitive to levels of humidity or change in air temperature, causing you to "overbreathe," or feel as if you are hyperventilating at times. Adding to your change in breathing is pressure on the breathing muscles (diaphragm and rib muscles) and lung space as your baby grows, making your lungs slightly smaller and less able to fully expand.

Temperature regulation is slightly impaired during pregnancy. Thicker blood and more red blood cells slow your body's natural cooling mechanism. Also, pregnancy hormones interfere with your normal thermostat that controls body temperature. This increase in temperature can be detrimental to a pregnancy, because research has shown that a fetus can develop abnormally if body temperature stays elevated for long. Therefore, you must avoid a rise in body temperature by not exercising in heat, wearing light clothing, and drinking cool fluids during exercise. If you have trouble judging your body temperature, check it with a thermometer while exercising; it should not go over 100 degrees. Exercising in heat also increases your risk of dehydration. Overheating should be avoided at all times, not just while exercising. It is for this reason that saunas, Jacuzzis, and hot tubs are prohibited during pregnancy.

Drinking more fluids is one of the most important changes you need to make to accommodate to pregnancy for many reasons, including preventing constipation, temperature regulation, maintaining increased blood flow, and higher breathing rate. Fluids are lost at increased amounts through digestion, sweat, in urine and stool, and through the lungs. Because your body system requires much more fluid when you are pregnant, it is very important to stay well hydrated.

During pregnancy, your body uses up its supplies of glycogen (stored energy) faster. The hormone changes of pregnancy require that you use carbohydrates as an immediate energy source during exercise, especially when exercise lasts longer than 45 minutes. With regular exercise, you need at least 400 to 500 more calories per day after the first trimester than you were eating before.

Body System Changes During Pregnancy

BODY SYSTEM	CHANGE
Heart	Increased rate
Lungs	Increased breathing rate, decreased lung space
Blood	Increased cells, thickness, volume
Blood vessels	Increased size and number
Metabolism	Increases
Body temperature control	Impaired
Glucose supplies	Used more quickly

WARNING Dehydration can cause decreased oxygen and nutrient supply to the baby, overheating, and early labor.

Your growing baby experiences the same responses to exercise you do: heart rate and temperature go up and blood sugar supply goes down. Remember this as you are exercising and considering whether to run that extra mile in the heat (don't!). Also, when you exercise, more of your blood is going to the muscles to allow them to work, taking some away from your baby. Therefore, if you are a competitive or professional athlete who wants to stay as fit as possible, it is recommended to split your workout into two 30- to 45-minute sessions at two different times of the day to decrease an overload of stress on the baby.

Exercise Guidelines During Pregnancy

Be able to say three sentences in a row without getting short of breath.

Do not allow yourself to feel hot for more than a few minutes.

Make sure you have carbohydrate snacks available for each 30 to 45 minutes of exercise.

Drink at least ½ cup of fluid for every 10 minutes of aerobic exercise or 15 minutes of light exercise.

Be aware of changes in balance and increased fall risk; avoid uneven or slippery terrain.

Rest if you have pain or feel weak or tired.

Always cool down for 5 to 10 minutes before resting completely.

During the last trimester, do not lie on your back for more than five minutes.

Muscles and joints change during pregnancy. They become looser and more stressed by your added weight and increased fluids in the body. Ligament looseness and increased joint flexibility occur because of the pregnancy hormones relaxin and progesterone. Also, as the baby grows, your center of gravity and sense of balance can be thrown off. This, along with ligament looseness, can lead to falls and ankle sprains as the joints lose stability, making racket sports, field sports, and running, jumping, or lunging sports more of a challenge and risk. Bouncy and forceful stretching should not be done to avoid overstretching or possibly tearing muscles, tendons, or ligaments.

Contraindications to Exercise

Medical problems that might restrict your exercise in pregnancy include heart or lung problems, infections, anemia, metabolic diseases, high blood pressure, bleeding, and problems with your cervix. If you have an eating disorder or trouble keeping weight on, your exercise should be limited. Problems with prior pregnancies or history of miscarriages might also impose restrictions on workout activity. Also, high levels of physical activity at work or home can limit exercise.

Reasons *Not* to Work Out in Pregnancy, as Determined by Your Doctor

Medical problems—high blood pressure, breathing problems, thin bones

Problems with previous pregnancies—more than three miscarriages, pre-eclampsia, pre-term labor

High-risk pregnancy—incompetent cervix, medical complications, high blood pressure, multiples

High level of physical activity at work or home

Warning signs to stop exercising completely include bleeding or fluid from the vagina, unusual swelling of the arms or legs, headache, dizziness, light-headedness, stomach pain, back pain, nausea and vomiting, contractions, heart palpitations, and severe shortness of breath. If these symptoms continue after resting for one hour, call your doctor right away.

Warning Signs to Stop Exercising

Vaginal fluid leakage or bleeding

Unusual swelling of arms or legs

Headaches, dizziness, light-headedness

Stomach pain, nausea, vomiting

Back or pelvic pain

Contractions

Heart palpitations

Being unable to catch your breath

Specific Sports Recommendations

The bottom line with regard to sports participation is preserving you and your baby's health. You must consider risk of falls, not only because this can affect the pregnancy, but also because x-rays, medications, and surgeries needed to evaluate and treat injuries can be harmful to the pregnancy. Repeated forceful impact can disrupt the placenta and put the pregnancy at serious risk. Environmental conditions such as high altitude and severe temperatures can interfere with the flow of oxygen and blood to supply the baby. These risks are relative to skill level and what your body is used to—for example, skiing at a high altitude is not recommended for most, but for a woman who lives at a high altitude and skis without falling, it can be done with caution due to other falling into her. General recommendations for sports are avoiding risks of falls and trauma, especially abdominal injury due to contact and impact. Falls should especially be avoided because impact can cause placental abruption, and orthopedic care of injuries such as x-rays or surgery can be risky to the fetus.

Activities Not Recommended/High-Risk Sports

INCREASED POTENTIAL FOR FALLS/TRAUMA	INCREASED RISK OF ABDOMINAL INJURY
Downhill and waterskiing	Hockey (field and ice)
Hang gliding, sky diving	Basketball
Horseback riding	Soccer
Skating	Boxing
Gymnastics	Wrestling
Rock climbing	Football
Scuba diving	Martial arts involving fighting/contact

Environment is very important to the health of your pregnancy. Vacationing or exercising at altitudes above 8,500 feet is not recommended due to lower oxygen content (unless you already live there, in which case your blood has adapted to this). If you are planning a ski or hiking trip, stick to the lower-altitude resorts. You can also be more prone to altitude sickness than when you are not pregnant, so beware of symptoms of light-headedness, headache, nausea, insomnia, poor appetite, or fatigue, and drink even more fluids than usual. As with any change in climate, take a few days to let your body adjust to the new altitude before beginning physical activity in the new environment. Temperature, as previously discussed, is a major consideration. Avoid exercising in temperatures above 80 degrees Fahrenheit.

Specific Sport Guidelines for Exercising During Pregnancy

Most sports can be continued with modifications. If you have any questions check with your doctor before participating. For all standing and weight-bearing exercises, make sure your shoes fit comfortably and are not too tight; it is common for feet to become swollen, so purchase shoes to accommodate. Also, make sure you have good cushioning to accommodate your added weight. Your exercise shoes should be replaced at least every three months. The following are generally recommended activity modifications:

- *Aerobics*—Avoid crowded, overheated rooms, and avoid advanced step or kickboxing classes to prevent falls or injury. After the second trimester, avoid bouncing movements and more than five minutes of lying on your back; do not do exercises lying on your stomach. Be careful that stretching is not done quickly or forcefully. Low-impact and water aerobics are less likely to cause injuries.

- *Cycling*—Changes in body weight, posture, and center of gravity can affect balance. A stationary bicycle is usually a safer choice. Elite-level cyclists might want to change from a racing bike to a mountain bike for more shock absorption and an upright position for increased comfort and visibility.

- *Racket sports*—As pregnancy progresses, decrease the aggressiveness of play to avoid falls and ankle sprains due to changes in center of gravity and coordination.

- *Running / jogging*—It is not recommended that you begin a running program during pregnancy, but if you have been running prior to your pregnancy, jogging can continue at shorter distances as long as you are physically comfortable, drink plenty of fluids, and stay cool.

- *Skiing/snowboarding*—Downhill activities should only be done if you are very experienced and do not fall. Cross-country skiing is much safer due to its much lower risk of falls. Special attention must be paid to fluid intake, as the cold weather makes you feel that you are not sweating, but you are. Follow the same fluid recommendations for any aerobic activity. Unless you already live at high altitude, you should not go above 3,000 feet. Most doctors prohibit skiing and snowboarding at all stages of pregnancy.

- *Swimming*—Swimming is one of the favorite pregnancy exercises, especially in the third trimester, when floating takes pressure off your spine and joints.

Do not dive or jump in the water, and extremes of water temperature need to be avoided. Swimming is not advisable if there is any vaginal fluid leak.

• *Weight training*—The goal of weight training in pregnancy is to maintain, not gain, strength. Routines should be modified with lighter weights and fewer repetitions with no straining. Proper breathing technique is important to avoid breath holding, which increases blood pressure, decreasing blood flow to the baby. Positions should be modified to avoid lying flat on your back in the third trimester. Avoid lifting weights so heavy that you would normally require a spotter.

Tips for Safe Jogging While Pregnant

Jog in the coolest part of the day.

Jog in air-conditioning if the temperature is above 80 degrees or humidity is above 90 percent.

Make sure you are always comfortable, not overexerting yourself, but feeling well.

Consider wearing a maternity support after the 5th month (see figure 15-1B).

Wear well-cushioned athletic shoes that are wide enough and fit well.

Wear an athletic bra with extra support.

Wear layered clothes that can be removed as you warm up.

Take water with you.

Stay within a 15-minute radius of home.

Consider jogging on grass to lessen impact.

Take a cell phone with you in case of emergency.

Be flexible with your workout goal and ready to decrease distance if you do not feel well.

Avoid strenuous hills.

Stick to populated areas.

Avoid sprinting.

Walk if you feel uncomfortable.

Wear a heart rate monitor and do not let your rate go over 150; 140 if you are over 40.

Spend the last 10 minutes walking to cool down.

Tips for Safe Swimming While Pregnant

Avoid crowded pools in which you might be kicked.

Avoid pools that feel too warm.

Keep a water bottle poolside and finish it by the time you are done.

Skip your "no breathers" until after pregnancy.

Stop and rest if you are short of breath.

Wear swim fins if you are having trouble moving through the water.

Stand in the pool or sit at the pool side for five minutes after swimming to avoid light-headedness or dizziness.

Avoid flip turns if they feel uncomfortable or lead to dizziness.

Tips for Safe Exercise Class Participation While Pregnant

Avoid crowded classes where you might bump into your neighbor.

Leave if the room becomes too hot.

Have water available, and drink every 10 minutes.

Work at your own pace, do not push yourself past what makes you comfortable.

Avoid advanced step or kickboxing classes due to risk of falls.

Do not participate in any repetitive bouncy or quick-stretching motions.

In the third trimester, do not lie on your stomach.

In the third trimester, lie on your side instead of your back whenever possible.

Use your own towel and wash your hands to prevent illness.

To date, no doctors or researchers can draw a specific line on what activities can and cannot be done during pregnancy. Everyone is different as to what they and their pregnancy can tolerate. However, to be sure, use the safe tips above and remember the following points: Make sure you are slowly gaining weight after the first trimester, about one pound per week; maintain your exercise activity at a *lower* level than you were doing before; make sure you are comfortable at all times during exercise. Remember that pregnancy changes actually improve your fitness level on its own. Your lower level of exercise will leave you extremely fit after pregnancy. Four to six weeks after a normal pregnancy and delivery, you should feel able to gradually return to your prior exercise routine and be back to feeling fit in two to three months.

Nutritional Demands

In active, athletic women, excess weight gain is rarely a problem. Guidelines for weight gain are about 3 to 5 pounds in the first trimester, then 1 pound per week thereafter after the first 3 months of pregnancy for a total of 25 to 35 pounds weight gain overall. Weight gains are adjusted slightly based on starting weight parameters: Underweight women can gain 30 to 40 pounds, normal weight women can gain 25 to 35 pounds, and overweight women can gain 15 to 25. Do not be concerned about this weight gain: It is necessary for your baby. It might sound like a lot because the baby weighs between 6 to 10 pounds, but the additional weight is essential for the health of your baby. This includes increased blood volume, amniotic fluid, the placenta (a bed of nutrition for the baby), and enlarged breasts. This weight is usually lost within the first few months after pregnancy, especially as you continue to exercise.

During pregnancy, you should eat three meals a day with a few snacks to keep your blood sugars stable and accommodate for the limited room your stomach has to expand as your baby grows. Eating smaller, more frequent meals also helps manage nausea during the first trimester. You should not diet or limit carbohydrates or fats or be on any type of restrictive diet, unless recommended by your doctor. You need the calories and fat in a well-balanced diet to feed your growing baby.

The exception to nutritional foods that should not be eaten in pregnancy includes foods that can become easily colonized with listeria. This is a bacteria that can lead to gastrointestinal, intrauterine, and cervical infections either with or without fever, nausea, vomiting, and diarrhea. It can also cause meningitis. In pregnant women, it is particularly dangerous, as listeria can cause miscarriages and stillbirths. Foods at risk of contamination with listeria include soft cheeses (brie, feta, Mexican cheese), unpasteurized dairy products, poorly stored deli meats that have not been heated to steaming, raw poultry, raw fish, raw meats, and smoked fish. Although fish is beneficial to the baby's developing nervous system, fish with a high content of mercury should be avoided. These include swordfish, large tuna steaks (albacore and most canned tuna is fine twice a week), tilefish, shark, and mackerel. Oysters and raw shellfish should be avoided due to other risks of diseases, including hepatitis A.

Foods That Should Be Avoided in Pregnancy

Soft cheeses—brie, camembert, feta, Mexican cheese, blue, or gorgonzola

Hot dogs, deli meats, meat spreads that have not been heated to steaming

Unpasteurized dairy products

Raw meat and poultry

Raw and smoked fish and shellfish

Swordfish, tuna steaks, mackerel, shark, and tilefish

Also, try to avoid processed and artificial foods. These include saccharine, which can cause cancer, and monosodium glutamate (MSG), which can raise blood pressure and cause diarrhea and allergic reactions in some people. MSG is found in many packaged products, including chips, cheesy crackers, gravies, soups, Chinese food, meat tenderizer, and some spice mixes. Other artificial sweeteners, such as Nutrasweet and Splenda may be used in moderation in pregnancy, as there has been no specific research proving their harm. Caffeine is not recommended at more than the equivalent of two six-ounce cups of coffee a day (or four eight-ounce servings of caffeinated soda or six-ounce cups of tea), as higher amounts might contribute to miscarriages. To be as safe as possible, eat natural foods and try to avoid chemical ingredients, other than vitamins and minerals, altogether.

Proper nutrition can sometimes be a challenge. During the first trimester, when morning sickness or general nausea peaks due to the rapid hormone changes of pregnancy, it might be hard to eat a well-balanced diet. During this time, try to get enough calories and fluids and take your prenatal vitamin. If the prenatal vitamin is making you feel sick or constipated, ask your doctor for a different brand. Until then, take calcium tablets and a multivitamin along with an extra 400 mg folate. Vitamin-fortified cereals, food bars, or drinks can also provide extra nutrients (read the labels). You might have to stop exercising for a while if you are unable to eat enough calories. After the first trimester, this should improve and you should be able to tolerate more foods along with your prenatal vitamin.

If you have severe problems with morning sickness, or nausea and vomiting during the day and night there are many things you can do to try to ease and even prevent it. These include smelling or tasting a lemon, ginger, or lavender; snacking on crackers or cookies; eating a small meal every two hours; and sipping very cold lightly sweetened or carbonated beverages.

Because nausea and vomiting can often last all day and even at night, be prepared with scents, foods, and drinks that work for you. If you are vomiting, try to take in as much fluid as you can. Sports drinks are recommended throughout the day to replenish lost electrolytes.

Tips to Help with Pregnancy Nausea

Lemon candies, scents, gum, or lemonade

Fresh ginger, ginger tea, candy, or gingerale

Peppermint tea, scents, and candy

A very cold drink or Popsicle

Essential oils that relieve nausea, including citrus, ginger, and lavender scents

Eat several small meals throughout the day

Have a carbohydrate snack every two hours between meals

Keep cookies, crackers, energy bars, or some cereal by your bed to snack on at night

Have a few bites of these foods when your alarm goes off; stay in bed another 15 minutes

Keep an icy cold drink at bedside to sip at night

Avoid strong-smelling food, caffeine, smoke, and garlicky, spicy, or fishy smells

Avoid fatty or spicy foods

Avoid large amounts of fluid on an empty stomach

Try a "Sea-Band" wristband, which works through acupressure points (available at pharmacies)

If you have a poor appetite, try shakes, smoothies, mashed potatoes, soups, cereal, and frozen yogurt

After the first three months, you must eat at least 300 calories more than when you were pregnant; if you are maintaining athletic activity, this increases to 500 calories. It is recommended that you increase the amount of protein you eat; consider doing this by adding an extra portion of lean red meat, which is an excellent source of iron. Dairy products are also an excellent choice to meet your increased calorie demands, as they contain not only protein but also calcium. Balance out your diet with nutrient-rich fruits and vegetables.

For exercisers in particular, taking your daily prenatal vitamin is extremely important, as you especially need additional B vitamins, calcium, and iron to support your active lifestyle. Folate is the B vitamin essential to pregnancy. Do not take any other vitamins or supplements not recommended by your doctor, as these can be harmful to the baby. You must be especially careful of vitamins A and K, which at high doses can contribute to birth defects.

Daily Nutritional Needs of Active Pregnant Women	
Iron	50 mg
Calcium	1,500 mg
Thiamine (B$_1$)	1.5 mg
Niacin	18 mg
Riboflavin (B$_2$)	1.6 mg
Pyridoxine (B$_6$)	2.3 mg (3)
Cyanocobalamin (B$_{12}$)	6 mcg (6)
Pantothenic acid	6 mg
Folate	600 mcg
Vitamin C	70 mg
Magnesium	360 mg
Vitamin D	400 Iu
Vitamin A	2800 Iu
Vitamin E	30 Iu
Zinc	20 mg

Fluid needs are extremely important, particularly with athletic activity. Losing and not replacing just 1 percent of your bodyweight through heavy breathing and minimally sweating—an amount of fluid lost before you even sense thirst—can disturb temperature control of the fetus. (If you weight 140 pounds, 1 percent is just 1.4 pounds!) Losing three to five times this amount in body water decreases oxygen supply to your baby. Therefore, you must not wait until you are thirsty to drink. Also, weigh yourself before and after exercise without clothes on to make sure you have consumed enough fluid during exercise. Dehydration during the last few months of pregnancy is also very risky, as this can lead to early labor. In general, two cups of fluid is required to replace each pound lost.

HEALTH TIP Flavored waters are a tasty alternative to plain water and will encourage you to drink more. You can make your own by putting a few pieces of cut-up fruit, cucumber, or citrus slices in refrigerated water for an hour.

Other Challenges of Pregnancy That Can Interfere with Being Active

Diabetes

Having gestational diabetes (diabetes in pregnancy), does not prohibit exercise. With your doctor's guidance, exercise at low and moderate levels is recommended to maintain blood sugars and insulin balance. You should have two doctors monitoring you, your obstetrician and your diabetes doctor (usually your internist, endocrinologist, or diabetologist). Blood sugars should be closely monitored when first starting the exercise, and you should have a snack available at all times. If you have diabetes, exercise sessions should not last more than 30 minutes unless you check and maintain normal blood sugars. Scheduling an appointment with a nutritionist who is a certified diabetes educator (CDE) is recommended to assist with evaluating and meeting your nutritional needs. This service is usually covered by health insurance. Drinking plenty of fluids is also especially important in diabetes and pregnancy.

Numbness

Numbness is a symptom that can occur in different areas of the body, including wrists and hands, feet, and occasionally the stomach and thighs. Patterns of numbness follow the path of nerves. Carpal tunnel syndrome, one of the most common causes of numbness, is hand and finger numbness, tingling, and pain. It is not known exactly why this occurs during pregnancy, but fluid retention is thought to contribute. To make sure these symptoms do not worsen, see a specialist if you have numbness with pain or problems lasting longer than one week. Wearing a wrist splint at night and during daily activities might be all you need to solve the problem. Carpal tunnel syndrome of pregnancy also responds to icing, stretching, and occupational therapy if the symptoms are severe. Additional vitamin B$_6$ can also help (ask your doctor before taking this). Carpal tunnel syndrome usually resolves a few months after pregnancy, although it can sometimes be made worse with child-care activities.

Leg Cramping

Leg cramping at night can be a common irritant during pregnancy. As long as the cramping goes away and is not accompanied by severe back pain or cramping elsewhere, leg cramps are not a sign of anything serious. Stretching or getting up and walking around usually relieves them. Stretching your legs before bed also can help. Sometimes, cramping is a sign that you are not eating enough salt, potassium, or calcium (see chapter 13, "Exercise Problems and Injuries"). Sports drinks are a good source of potassium and salt. You can also try taking an extra dose of calcium at bedtime.

Sore Breasts/Nipples/Belly Button

Tender and swollen breasts can occur early in pregnancy and cause discomfort during exercise and activities. Make sure you wear a supportive, well-fitting athletic bra to prevent irritation. As the pregnancy progresses, soreness of the belly button can also occur and cause discomfort when it rubs against your clothes during activities. Applying a large Band-Aid to belly button can help. If you are nursing, wear your supportive maternity bra and use lanolin on your nipples to ease the dryness.

Varicose Veins/Leg Swelling

Varicose veins can be common in pregnancy, although regular exercise makes them less likely. They can cause both lower leg and thigh tightness and pain, especially when standing. If varicose veins and swelling are a problem, consider taking up swimming (with a flutter kick). Moving your feet up and down and in circles throughout the day and elevating them as much as possible is also helpful. Support stockings not only help with symptoms but also prevent worsening of the varicosities. Under no circumstances should you take diuretics!

Poor Sleep

During the first and third trimester, pregnancy is infamous for interfering with sleep. Factors include breast and abdominal discomfort, leg cramps, baby's movements and having to go to the bathroom frequently during the night. This, along with the fatigue that is present in general, can lead to a stressed, emotional, exhausted expectant mother. Do not try to exercise on the days you have not slept well. You might also notice increased nausea on those days. Try to take naps if you can, and go to bed earlier at night.

Back and Pelvic Pain in Pregnancy and Exercise

Back and pelvic pain in pregnancy is very common and can be a significant concern in athletic pregnant women. Most pregnant women experience some type of back or pelvic ache or pain at some point in their pregnancy. Occasionally, pregnancy-related back or pelvic pain can continue beyond pregnancy; therefore, it is best to do the most you can to prevent it from becoming severe. Fortunately, as an active, strong woman, you are at less risk of serious back pain.

There are many types of back pain in pregnancy. Most is felt low in the middle back and pelvis, although it can be one sided or in the middle back. Some only get pain in the evening or at night. Back and pelvic pain is related to hormones, biomechanics, circulation, posture, and activity level.

Pregnancy hormones have multiple roles in the cause of back pain. They cause water retention in the tissues and ligaments, putting pressure on not just these structures but the joints as well. Also, the hormone unique to pregnancy, relaxin, leads to the pelvic loosening that is needed for childbirth. This hormone and the increased movement in the pelvis that occurs can cause pain at the sacroiliac joint and in other ligaments of the spine. Occasionally, the abdominal muscles can split (diastasis recti), compromising spine and abdominal stability. Stability problems in the back and abdomen can lead to increased risk of back pain. Strengthening surrounding and supporting muscles before and throughout pregnancy protects these looser structures and can prevent pain related to changes in stability.

Relaxin, the Hormone of Pregnancy

Causes loosening of ligaments and joints

Increased flexibility starts in the second trimester

Remains in the body for four to six months after pregnancy

Posture is a factor of back pain that can be modified. Maintaining good posture reduces the increased arch in the lower back that is so common to pregnancy. Muscles can get fatigued trying to hold certain positions, causing increased pain at the end of the day. Toward the end of pregnancy, you might walk a little differently or get out of a chair by leaning farther forward or twisting. Strengthening exercises to keep the spine and abdominal muscles strong will prevent body positions that cause more problems. Keeping your legs and core as strong as possible will prevent compromising movement patterns.

Symptoms of Back or Pelvic Pain Due to Ligament Looseness at the Pelvis

Pain stepping off a curb

Pain turning in bed

Pain climbing or descending stairs

Pain walking on uneven surfaces

Feelings of looseness or sliding in your joints

Diffuse middle and lower back pain is usually due to muscle spasms, strain, and fatigue. This dull and achy pain can be made worse bending, lifting, and sitting or standing for a long time. Sometimes, it can be sharp with sudden movements, and it is often worse at the end of the day. Weakness of the core stabilizing muscles, including the abdominal muscles, contributes to this discomfort. Middle and lower back pain of this nature usually is relieved with massage and stretching.

Symptoms of Back Pain Due to Muscle Strain

Dull, achy

Worse at the end of the day

No specific area that hurts

Better in the morning

How to Prevent Back Pain in Pregnancy

Begin an abdominal- and spine-strengthening program before becoming pregnant.

Allow yourself to recline when your back muscles feel tired (lay on your side on the 3rd trimester).

Wear comfortable, well-cushioned shoes when walking or standing.

Do gentle back stretches daily (see the end of this chapter).

Do strengthening exercises at least three or four times a week.

Avoid bending, lifting, twisting (no "BLT").

Consider swimming or water aerobics to unload the spine.

Less frequent types of back pain during pregnancy include sciatica, night pain, and bone pain. Sciatica, or leg pain related to back pain, can occur but is very rare. If you are having leg pain, weakness, or numbness in the legs or pelvis, see your doctor as soon as possible. Back pain at night is often attributed to sleeping position and can also result from day-long fatigue and gravity-related biomechanical stress. Sleeping on your left side is more comfortable and also ensures the best blood flow to both you and your baby. Osteoporosis can sometimes be a cause of back and pelvic pain in pregnancy, and although rare, is another reason for taking calcium supplements and vitamin D and making sure you have a healthy diet with enough protein, fat, and calories.

Severe, continuous back pain can be a sign of fetal distress. If back pain is associated with fever, bleeding, severe cramping, or fluid leaks, call your doctor at once. Other internal causes that can lead to back pain include urinary tract infections; stomach or digestive disorders, including constipation; lung or heart problems; or other organ problems. Having pain that is persistent and not relieved by changing position, activity, or rest needs to be evaluated by your doctor. Neurologic symptoms including numbness, weakness, and loss of reflexes require close medical supervision. Do not exercise if you are experiencing any of these dangerous symptoms.

WARNING Call your doctor immediately if you have severe back pain, bleeding, severe cramping, or fluid leaks.

Most back pain can be relieved with modifications in posture, positioning, and activity schedule. Avoid bending, lifting, and twisting without bending your knees and stabilizing your spine (suck in your lower belly with these movements). Avoid activities that make the discomfort worse (such as jogging). Do not wear high heels, and preferably wear walking shoes with extra cushioning. Be aware of sitting, sleeping, and activity positions and posture, and use lumbar cushions and pillows as needed. Using a wedge-shape pillow to support you abdomen while lying on your side can be helpful to relieve back and pelvic pressure. Relaxation techniques and 10 minutes of ice or heat packs to the painful area (not over the front of the abdomen or pelvis) can be helpful. Exercising or swimming in a pool can be very effective to prevent and treat back pain. An SI brace can be helpful with back and pelvic pain due to ligament looseness; a more supportive maternity brace can be worn for general back pain due to postural and muscle strain (see figures 15-1 A,B). The supportive "mother to be" brace may also be worn while exercising to prevent jostling.

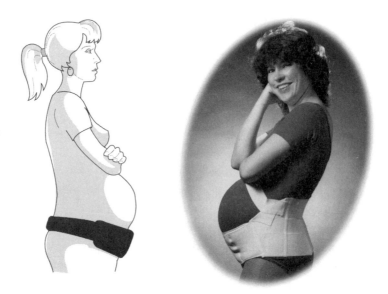

FIGURE 15-1 A: Maternity SI-LOC, side view. This brace is worn low under the baby to provide stability to the pelvis. B: Mother to be brace (this brace has an optional plastic back support). These are two of many types of braces such as this available for expectant mothers. (Photos courtesy of OPTP. See the resources at end of the book for purchase information.)

More aggressive, active treatment for back pain in pregnancy includes physical therapy, which is recommended for back pain that persists for more than a few weeks, seems to be worsening, or interferes with sleep or activities. Accepted alternative therapies include acupuncture, acupressure, and gentle manipulations. Do not use whirlpools, saunas, or heat over the abdomen and pelvis. The safest medication to take for pain relief is Tylenol; do not take any other medications, even those without a prescription, unless you ask your doctor first.

Management of Back Pain in Pregnancy

Posture maintenance

Lumbar and support cushions for sitting

Wedge-, J-, or C-shape pillows for sleeping on your side

Frequent repositioning

Sacroiliac belts or maternity supports

Ice packs

Lukewarm baths with Epsom salts

Relaxation

Physical therapy

Moderate exercise

Pool exercises

Stretching programs

Massage on your side or in a chair

Occasional Tylenol (acetomenophen) tablets

If back pain continues after pregnancy, more aggressive treatments can be helpful and curative. See a sports medicine or back doctor (orthopedist or physiatrist) as soon as possible to prevent the pain from becoming chronic. You might need x-rays or an MRI to evaluate the cause. If you are breastfeeding, check with your pregnancy-care physician or pediatrician before taking medications for pain.

Exercise Equipment and Clothing

To accommodate for temperature changes during exercise, you should wear layers of loose, breathable clothing. The newer synthetic materials are excellent to exercise in as they "breathe," preventing heat from getting trapped inside the clothes. Be aware that wearing a hat keeps heat in. Switch to a visor to keep the sun out of your face but let your heat out.

As your breasts increase in size, you will need more support. Most athletic stores have a range of sizes of supportive athletic bras; you can also order from the manufacturers (see the resources at end of the book).

Your shoes should be well cushioned and supportive. You might need a half or full size larger to accommodate to fluid retention. Too tight shoes can cause unnecessary numbness, tingling, and pain. Be careful not to have shoes that are too big, however, as shoes that are loose can cause you to trip and fall. Getting a few bigger-size pairs of shoes in pregnancy is a very worthwhile investment. If you have trouble finding wider sizes, consider looking in the men's or boy's department, as their shoes are wider throughout.

Special Situations in the Third Trimester

> WARNING **Lying on your back for more than five minutes in the third trimester can compromise blood flow to the baby.**

During the third trimester, your body size is growing to its maximum. Due to your expanding size, you might find engaging in high-impact activities or brisk walking uncomfortable. It can be more difficult to get around as quickly as you did before, so slow down! You should eliminate any activities in which you might fall or where quick stops and starts are needed such as in tennis or field sports. Balance is challenged by your new size, looser ligaments, and loss of sight of your feet. Your added weight can further stress your joints in your feet, ankles, knees, hips, and, of course, back.

Organs can become crowded by the size of your baby. Because the space for your lungs is compromised, you might feel more easily short of breath. Your bladder cannot hold as much urine as before, and pressure from the expanded uterus might cause you to urinate more frequently. You might have trouble holding in your urine with coughing or if your bladder gets too full. Do not let this stop you from drinking enough fluids. Even if you have to go to the bathroom every 30 minutes or wear mini pads, keep drinking.

Sleeping can become a challenge due to difficulty getting comfortable and frequent urination. Let yourself take naps, and remember that rest is essential to your and your baby's health. Try to lie on your left side as much as possible; not on your back. If you are too tired to exercise due to a bad night's sleep, rest.

Braxton-Hicks contractions are mini-contractions that help reposition the baby, but if they become frequent, they are a sign that you need to rest. If you get them while being active, stop and rest. Drink an extra glass of water, and if they do not stop, lie on your left side. If they last longer than 30 minutes or are closer than 10 minutes apart, call your doctor.

After Childbirth

After childbirth, your body needs about six weeks to return to its normal anatomy and physiology. Most precautions at this time are to protect the uterus; it is still enlarged and healing, and the cervix is still open. To prevent bacteria from entering the uterus, you should not use tampons for bleeding in the first month after childbirth. If you had a cesarean section, you might need longer before beginning activity to allow the incisions to fully heal. Check with your doctor for more specific guidelines.

Impact activities are not recommended during the time immediately after delivery, as this can cause increased uterine bleeding and stretching of the ligaments that hold up your uterus. Swimming should also be avoided until vaginal bleeding or episiotomy tears have healed. A healing episiotomy also limits cycling, although riding a recumbent bike with padded shorts is possible as long as it is not irritating the area.

You should gradually return to exercise. If you find that you bleed heavily after a workout, rest for a few days then try again at less intensity. Also be aware that your ligaments throughout your body are still loose, and you can be prone to ankle or ligament sprains. Because breasts remain enlarged throughout breastfeeding, continue to wear your extra-supportive athletic bra; this also prevents nipple irritation. You might need to put gauze over your nipples if they are sore, and wear nursing pads to prevent leakage. If you are breastfeeding, you still need to follow pregnancy guidelines for nutrition, including extra calories and fluids.

Having trouble controlling urine, or incontinence, is a common problem after childbirth due to the stretching of all structures. This improves over time and with Kegel exercises. If you are still having difficulty with incontinence after two months, speak to your doctor about it. If you have associated burning, funny odor, or are urinating often, you might have a urinary tract infection.

Kegel Exercises

These are exercises to strengthen the muscles at the base of your pelvis and help support your urinary muscles. Kegels are done by squeezing the vaginal muscles as if you are stopping your flow of urine. Hold each contraction for 5 to 10 seconds. They should be done 10 to 20 times 3 to 5 times a day. They can be done anywhere, and no one can see you doing them.

Fatigue is very common after childbirth for many reasons. You are probably not sleeping through the night with the challenges of baby care, and your body is healing. You might also be slightly anemic after delivery, which contributes to tiredness. Listen to your body and let it rest and heal as best you can. This will make you a better mother and preserve your health and fitness in the long run. If you are too fatigued for daily activities, speak with your doctor.

In Summary Remember:

1. Pregnancy is not the time to try to take on a new program, improve your fitness level, or increase your exercise program. Your goal should be to maintain a healthy level of fitness at moderate levels of intensity. After you give birth, this will translate into healthy fitness at higher levels of intensity.

2. You should discuss your exercise program with your doctor and be aware of any special risks or precautions.

3. Remember you need more calories, vitamins, and fluids.

4. Do not allow yourself to overheat.

5. Breathable athletic wear with a supportive bra should be worn. Shoes might have to be bigger than when not pregnant to accommodate for swelling.

Just as pregnancy is a time for growth of a baby, it is a time to preserve and maximize your own health. Regular exercise is an integral part of that, but it should be *healthy* exercise, not exercise to exhaustion. You should be eating well, including enough calories and a well-balanced diet. You should be in tune with your body and call your doctor if you have any questions or notice strange symptoms. Allow yourself rest if you are feeling tired, sore, or ill. Remember that pregnancy actually improves fitness and metabolic performance; you can maintain your high level of cardiovascular fitness with less exercise.

Recommended Exercise Routine to Keep You Fit and Healthy Four to Six Days a Week

Monday, (Wednesday,) Friday
Walk 20 to 40 minutes

Have a small (100 to 200 cal) carbohydrate snack plus (at least) 12 ounces of fluid

Upper body strengthening, using 3- to 8-pound weights (choose four to six exercises from chapter 7, figures 10–16, 18, 19, and chapter 8, figures 15–17), varying exercises on different days.

Two sets of 10 hands and knees trunk stability (see chapter 9, figure 17)

Two sets of 10 bridges with a Kegel exercise held through each up motion (see chapter 9, figure 9). In third trimester, do 2 sets of 5 and lie on your side in between

Three sets of 10 Kegel exercises with each of 3 standing balance exercises (see chapter 12, figures 7 through 9)

Cat and cow (see chapter 9, figure 16)

Stretch upper body (see chapter 7, figures 20 through 23 and chapter 8, figure 14)

Stretch back (see chapter 9, figures 28 through 30)

Tuesday, (Thursday,) Saturday
Swim, stationary cycle, cross-country ski, or elliptical machine, 20 to 40 minutes (or walk)

Have a small (100 to 200 cal) carbohydrate snack plus (at least) 12 ounces of fluid

Lower body strengthening (choose four to six exercises from chapter 10, figures 7 and 8, and chapter 11, figures 6 through 9 and 11), varying exercises on different days

Two sets of 10 crunches (see chapter 9, figure 6; during third trimester on ball, figure 8)

Two sets of 10 wall seats with a Kegel contraction during the seated hold (see chapter 11, figure 15)

Two sets of 10 double ball obliques (see chapter 9, figure 22)

Two sets of 10 ball roll-outs with a Kegel contraction as you hold the ball out (see chapter 9, figure 19)

Stretch lower body (choose 6 stretches from chapter 9, figures 23 through 27, chapter 10, figures 25 and 28, chapter 11, figures 16 and 18, and chapter 12, figures 20 through 22). Vary stretches on different days.

Do lying stretches on your side in third trimester.

Back stretches (see chapter 9, figures 28 through 30)

Sunday—REST!!!

Optional: Substitute one to three workouts a week with a prenatal exercise class, yoga class, or water aerobics class.

For advanced athletes, replace walking with jogging or another aerobic sport if it is comfortable for you. If your aerobic portion is more than 40 minutes, eat 100 to 200 calories of carbohydrates every half hour and drink two cups of fluids each half hour.

Remember to take the day off or cut back your exercise time if you are too tired.

CHAPTER SIXTEEN

Sports-Specific Injuries

Playing style, technique, rules of play, equipment, level of contact, level of competition, and level of training can all contribute to risks of injuries. There are many injuries common to particular sports and activities such as swimmer's shoulder, tennis elbow, golfer's elbow, skier's thumb, runner's knee, turf toe, and dancer's fracture. Contact sports such as team court and field sports are associated with more traumatic injuries. Sports and athletic activities requiring explosive bursts of speed, cutting and turning maneuvers, and jumping and landing increase risk of injury to the lower body.

There are other factors less predictable that contribute to injury risks. These include weather conditions, playing surface conditions, and faulty equipment. Past pain or injuries can suddenly reoccur during play. Weakness that was not noticed can cause injury if the area is stressed and falters. Overuse of a joint or muscle group always can lead to pain and injury.

In general, sports injuries can be classified as either due to accident (trauma) or wear and tear (overuse). Regardless, there is a lot that can be done to prevent injuries. Knowing what you are at risk for is half the battle. Following is a description of the most frequent injuries related to each fitness activity. In preventing these injuries, a focus is also placed on maintaining overall health and conditioning, as this can often be overlooked in a highly competitive environment.

Sports-Specific Injuries

Aerobics, Circuit, Kickboxing, and Exercise Classes

Although these activities are fun and usually offer a great cardio workout, the repetitive motions can lead to a variety of overuse injuries, especially if techniques are poor. Instructors should be well trained on enforcing proper form and instruct activities that do not cause injuries, but it is often difficult for them to watch everyone in class closely enough. Occasionally, they themselves do not demonstrate proper technique.

The faster the pace of a class, the more equipment used, and the larger the range of repetitive movements, the more likely an injury. Improper posture, poor balance, and quick, uncontrolled movements can lead to ankle sprains, shoulder tendinitis, knee bursitis and tendinitis, and muscle sprains. Squats, lunges, and dead lifts, common exercise class moves, often cause knee or back stress, pain, and injury. Repetitive quick twisting and kicking motions in kickboxing classes are risky to backs and legs. Weights that are gripped too tightly or too heavily can lead to wrist, arm, and shoulder injuries. Foot injuries can also be due to shoes that have insufficient support or have lost their cushioning or support from overuse. Ankle sprains, plantar fasciitis, and calf injuries are common.

To prevent injuries in exercise classes: Do not take more than three of the same class a week, alternating days with other activities or rest. Do not do any movements or activities or use weights or equipment you are uncomfortable with, and especially avoid those that cause pain. Ask your instructor if you have questions regarding techniques. If you do not feel you get a reasonable answer, take a class with a different instructor. Make sure you get new shoes every three to six months, especially for high-impact, jumping classes.

Factors Increasing Risk of Exercise Class Injuries

Faster pace of class	Large motions
More types of equipment used	Quick, repetitive movements

Basketball

The most common injury to a basketball player is an ankle sprain. Knee injuries to the ACL and meniscus can also be common, along with finger dislocations, jams, and fractures. Contact injuries and falls can result in more serious injuries. Overuse injuries can lead to sprains, strains, and tendinitis, including jumper's knee (patellar tendinitis).

> ACL injuries can occur three to six times more in female than male basketball players. ACL tears usually require surgery and three to six months of recovery time.

To prevent injuries in basketball: Knee injuries can be prevented with quad and hamstring strengthening, balance activities, and improved jumping and landing techniques. An excellent conditioning program includes cutting maneuvers, skill drills, and single-leg jumping and landing techniques. Box jumping, side stepping, running cones, and jumping rope on one leg is great practice.

Bowling

Bowlers can get back, knee, elbow, wrist, and finger sprains. Most injuries are soft tissue sprains or tendinitis, although occasional injuries occur related to falls or dropped balls.

To prevent bowling injuries: Bowlers should do general strengthening and stretching exercises for the back, legs, and arms. Wrist- and upper-arm-strengthening exercises are also recommended. Bowlers should also add 30 minutes of cardiovascular activities to their workout schedules 3 to 5 days a week.

Boxing

Besides expected contact injuries, boxers tend to suffer upper extremity injuries, including wrist, elbow, and shoulder sprains. Shin splints, Achilles tendinitis, plantar fasciitis, and knee and leg tendinitis can occur due to repeated short, quick steps and jump-rope training.

To prevent boxing injuries: Upper body strengthening is recommended, particularly to the wrists and shoulders. Proper punching, jabbing, and defensive techniques are crucial to avoiding overuse injuries. Wrapping should be done correctly to protect the fingers, hands, and wrists. Protective gear, including headpiece, mouthpiece, chest guards, and groin protectors, should be adequate and fit properly so they are optimally functional. It is suggested to wear well-cushioned, supportive cross-training shoes when training to prevent overuse injuries in the legs, ankles, and feet.

Cheerleading

With advanced cheerleading there is a risk of serious traumatic injuries and fractures due to falls. Jumping and landing can cause ankle and knee injuries. Wrist, elbow, and shoulder injuries can occur from repetitive quick motions. Because cheerleaders are usually thin, they are at higher risk of eating disorders and stress fractures (see chapter 4, "Weight Concerns and Body Image").

To prevent cheerleading injuries: General strengthening of the upper and lower body should be done two to three times a week. Stretching should be done daily to maintain flexibility. Balance training is helpful to prevent ankle sprains and falls.

Climbing

The upper body is susceptible to injuries in climbing. Handholds can result in finger tendon injuries; tendinitis and nerve injuries can also occur from the strain and stretch of climbing holds. To prevent catastrophic injuries, climbing should never be done alone, and preferably with a very experienced climber. Wearing a helmet is recommended to prevent head injuries due to accidents or falling debris.

To prevent climbing injuries: Climbers should do general body strengthening two to three times weekly. Wrist-strengthening and balance exercises are excellent injury prevention measures. Learning proper technique and having working and correctly used equipment is crucial to safety and injury prevention.

Cycling

Cycling often leads to repetitive motion injuries, particularly knee pain. Tendinitis of the knee, Achilles, and hip can occur. Nerve injuries can occur across the wrist and in the feet due to positioning and pressure on these areas. Neck pain is common and can occasionally be serious, with disc herniations leading to pinched nerves. Thigh and genital irritation can occur with long rides in the heat. Falls can lead to severe abrasions, fractures often to the collarbone, and head injuries.

To prevent cycling injuries: Always wear a helmet, and ride a bike appropriate for your size. Padded gloves can prevent hand pain. A comfortable or cut-out seat and padded shorts will protect the genital area. You should be extremely familiar with clicking in and out of cleats and know how to shift without looking down. Biking alone is not recommended; having a cell phone is an excellent idea in case of emergency. Because cycling is easy on most joints, correcting seat and bike alignment usually corrects pain in the knees, hips, or neck. Stretching in the opposite direction of the crouched cycling position should be done after riding with extension exercises (arched head, neck, and back) to improve posture. Yoga twice a week would be an excellent way to prevent posture problems and establish core strength and stability. Weight-bearing exercises such as walking, hiking, or jogging with upper body strengthening should be done two to three times a week to protect bones.

Dance

Injuries vary between types of dance. In general, hip, lower leg, and back pain is most common due to a frequently arched back. Ankle, foot, and toe problems can result from *en-pointe* exercises. Poor turnout can lead to hip problems. Knees can be strained and cartilage torn from twisting, rotation, squatting, jumping, and landing, resulting in knee, foot, and ankle tendinitis. Stress fractures and dancers fractures (foot) can also occur, especially in thin dancers who also are at risk of eating disorders.

To prevent dance injuries: Proper technique and flexibility is crucial. Rest is essential to prevent overuse injuries. Proper nutrition with adequate calories and calcium is necessary to prevent stress fractures. Abdominal or core strengthening should be done at least three times weekly to prevent back pain and injury.

Diving

Neck and back injuries can be common from high-velocity movements and impact of water entry. Shoulders can become unstable and painful. Repeated high-velocity water impact can cause wrist tendinitis and chronic sprains. Back injuries, including spondylolisthesis, can occur. Jumping results in overuse ankle and lower leg injuries. Other traumatic injuries include contusions and lacerations and occur more often in 10 M platform diving. Divers can also develop problems with their ears or repeated dizziness.

To prevent diving injuries: Overall strengthening along with core stabilization such as pilates should be done three times weekly. The focus should be on back, abdominal, shoulder, and wrist strengthening. Stretching should be done daily to maintain necessary flexibility. Lower leg strengthening and stretching should be done three times weekly to prevent calf, ankle, and foot pain and injury. Proper nutrition and adequate calories are crucial, as divers are at high risk of eating disorders leading to poor bone health.

Fencing

Activities in fencing are done primarily on one side of the body, leading to overuse injuries on that side. Leg overuse injuries include iliotibial band syndrome and plantar fasciitis. Ankle sprains, foot injuries, knee ligament sprains, meniscus tears, and wrist and hand tendinitis can also occur. Lumbar sprains, along with other causes of back pain, can be common due to the forward posture. Traumatic injuries are a risk from the weapon.

To prevent fencing injuries: Leg and spine strength and flexibility is essential. To maintain posture and promote body balance, core strengthening and stretching such as yoga should be done at least twice weekly.

Field Hockey

Like most field sports, ankle sprains are most common. Spine pain and even disc herniations can occur due to bending and rotating required during play. Knee injuries of all types can be frequent. Hand, wrist, and elbow sprains can occur. Due to the contact nature of the sport, as well as the use of sticks and balls, fractures, shoulder and knee trauma, and head and face injuries can occur.

To prevent field hockey injuries: Balance drills and overall body strengthening and stretching should be done three times weekly. Proper technique is important in stick and ball handling to prevent overuse injuries of the wrists and back, and equipment should be properly sized.

Golf

Improper conditioning and technique can lead to overuse injuries, such as shoulder impingement and epicondylitis (golfer's elbow). Back pain and injury is most common and can be chronic and problematic. Wrist pain and tenosynovitis along with trigger fingers and wrist ganglia can occur. Stress or impact fractures can include those in the wrist, ribs, and spine.

To prevent golf injuries: Conditioning exercises including wrist and shoulder exercises and back and abdominal strengthening should be done three times weekly. Stability ball exercises, including rotational torso maneuvers, are quite popular among golfers. Regular golfers should do spine and upper body flexibility exercises. Technique is crucial to reducing overuse injuries.

Gymnastics

As a sport that challenges entire body strength, balance, and flexibility, both chronic and acute injuries can occur. Repetitive spine movements in many planes can contribute to spondy and disc problems. Wrist pain and injury is also quite frequent, including stress fractures, tendon tears, ganglion cysts, and chronic tendinitis. Elbow and shoulder problems can also be common. Due to constant jumping, running, and landing, ankle and knee injuries are also frequent. Body image problems and eating disorders are common to gymnasts.

To prevent gymnastic injuries: Training sessions should be no longer than two hours with plenty of fluids available throughout practice, and there should be at least one day of rest a week. Proper nutrition and adequate calories are essential to health and optimum performance along with prevention of stress fractures. Overall strength and conditioning should be done in addition to technical training three times weekly.

Horseback Riding

Overuse injuries include inner thigh sprains and hip and pelvic bursitis. Low back pain can occur, with possible disc injuries. Traumatic falls are the most threatening and can include head, spine, and limb injuries and fractures. Fractures to the collar bone, upper arm, elbow, and wrist and hand are most common. Asthma can also be problematic due to environmental allergies.

To prevent riding injuries: Spine and leg strength and flexibility should be optimal. Riders should incorporate weight-bearing exercises along with upper body strengthening three times weekly to protect bone health and overall health and fitness. Because of the seriousness of accidents that might occur, technique and equipment is crucial; a rider should never go without a bit to control the horse. Saddles and stirrups should fit both horse and rider properly. A helmet is essential.

Ice Hockey

Lower body injuries are most common, particularly hamstring, groin, and inner thigh sprains and tears. Knee ligament and meniscus tears and sprains can also occur, along with ankle and foot injuries. Traumatic injuries include cuts and bruises, concussions, spine injuries, shoulder separations, and fractures to the upper and lower body. Skin rashes can sometimes occur due to ill-fitting or wet, moldy padding.

To prevent hockey injuries: Inner thigh and groin stretching should be done prior to going on the ice. Overall leg and spine conditioning should be done three times weekly. Upper body strengthening should be added to promote overall fitness. Equipment including chest plates, head and mouth gear, and skates should fit properly and be allowed to air and dry out regularly.

Military Training/Obstacle Course

Due to explosive bursts of speed, climbing, cutting, and jumping, both major and minor traumatic injuries are possible. Overuse injuries occur such as march fractures (stress fractures of the metatarsals), Achilles tendinitis, and plantar fasciitis. ACL tears have been studied as occurring nearly 10 times more frequently in female military personnel than in males. Other knee, shoulder, wrist, and hand injuries can also occur.

To prevent military training and obstacle course injuries: Overall body conditioning is essential, including balance exercises, core stability, and shoulder and leg strengthening. Lower body stretching should be done daily. Technique should be optimal and special care taken when fatigued so as not to fall.

Mountain Biking

Along with common cycling injuries, wrist, elbow, and shoulder tendinitis, sprains, and stress fractures, and pelvic, hip, and knee bursitis can occur. The greatest risk of mountain biking is due to falls; collar bone fractures are most common.

To prevent mountain biking injuries: Ride within your abilities with equipment you are comfortable with. Your bike should be properly fit with brakes and gears working optimally. Helmets are essential and should fit snugly. Shoe clips should be adequate, and you should know how to easily get in and out. Riding alone is not recommended! Carrying a cell phone is an excellent idea in case of emergency.

Rowing

The repetitive high-resistance movements of rowing can lead to many overuse injuries. Mid and lower back pain is frequent; rib stress fractures and disc disorders can also occur. Bursitis of the hip and pelvic areas can also occur. Forearm and wrist tendinitis, DeQuervain's tenosynovitis, and extensor tendinitis are common due to feathering (rotating) the oar. Traumatic injuries can occur from lifting the boat, or "catching a crab," in which the oar gets pulled under the boat. Cross-training can also lead to injuries, as weight training is usually strenuous. Knee problems such as patellofemoral and iliotibial band syndromes can occur secondary to hill and squat training. Palm and finger blistering is frequent and can lead to infection if not properly managed.

To prevent rowing injuries: The most important conditioning exercises are spine and abdominal strengthening and wrist strengthening. Proper technique, especially initiating each stroke with the legs, is crucial to protect the back and arms from injury. Coxswain commands and stroke pace are important to prevent catching crabs. Conditioning exercises should avoid high-velocity, repetitive motions and protect the back and knees from repeated stress. Rest is important. To manage blisters, antibiotic ointments applied while sleeping helps promote quick healing.

Rugby

Because rugby is a high contact sport, shoulder dislocations, sprains and instabilities, ACL tears, face and eye injuries, and collarbone, rib, and finger fractures are possible traumatic injuries. Quad and hamstring strains, hip pointers, and lower leg injuries can also occur due to both overuse and trauma during field play. As in all field sports, ankle sprains are the most frequent injuries.

To prevent rugby injuries: Rotator cuff strengthening should be done three times weekly. Stretching of the spine and legs should be done before and after play. Balance and agility drills should be done three times weekly to prevent knee and ankle injuries. The playing field should be well maintained so the surface is even.

Running

Both endurance and sprint training lead to overuse leg injuries, the most common of which are iliotibial band syndrome, plantar fasciitis, metatarsalgia, Achilles and tibial tendinitis, and shinsplints. Sprinters frequently suffer hamstring sprains. Knee pain can also be common; runner's knee is patellofemoral syndrome; patellar tendinitis or jumper's knee can also be problematic. Meniscus injuries can occur from running on uneven terrain. Bursitis of the pelvis, hips, and knees can occur also as an overuse injury. Shinsplints are overuse injuries also associated with improper foot alignment in the shoe and also lower leg weakness. Morton's neuromas, tarsal tunnel, and bunions and blisters can also occur frequently in women due to improper shoe size worn while running and uncomfortable-fitting dress shoes. Compartment syndrome and stress fractures are the most serious running injuries. Eating disorders are more common in runners who desire to maintain an ultra-light frame.

To prevent running injuries: Conditioning should include hip, knee, and lower leg, ankle, and foot strengthening three times weekly, with stretching daily. A stretch-out strap or rope is recommended to promote optimum hamstring, calf, and foot flexibility. Proper shoe fit, arch support, and cushioning can also prevent shinsplints and foot pain. Shoes should be replaced every 300 miles in frequent runners, and rotated through two pairs if running is done daily. Banked running surfaces should be avoided, or running directions alternated if unavoidable. Adequate fluid and nutritional intake is essential for optimum performance and best health. The diet should contain recommended amounts of calcium to protect the bones and iron to prevent anemia.

Tips to Prevent Running Injuries

Shoes should be replaced every 300 miles.

Shoes should have adequate arch supports.

Avoid uneven and banked running surfaces.

Stretch after running.

Do toe curls and calf stretches daily.

Ice after a run if you have pain and take a day or two off until it feels better.

Scuba Diving/Snorkeling

It has been speculated that women are more susceptible to decompression sickness, but this is still under debate. Pregnancy is a contraindication to diving. Injuries are not frequently reported but are often secondary to equipment, marine life, and terrain. Hypothermia is a concern.

To prevent scuba diving injuries: Knowledge of terrain and equipment is most vital. Scuba diving should never be done alone. Having proper vision, swimming skills, and wet suits will prevent many injuries.

Skating

Figure skaters, like dancers, can suffer from back pain due to spondy, sprain, and disc injury. Thigh pain due to hamstring sprains and adductor tears and pulls can be chronic. Knee pain is also common secondary to bursitis or ligament sprains. Achilles tendinitis, foot tendinitis, and chronic injuries can also be problematic; even blisters can lead to other problems as position changes for pressure relief. Collisions, falls, and jumping and landing can result in fractures of the ankle, tibia, distal radius, femur, and patella, along with wrist sprains, shoulder separations, and knee and wrist ligament tears. Head injuries also occur. Figure skaters are at high risks for eating disorders and stress fractures.

To prevent skating injuries: Core strengthening should be done three times weekly, along with leg and knee strengthening. Flexibility is crucial, and stretching should be done daily. Proper technique will also prevent injuries. Skates should fit perfectly and not cause pressure on any one area of the foot or ankle. Rest is essential, as is adequate nutrition and calorie intake. Addressing injuries early is very important to prevent the injury from becoming chronic or causing other problems.

Skiing

Skiing is notorious for knee injuries. ACL injuries occur more frequently in women. Meniscus and collateral ligament sprains and tears can also occur, along with patellar dislocations. Falls and caught poles can cause skier's thumb (a ligament tear) and shoulder injuries. Traumatic injuries include fractures of the arm, shoulder dislocations and separations, and thigh, pelvic, thumb, and wrist fractures. Collisions with other skiers, objects, and ski and lift equipment raises the risk of traumatic injuries. Environmental hazards include terrain, trees, tree wells, and ice; deep, heavy snow can increase knee injury risks also. Head injuries can be deadly. Traumatic injury risks decrease with Nordic and cross-country skiing.

To prevent skiing injuries: Quadriceps and hamstring strengthening should be done three times weekly. Core strengthening and balance drills help prevent falls. Equipment suited to skill level with bindings adjusted to release properly is crucial to injury prevention. Skiing within your skill level and being aware of terrain and conditions that might be threatening such as ice, poor visibility, or avalanche risk is essential. Helmets are advised, especially if tree skiing. Tree wells must be avoided. Nutrition is important, with adequate calorie and fluid intake; iron should also be adequate to prevent the anemia documented in female skiers. In skiing and mountain sports, heed the rule of threes: most injuries are likely to occur on the third day, after 3 P.M. and over 3,000 feet.

INJURY PREVENTION **Listen to your body and rest when you are tired—skiing injuries occur more often at the end of the day when you are tired.**

Snowboarding

Because of the daring nature of flips, jumps, and obstacle riding, traumatic injuries occur most in freestyle snowboarding. Common injuries are to the wrist and forearms including sprains, tendon tears, and fractures. Shoulder dislocations, chest injuries, rib fractures, and head injuries can also occur. Snowboarder's ankle is a fracture of the top of the ankle, most often caused by a fall.

To prevent snowboarding injuries: Knowing your terrain and riding within your limits is most important to prevent serious injuries. Abdominal and core strengthening can prevent falls. Educated falling with arms in, not outstretched, will prevent shoulder separations and dislocations, along with wrist and arm fractures. Helmets should be encouraged to prevent head injuries, due to the likelihood of backward falls. Tree wells must be avoided.

Soccer

A variety of soccer injuries can occur due to field play, sprinting, kicking, and contact injuries. Ankle and knee sprains and injuries are most common, followed by back injuries, thigh and calf contusions, tears, and sprains. ACL tears are up to five times more common in female soccer players than in males. Goalkeepers are at more risk of arm and shoulder sprains and tendon injuries. Meniscus, ligament injuries, and patellar syndromes also occur. Turf toe, footballer's ankle, a pinched nerve in the ankle, inner thigh and hamstring sprains and tears, foot sprains, and stress fractures can also be problematic. Heading the ball can cause head and neck injuries.

To prevent soccer injuries: Balance and agility training is crucial for knees and ankles. Hamstring and quadriceps strength is important to prevent ACL injuries. Fields should be maintained and level. While cross-training, well-cushioned shoes should be worn. Core strength prevents abdominal and back injuries while promoting more powerful kicks. Kicking techniques should be optimum to prevent foot and ankle injuries.

Softball, Baseball, and Fast-Pitch Softball

Shoulder, elbow, wrist, and finger injuries are common due to both overuse and trauma from striking the ball, sliding into bases, or collisions. Ankle sprains are common. The foot-first sliding technique can result in ankle, foot, and knee ligament sprains, tears, and fractures. Sprinting can lead to hamstring and quadriceps sprains and strains. Pitching injuries include shoulder instability, inflammation, and tears, along with Little Leager's elbow, a stress-related bone or ligament injury. Hitting can lead to abdominal muscle tears, back injuries, or rib stress fractures.

To prevent softball and baseball injuries: Upper body strengthening should be done three times weekly, including wrist, elbow, and shoulder muscles. Stretching of the hips, thighs, and legs should be done before and after play. Core strengthening helps prevent hitting injuries. Balance and agility drills should be done to prevent ankle and knee injuries. Proper technique in catching, hitting, throwing, and sliding is essential to prevent traumatic and overuse injuries. Pitchers should be rotated and allowed to rest some games to avoid overuse injuries.

Swimming

Swimmer's shoulder is the most frequently occurring overuse injury with components of impingement, tendinitis, bursitis, and instability. Breast-strokers can develop knee pain, including patellofemoral pain and MCL strains and sprains. Butterfly kicking can lead to back pain and spondylolis-thesis. Finger jams can occasionally occur from striking lane lines or other swimmers. A frequent medical problem is swimmer's ear. Exercise-induced asthma can be irritated by the chemicals used in pool maintenance. The heavy training schedule and focus on body shape contributes to eating disorders. A relatively safe sport with no real risk of trauma, overall body injuries from improper cross-training occur almost as frequently as those due to overuse injuries in swimming.

To prevent swimming injuries: Rotator cuff strengthening is the number one recommended exercise and should be done at least three times weekly. Overstretching of the shoulders should be avoided, as swimmers are already prone to loose shoulder joints. For breaststrokers with knee pain, patellofemoral exercises should be done three times weekly. Abdominal and core strengthening is also important, especially in long-distance swimmers and stroke swimmers. Other swimming injuries have been attributed to nontraditional cross-training exercise. Overuse injuries are the most common, and rest is essential at least one day a week. Older swimmers should cross-train with land weight-bearing exercise to prevent osteoporosis. Swimmers should also perform balance exercises, as this is a common deficit in swimmers.

Tennis

Overuse injuries of the wrist, shoulders, spine, legs, and feet, along with acute injuries, are common in tennis due to the quick, multidirectional, explosive nature of the sport. Tennis elbow (outer elbow pain) is the most widely known due to improper racket grip, tension, and poor technique. Other types of shoulder, wrist, and elbow tendinitis are also quite common. Core muscle sprains and tears can occur, along with back pain due to lumbar sprain, sacroilliitis, and disc problems. Tennis leg, calf muscle tears, Achilles tendinitis, and plantar fasciitis is also quite common. Ankle sprains occur frequently. Turf toe and tennis toe can also occur.

To prevent tennis injuries: Shoulder and wrist strengthening should be done three times weekly in the frequent tennis player. Calf and leg stretching after a short warmup is recommended before play. Balance drills prevent ankle sprains; core strengthening prevents abdominal muscle and back injuries. Equipment should also be appropriate; shoes should provide adequate cushioning and multidirectional support. Racket grip and string tension should be appropriate, partic-

ularly in players prone to tennis elbow. Correct technique and form, including hitting the ball in front of the body and minimizing wrist use, will prevent overuse injuries in the arm and shoulder.

Triathlon

Races combining swimming, biking, and running require many hours of training and result in overuse injuries associated with each sport, along with the traumatic injuries associated with biking. Specific to triathlons, the combination of open water swimming and cycling can cause chronic neck and shoulder pain, including nerve and muscle impingements. Running injuries are common and include plantar fasciitis and iliotibial band syndrome. Patellofemoral pain can develop due to running and cycling at intense levels. Eating disorders can be common, along with dehydration, anemia, and low sodium levels, secondary to the endurance nature of training and events.

To prevent triathlon injuries: Rest and flexibility is crucial. For ultra and endurance events, it is better to be slightly undertrained than overtrained, to reduce the incidence of chronic, overuse injuries. Event training should be seasonal, with at least a few months off a year to allow the body to heal and rest. The triathlete should rest at least one day a week and eat enough calories with slightly higher protein, iron, and B vitamins due to heavy endurance training. Calcium and dietary fat should be adequate to protect bones. Triathletes must also drink plentiful amounts of fluids, including electrolytes throughout training and throughout the day to replace what is lost. Proper equipment, cycle positioning, and frequent replacement of running shoes with proper support is essential. Thorough stretching two to three times weekly is important to prevent limited motion and pain.

Volleyball

Jumping, overhead motions, and the contact nature of volleyball leads to a variety of injuries, the most common of which is ankle sprain, followed by knee and finger injuries, including dislocations, jams, and fractures. Wrist sprains and tendon tears, along with shoulder overuse syndromes, including rotator cuff tendinitis, impingement, sprains, and chronic impingement as well as lower spine injuries are common. Knee injuries have been well studied and include ACL tears, patellar tendinitis (jumper's knee), and patellofemoral pain. Stress fractures can also occur in the lower leg.

To prevent volleyball injuries: Flexibility, core strength, and balance is crucial. Hamstring and quadriceps strength along with jumping and landing skills should be worked on three times weekly. Shoulder and rotator cuff strength should also be a focus of conditioning. Proper ball strike technique should be established to reduce stress on the wrists and hands and prevent finger injuries.

Waterskiing

Hamstring, quadriceps, and knee strains or tears can occur. Ligament tears can occur secondary to rotational injuries and jumps, which can also cause fractures and ankle injuries. Neck, middle, and low back injuries can occur both as overuse and acute injuries. Forearm, wrist, and hand injuries can occur, including tendinitis, tears, and chronic sprains. Traumatic injuries occur from impact with the water (or objects) and include shoulder dislocations, rib fractures, ruptured eardrums, and head injury.

To prevent waterskiing injuries: Proper technique, equipment, and a safe and experienced boat driver is essential. Posture and foot and arm alignment can prevent strains and muscle pulls. The use of gloves allows for more effective grip. Flotation vests or bright-colored wet suits are essential to identify a skier after a fall. Conditioning exercises should include the upper body, especially wrist and shoulder strengthening. Weight-bearing aerobic exercises should be done three times weekly to maintain bone strength.

Weight Lifting

Injuries occur due to lifting either too much weight, too frequent training, or poor technique. Injuries include neck and back sprains, disc herniations, shoulder sprains, and tendinitis, including AC joint sprains, rotator cuff injuries, pectoralis rupture and instability, lateral epicondylitis, flexor carpi radialis and DeQuervain's tendinitis, and knee sprains, including patellofemoral and meniscal pain and patellar tendinitis. The tendency for these athletes to use muscle-building supplements and performance-enhancers can cause permanent internal problems in liver, kidneys, and with fertility. Bodybuilders are at a high risk of eating disorders due to restrictive diets.

To prevent weight lifting injuries: Do not increase weight too rapidly. Rest is important, and similar muscle groups should not be strength trained two days in a row. Quick, thrusting, and twisting motions can lead to injury, so pace should be slow and comfortable. Technique is equally important to prevent injuries; weights should not be lifted behind the plane of the body to protect the shoulders from injury. Alignment of arms and wrists should be straight, and alignment and direction of weight movement should be straight and controlled. Squats, lunges, and dead lifts should also be controlled and in proper form. In women with knee problems, squats and lunges should be avoided. In women with back problems, dead lifts and loaded squats should be avoided.

Windsurfing

Back pain and injury can be common due to poor positioning, carrying, and lifting equipment, along with uphauling. Shoulder dislocations occur from falls, along with foot sprains and fractures if feet are strapped in. Cuts, bruises, and head injuries can occur from falls on the fin, mast, boon, or rocks or corals.

To prevent windsurfing injuries: Proper technique of foot placement, balance, and sail maneuvering and knowledge of wind and currents is essential to preventing serious problems. Headgear is available and should be worn while surfing in rocky areas. General strengthening, especially to the back, abdominal muscles, and shoulders, should be done three times weekly. Stretching and balance exercises should also be done three times weekly, along with weight-bearing aerobic activity.

Yoga

Injuries from yoga are most frequently overuse injuries or from pushing a position beyond comfort. Postures held in unbalanced positions or beyond fatigue can stress and injure the ligaments, tendons, and joints of the knees, wrists, spine, and shoulders. Hamstring and inner thigh sprains and occasionally tears can be common. When movements are quick, as in a few types of yoga classes, it is possible to suffer knee, wrist, or back sprains. Shoulder injuries can occur from inversions or postures where the hands are behind the head and trunk.

To prevent yoga injuries: Make sure you feel balanced, you have drunk enough fluids, and you feel strong enough to hold postures. If your muscles are trembling and you are uncomfortable with a maneuver, perform a modified posture. Yoga classes involving quick movements and highly heated rooms (Bikram) can be dangerous to an unconditioned person. Bikram should never be done if pregnant, and water should be drunk every 15 minutes to prevent dehydration in these classes. Do not push a position through pain; instead, release the pressure and stretch a painful area.

————

Many sports-related injuries can be avoided with proper conditioning, including strengthening and stretching muscles most frequently used. Rest is an essential component to avoiding overuse injuries, which can become chronic and lead to other problems. Proper skills and technique decreases risks of injuries, and you should not play above your skill level to avoid serious injuries. Equipment should fit well and be appropriate to the sport. Listening to your body signals, resting when you feel fatigued or pain, and maintaining overall strength and balance is key to enjoyment and success in your sport.

CHAPTER SEVENTEEN

Achieving Maximum Health and Fitness

One of the greatest goals for every girl and woman is to achieve maximum health and fitness. This includes doing the best you can to optimize strength, flexibility, mental and physical well-being, and prevent illness and injury. The levels at which these goals are achieved are slightly different for everyone, but strategies and techniques are similar. Maximizing fitness in an athlete results in faster performance with less fatigue and pain and greater strength and endurance. Maximum health allows maximum fitness, as there are fewer illnesses and injury and fewer limits to training and performance activity.

As we all become more knowledgeable from research and experience, we improve our likelihood of being free of illness and injury. This allows us to exercise daily and embrace competitions and life events as welcome challenges. Strategies include a proactive and preventive approach to decrease risks of problems. Reducing our health and injury risks by even a small amount can make a significant impact on maximizing health.

Strength Training

S trength training is done to increase muscle size and strength, improve endurance, and decrease fatigue, ultimately increasing performance. It also improves body image and appearance and prevents muscle, ligament, and bone injury. Health benefits of strength training include improved posture, improved lung capacity, decreased injuries, improved circulation, improved muscle tone, and less risk of obesity.

Fitness and Health Benefits of Strength Training

FITNESS BENEFITS	HEALTH BENEFITS
Increased muscle size	Improves posture
Increased muscle strength	Improves lung capacity
Increased endurance	Decreases injuries
Prevents muscle injury	Improves circulation
Prevents ligament injury	Improves muscle tone
Prevents bone injury	Prevents osteoporosis
Prevents fatigue	Lowers diabetes risk Prevents obesity

The recommended amount of strength training is 20 to 30 minutes, 2 to 3 times per week for most athletes and active women. For those involved in power and strength-dependent sports, strength training may occur five days a week as part of training, but muscles should be alternated day to day to allow recovery. The heavier the weights and quicker the movements, the greater the risk of injury.

Personal training is a very popular method of strength training. Trainers should be well qualified to design a program for you, listen to your needs and accommodate for the way your body performs, and guide you through a safe exercise program. It is recommended that you have a trainer who is certified, although there are different qualities and requirements for certification. The highest recommended certification types are through the American College of Sports Medicine (ACSM), National Strength and Conditioning Association (NSCA), American Council on Exercise (ACE), and National Council of Strength and Fitness (NCSF). These require testing and updated continuing-education credits. Health-care professionals can also make excellent personal trainers, including certified athletic trainers, physical therapists, exercise physiologists, and physical therapy assistants.

Qualities of a Good Personal Trainer

Certification or degree in exercise

Listens to your needs

Gives you full attention during workouts

Does not encourage painful activities

Works you at your level, not above it to impress you

Any muscle soreness after a strenuous workout should last no more than two days

Is motivating

You do not develop new or worsening pains

Workouts make you feel stronger and healthier

Also be aware of the importance of equipment used for strength training. The safest way to strength train is with correctly used free weights and your own body weight as resistance; done properly, this can be very effective and challenging. Exercise machines often make strength training simple; however, they are not for everyone. Because equipments and machines are designed mostly for men; small women might not fit in certain machines. Using a machine that is too big for you can result in injury as you stretch to try to reach the equipment. As you increase weight, do so only very gradually, no more than 10 percent each week. If you are feeling too much stress on your body with an increase to the next available level of weights, decrease the number of repetitions for the next few weeks. To avoid injuries while strength training, stop if you have pain. If the pain continues after you have stopped the exercise, apply ice to the area, take the next day off, and see a doctor if it does not get better. If the pain goes away, decrease the repetitions, weight, or range of motion as you begin the exercise again. Pain that returns every time you do the same exercise is a sign that you are doing something wrong.

Techniques to Avoid Injury While Strength Training

Gradually increase weight; no more than twice a month.

Keep motions slow and resistance low.

Stop the motion if you feel pain.

Do not train the same muscles two days in a row.

Keep your range of motion in a comfortable zone for your body.

If your muscle soreness lasts longer than two days, reduce the amount of weight and repetitions.

Stretching

Stretching is an essential component of many women's fitness and lifestyle regimes. Stretching is done to increase and maintain motion at the joints. It is rarely harmful, unless it is done in quick, ballistic motions. It should be a part of every woman's health maintenance and injury prevention program, as it reverses abnormal postures required in sports and in life activities that can cause pain and lead to tightness, weakness, and injury.

Maintaining normal motion prevents stiffness and subsequent weakness. In sports, full motion is necessary to achieve maximum power for most activities. There have been many studies done to evaluate the effects of stretching on preventing injuries, with some mixed results. Recent studies have suggested that stretching is not necessary immediately before competition; one study suggested that stretching before a speed event can actually slow you down, because muscles and ligaments may lose their "spring." Another study showed that the number of acute injuries (such as tears) sustained during athletic activities are similar whether stretching was done first or not. In regards to preventing pain and overuse injuries such as bursitis and tendinitis, however, stretching studies show positive effects. Stretching also has been found to increase strength gained during weight training.

Regular stretching after exercise will reduce muscle and ligament pain and soreness. Decreasing pain is essential to maintaining muscle and bone health, because pain is a sign of injury or weakness. Pain thereby limits full participation in training and performance. Stretching decreases the muscle spasms and tightness the body can develop after a hard workout. These spasms and tightness, if not reversed, can lead to weakness and decreased range of motion with ultimately poorer performance. Maintaining your full range of motion in muscles and joints allows the joint to function as it is designed without restrictions; this is crucial to sports that require large, powerful movements, including golf, softball, tennis, volleyball, and basketball.

Stretching is also an essential component of recovery from injury. The shoulder and knee joints are especially vulnerable to decreased motion after injury. Not using or moving the joint secondary to pain, swelling, or weakness can lead to a stiff, dysfunctional joint that is painful to move and difficult to recover from. This can reach a point of such tightness that the muscles become weak, causing a vicious cycle of pain, weakness, and limited motion, which can lead to further pain or overuse injuries in nearby or opposite joints as they try to make up for lost movement and strength.

Stretching the major muscle groups for at least 10 minutes a day, especially after exercise, is recommended for everyone. If you have an area that has been injured or is aching, more focused stretching to this area will prevent further pain, weakness, or injury. Effective stretching is done slowly. Breathing should be relaxed, and you should feel comfortable. Movements should be held with a gentle pull without pain. Stretching has its greatest benefit after working out, when the muscles and tendons are warm and more flexible.

Yoga is an excellent form of stretching, as it encourages maximum joint and muscle movement while also strengthening muscles as the positions are held. Yoga is generally very safe, although occasionally certain postures or styles of yoga (such as Kundalini, which includes quick, ballistic movements) can be too aggressive.

Benefits of Stretching After Exercise

Decreases pain and soreness

Decreases risk of overuse injuries

Allows full strength throughout the full joint movement

Increases flexibility and motion

Increases performance

Improves posture

Preventing Injuries

Injuries can be prevented. Overuse injuries that are addressed and treated early are less likely to turn into chronic injuries. Accidental injuries or severe, focal injuries can also lead to chronic, recurrent pain patterns. All injuries cause pain and limited motion and function in the injured area. If an injury lasts longer than one week, it can lead to other weaknesses and injuries, turning into a more complex problem. Icing an injured or painful area immediately after it occurs and for the next several days decreases inflammation and can prevent some injuries from causing problems with sports participation. Heat is not as beneficial because it can increase swelling.

PERFORMANCE TIP **When in doubt, after injury, or when in pain always apply ice.**

Many athletes feel that they have one weak side, often from one or several old injuries that were never properly strengthened after recovery. This weak side can continue to be vulnerable to injuries if it is not protected and strengthened with exercise and stretching. Injuries can also cause pain or trouble elsewhere, including joints and muscles not related to the injured area, or on the opposite side as these areas do more work to compensate. Common examples of this include the use of crutches, causing arm and wrist pain along with underarm skin irritation; limping can lead to back, hip, or knee pain, especially on the opposite side as it is taking most of the weight; neck injury leading to back pain, as that tends to become the site of more rotation and movement; and back pain contributing to knee pain as bending is avoided and squats stress knees more.

Injury Prevention Techniques

Seek medical care for pain or injury early in its development.

Use proper-fitting and working equipment.

Strengthen and stretch weak and overworked areas.

Stop the exercise if there is pain.

Ice the area for 10 to 15 minutes.

When an injury requires surgery, there can be complications. These can include infection requiring antibiotics, which can cause stomach problems and yeast infections. Surgery can also result in scar tissue, which can further lead to limited motion and pain. If there is trouble with healing from surgery, injury treatment might have to start over from the beginning.

If the injury is a bone fracture, this often takes you out of exercise for weeks to even months. Basic motion can be a challenge after a cast is removed, and muscles need a lot of time to regain their strength. In older women or women with other health problems, the complications of fracture can become more serious, including pneumonia, bleeding, and overall decreased stamina. This leaves a woman vulnerable to other medical problems as well, especially if a hospital stay is required.

The mental effects associated with injury can be very problematic. Decreased activity can lead to depression. Pain may interfere with sleep or enjoyment. Pain medications can be sedating and depressing. Fear of weight gain may cause anxiety. While these negative emotions are usually temporary, they can be difficult to manage.

Injury prevention education, such as jumping and landing training and sliding, falling, and rolling drills reduce risk of injury and should be included in practice, training and rehabilitation. Programs incorporating such training has been shown to reduce knee injury incidence in high school soccer and basketball players. Similarly, training workshops to teach techniques to avoid injury in skiing have been found to reduce knee injuries. Implementing safety regulations and modifying equipment, clothing, and rules in sports has been proven to reduce injuries. Examples include secure goalposts, breakaway bases, helmets, streamlined clothing, and releasable ski bindings. Fingernail extensions as well as jewelry should not be worn during athletic activity, as these can lead to finger, nail, and skin injuries.

Sports conditioning programs should focus on strengthening and stretching the muscles and joints most commonly used to improve performance and prevent injuries (see chapter 16, "Sports-Specific Injuries"). Making coaches, trainers, instructors, and athletes more aware of the risks and severity of certain injuries will help better establish protocols to reduce injury risk. Being aware that minor injuries, fatigue, poor nutrition, and poor fluid intake can increase injury risk will promote healthier behaviors. Making athletes better skilled in the best way to perform with least illness and injury is the greatest goal. Remembering that minor injuries can progress to major problems or lead to other injuries will hopefully encourage athletes to seek care earlier rather than later.

Because few sports condition the entire body, maintaining a conditioning program that incorporates all aspects of musculoskeletal health, including postural strengthening and correction, along with bone strength, flexibility, and balance is highly recommended. This also allows easier transition to other sports later on. Maintaining a well-rounded, fit musculoskeletal system is always beneficial in the long run.

Preventing Heart and Blood Vessel Problems

Cardiovascular disease is the term used to describe problems involving the heart (cardio) or blood vessels (vascular). The most devastating complications of cardiovascular disease are stroke and heart attack; these can often be fatal. In fact, cardiovascular disease is the number one cause of death overall in the United States; the statistics that one in five Americans has cardiovascular disease includes women.

Active, exercising women already have lowered their risk of cardiovascular disease, as exercise affords the best heart protection. The recommendation by the American Heart Association is 30 minutes of moderate to intense physical activity 5 days a week. Aerobic exercise, which raises heart rate and uses up oxygen, improves cholesterol levels and maintains the peak functioning efficiency of heart and blood vessels. It also trains the cells to carry oxygen more efficiently and improves the rate of oxygen uptake in breathing.

High blood pressure is a precursor to heart and blood vessel disease. Blood pressure is necessary to promote exchange of nutrients from the blood into the capillaries and into the body. If there are problems such as hardened arteries, slow or inefficient heart functioning, or increased body demands due to poorly trained muscles, blood pressure rises. Because regular exercisers do not usually have these problems, blood pressure remains low. This reduces the occurrence of bad side effects of blood pressure such as heart attack and stroke. Studies have recently shown that regular exercise of moderate intensity for one hour five days a week is as effective as medication in managing high blood pressure.

The unmodifiable factors that can also increase your risk of cardiovascular disease are family history of stroke or heart attack, especially in family members under the age of 50; high cholesterol or triglycerides; and diabetes. Modifiable factors include smoking, obesity, and inactivity. Less clear but risky lifestyle behaviors are high stress and poor diet (high sugar and saturated fat/high cholesterol/low fiber). If you have any of these increased risks, you should see your doctor to discuss prevention methods in addition to exercise. These may include an aspirin a day, a low-cholesterol, unsaturated fat, high-fiber diet, and medications.

Factors That Increase Risk of Cardiovascular Disease

High LDL cholesterol	Obesity
High triglycerides	Inactivity
Diabetes	Stress
Family history	Poor diet
Smoking	Older age

Because women who have been through menopause are at an increased risk of heart disease and stroke, and women taking oral contraceptives or hormone replacement can be at an increased risk of stroke and blood clots, if you are in these categories and have the risk factors mentioned above, consult with your doctor for the best prevention strategies. Other heart-protective dietary behaviors can include a high-fiber, low glycemic index diet, increasing amount of omega-3 fatty acids, adding soy products, and having (only) one alcoholic drink per day.

Health Benefits of Aerobic Exercise

Prevents heart disease	Decreases osteoporosis risk
Lowers blood pressure	Reduces depression
Reduces strokes	Reduces cancer
Prevents obesity	Reduces stress
Prevents diabetes	Improves sleep
Reduces cholesterol	

Preventing Illness and Disease

Without question, the most important positive action you can take to prevent illness and disease is exercise. Exercise prevents a long list of diseases that can cause chronic or severe illness, disability, and even death, including cancer, heart disease, stroke, high blood pressure, vascular disease, diabetes, obesity, and osteoporosis. Exercise also prevents mental health illness and disease disorders, including depression, anxiety, and stress. While some of these disease processes can be reversed with exercise and healthy lifestyle, some cannot. Preventing them from starting is the number one goal.

Not Smoking

The most negative lifestyle behavior is smoking. Smoking contributes to the development of almost all diseases, notably cancer, heart disease, high blood pressure, high cholesterol, diabetes, and asthma. Smoking has the following negative health effects: lowers immunity, making you more likely to get bronchitis, colds, and other infections; interferes with breathing by causing wheezing and asthma; causes snoring and sleep apnea; impairs fine motor skills, leaving you shaky and unable to control your hands. Athletes who smoke have decreased endurance and are more likely to suffer from exercise-induced asthma.

If you quit smoking before the diseases becomes chronic, you can reverse most of the effects smoking has on the body—breathing, snoring, immunity, and risk of cancer, heart disease, and high blood pressure all improves. Problems exist, however, if smoking has done permanent damage. Severe smoking-related diseases, including cancer, emphysema, and coronary artery disease, are permanent.

HEALTH TIP **The best thing you can do for your body is exercise; the worst is smoke.**

See Your Doctor

Because doctors and health professionals are trained to recognize, treat, and prevent illness, following their advice is recommended. Each person has different risks of diseases based on genetics and other health history; therefore health recommendations can be slightly different for each individual.

Still, following the basic recommendations outlined below will reduce your risk of severe diseases.

Recommended Medical Testing and Check-Ups

Yearly check-up (every other year if no health risks)

Yearly dental exam

Monthly breast self-exams

Yearly Pap smear/OBGYN visit after the age of 18 or when sexual activity begins

Mammogram initially by age 40; high risk by age 35

Colonoscopy initially by age 40; high risk by age 35

EKG as recommended by your primary physician

Disease Prevention Through Nutrition

The health benefits and risks of foods has been and will always be a source of excitement, controversy, and research. Although it might seem that dietary recommendations change frequently, the consistent findings are that getting adequate sources of vitamins, minerals, and antioxidants through foods are the best way to stay healthy. Eating a diet rich in fruits and vegetables, and moderate in everything else, has been consistently found to be most beneficial. A general rule is that the darker the color of the fruit or vegetable, the more nutritional value it has. Cancer-fighting chemical groups include phytochemicals and antioxidants. Some of the most beneficial foods, according to recent research include the following:

- *Tomatoes*—Tomatoes and tomato products contain vitamin C and lycopenes, antioxidant cancer-fighting chemicals that reduce digestive tract (and for men, prostate) and other types of cancer.

- *Broccoli*—Broccoli contains phytochemicals that are thought to make cancer cells less toxic (destructive). Also contains beta-carotene, vitamin C, calcium, and fiber.

- *Spinach*—Spinach is rich in folate, fiber, and iron—nutrients needed especially in women. Other similar beneficial vegetables include kale, Swiss chard, and collard greens.

- *Tea*—Tea contains phytochemicals, which are cancer-cell fighters. Green tea has been associated with a lower risk of stomach, esophageal, and liver cancers.

- *Nuts*—Monounsaturated and polyunsaturated fats in nuts improve levels of cholesterol by lowering triglycerides and LDL along with raising HDL, preventing heart disease and stroke. Nuts also contain fiber and Vitamin E, both of which prevent heart disease and cancer.

- *Oats*—Beta-glucan is the fiber in oats that helps eliminate cholesterol from the intestines before it gets absorbed and lowers blood pressure. Oats also contain vitamin E and antioxidants.

- *Fish*—Fish, especially salmon, herring, anchovies, and sardines, contain omega-3s, the magic fatty acids that prevent clumping of the blood platelets, preventing heart disease, hypertension, and stroke. They also reduce triglycerides and LDLs, bad cholesterol. Additionally, omega-3s have been suggested to protect the brain cells from diseases of aging, prevent autoimmune diseases like lupus and rheumatoid arthritis, and lessen depression and menstrual cramps.

- *Garlic*—Allyl sulfides and phytochemicals in garlic protect the heart, reduce cholesterol, and prevent blood from clotting (a big reason for heart attacks and strokes).

- *Blueberries and other berries*—Blueberries are noted to have the highest amount of antioxidants, including phytochemicals, which work against the free radicals that cause heart disease and cancer. Blueberries are also suggested to prevent memory loss and also prevent urinary tract infections in the same way cranberry juice does, by preventing bacteria from sticking to the bladder wall.

- *Wine and grape juice*—Red wine has its beneficial effects from the polyphenols in the skins of the grapes, which increase HDL and prevent hardening of the arteries. Wine also contains alcohol, which in moderation (one drink a day, for women) prevents heart disease and more serious outcomes of heart failure and heart disease. (Note: Alcohol can increase breast cancer risk and should be avoided in pregnancy.)

- *Soy*—Soy contains omega-3 fatty acids, which prevent heart disease and stroke. Soy also contains phytochemicals that prevent certain types of cancer. (Note: Soy should not be eaten in large amounts in women with certain types of breast cancer, and soy protein isolates at greater than 30 to 40 mg daily is not recommended.)

- *Water*—Drinking at least eight, 8-ounces glasses of water a day is recommended to prevent colon cancer, urinary tract infections, kidney stones, bladder cancer, constipation, obesity, and complications of dehydration. In active athletic women, more is often required.

Health Benefits of Proper Nutrition

BENEFIT	HOW	WHY
Provide fuel	Ultimately, all food is broken down into glucose, the energy source for all body cells.	You need fuel to function.
Lower cancer risk	Antioxidants combat free radicals, which are linked to cancer.	Studies suggest that women who eat a lot of fruits and vegetables have half the risk of cancer.
Prevent heart disease, stroke, hypertension	Antioxidants, fiber, and folate; omega-3 fatty acids	The healthiest foods for the heart are fruits, vegetables, fish, and nuts.
Cholesterol	Appropriate levels reduce risk of heart attack and stroke.	High-fiber, low-saturated fat and high monounsaturated and polyunsaturated fat foods lower cholesterol.
Diabetes prevention	Low glycemic index foods	Eating regular meals with minimal sugary foods can prevent adult-onset diabetes.
Vision	Fruits and vegetables can prevent macular degeneration and cataracts.	Fruits and vegetables can help prevent vision problems.
Healthy bones	Adequate calcium and vitamin D	Bone requires proper nutrients.
Maintain stable mood	Blood glucose supplies the brain.	Steady blood glucose levels steady mood.

General dietary recommendations include eating a high-fiber, medium to low glycemic index diet rich in fruits and vegetables and low-fat dairy sources. Choosing monounsaturated and polyunsaturated fats and avoiding saturated and trans-fats is the best way to naturally prevent heart disease, diabetes, obesity, cancer, and many other diseases (see chapter 3, "Nutritional Health").

Nutritional Supplements

Supplements are not only expensive; they can be dangerous. With the exception of calcium and a multivitamin, supplements are rarely needed or recommended. Taking handfuls of vitamins is not useful, and there is nothing "natural" about it. There are a few vitamins and minerals that, in an extra dose, can be helpful in certain situations; these should be discussed with your doctor (see chapter 3: "Nutritional Health").

Preventive Pills to Discuss with Your Doctor

Aspirin works as a blood thinner to prevent strokes and heart disease. Just one baby aspirin a day can reduce severity of heart attacks. Also, if you have high cholesterol (total over 240) and a family risk of heart disease or other risk factors, you should also be taking a cholesterol-lowering medication. The benefits of a multivitamin and calcium supplement are for girls and women of all ages.

Safe Preventive Pills

PILL	FOR WHO?	WHY?	COST	CAUTION
Multivitamin— one a day	Most everyone— those who do not have a perfect diet every day of the year	Provides essential nutrients of vitamins and minerals, preventing diseases and illness	$5/month	Check with your doctor if you take additional vitamin supplements to avoid overdoses
Calcium—600 to 1,200 mg daily	Most girls and women—those who do not eat at least four servings of calcium-rich foods daily	Provides bone building nutrient, prevents muscle cramps, and can help with PMS	$10/month	Calcium should be taken in divided doses with meals
Aspirin— one regular or baby aspirin daily	Women past menopause with risk of heart disease	Thins blood and prevents heart disease and stroke	$3/month	Take with food; check with your doctor if you are not sure

In some people with knee osteoarthritis, glucosamine chondroitin can reduce pain, stiffness, swelling, and maintain functional joint movement. You might need to take glucosamine chondroitin for up to two months to have an effect; then take it once daily. If you do not notice a difference in joint stiffness or pain after three to four months, stop taking it. Glucosamine chondroitin can sometimes raise cholesterol levels; have your cholesterol checked within the first six months of taking the supplement. This supplement should not be taken in people with allergies to shellfish, diabetics, or people who take several medications or have medical problems.

Weight Maintenance

Being both under- and overweight can cause health problems. Although most chronic disease processes are related to obesity, the health risks to women who are underweight cannot be ignored. Both extremes can be life-threatening. Staying active and eating a well-balanced diet with lots of fruits and vegetables, healthy protein sources, healthy fats, and healthy carbohydrates with one single serving "treat" per day should allow you to avoid weight problems. Avoiding fad diets is crucial to maintaining a healthy weight. Fad diets are not only unhealthy, they also slow your metabolism, making it more likely you will regain lost weight after the diet is over. Diet pills are dangerous and addictive and can lead to heart and kidney failure.

Obesity both causes diseases and makes underlying diseases worse. It increases risk of diabetes, heart disease, stroke, and poor blood flow. It also places unnecessary stress on joints. Those who are overweight have much higher rates of knee and hip arthritis. Being severely underweight is also unhealthy, as this can result in osteoporosis, malnutrition, and in certain cases, heart problems.

Stress Management and Relaxation

Not only do stress management and relaxation allow for better training and athletic performance, they help prevent illness and injury, and most important, allow for a happy and fulfilling life. Stress that is out of control makes pain worse, interferes with mental clarity and mood, and causes numerous health problems, especially digestive and heart problems, along with high blood pressure. This takes a large toll on your body, leading to chronic fatigue and depression. Your body can react by tensing muscles in your head, neck, and back, causing pain and poor posture.

Beware of chest pain, shortness of breath, or abdominal symptoms, which can be both signs of stress or signs of illness. If any of these interfere with activities or sleep, or are accompanied by chest pressure or heaviness, see a doctor immediately. Talk about unusual body symptoms with your doctor or health-care provider, or if you can identify stress as the cause, schedule healing sessions into your day—massage, yoga, deep breathing, stretching, or a warm bath. Take deep breaths when you feel tense. Close your eyes and remind yourself that you are in control of your feelings and reactions. Relaxation and stress management are essential components of your health and wellness. Whatever can be done to decrease stress will have a long-lasting, positive effect on many body systems (see chapter 2, "Stress and Sports Psychology Techniques").

Relaxation is the number one way to decrease stress at any minute. There are many types of relaxation techniques to enhance performance, sleep, and overall health, and ultimately, to decrease stress. Just as the body needs rest to repair itself, so the brain needs to relax to allow it to function. Being able to relax is essential to any success. Fine motor skills, accuracy, agility, and coordination is optimal when the mind is relaxed and in control. Without being able to relax sleep is worse, muscles are tight and more prone to spasm and weakness, and nutrition tends to be poor. All this influences not only sports and athletic performance, but also health. Relaxation should be incorporated into every day. Common relaxation techniques are outlined on page 357.

Often, simply being aware that stress is the cause of these symptoms is enough to bring some relief. Allowing yourself between 7 and 8 hours of sleep a night helps significantly, as does allowing 30 minutes each day to indulge in a relaxation activity. Regular exercise is crucial to stress management, but also be aware that overtraining can also cause stress.

People who manage stress well are happier, healthier, and more productive, as they do not let the stress interfere with their activities. They also tend to be less overweight and suffer fewer chronic illnesses such as heart palpitations, thyroid dysfunction, chronic fatigue syndrome, fibromyalgia, painful arthritis, back and neck pain, bowel problems, and frozen shoulders. Lower levels of stress can also reduce allergies, immune diseases, and even cancer. Athletes who have less stress are more likely to be focused on tasks and less prone to accidents and injuries.

Relaxation Techniques

TECHNIQUE	DESCRIPTION	BEWARE OF	COST/ AVAILABILITY
Massage	Someone rubs and soothes your muscles, back, neck, and head	A masseuse who makes you uncomfortable	High cost, appointment usually needed
Meditation	Learning to put your mind in a focused but relaxed state	Distractions, feeling too pressured to meditate; this is not for everyone	Free, portable
Yoga	Spiritual deep breathing, stretching, and holding strengthening postures	Uncomfortable postures, pain with activity, pushing yourself too far	Medium cost; at-home tapes inexpensive; need small space and comfortable clothing although mini-yoga moves can be done anywhere
Deep breathing	Using mantras or counting to breathe in good and exhale bad thoughts or simply relax the body and mind rhythmically	Holding your breath too long, becoming light-headed	Free, portable
Conversation with a friend or understanding family member	Discussing what makes you stressed or simply being with someone who makes you feel at ease	Negative comments, questions	Free, can be done by phone anywhere
Visualization	Picturing a relaxing scene such as a beach	Letting other thoughts in that are not relaxing or stressful	Free, portable, effective
Water therapy	Floating, swimming, taking a bath	Uncomfortable temperatures	Inconvenient but can be inexpensive
A nap	A catnap is less than 30 minutes	Oversleeping can ruin your sleep schedule	Free, sometimes inconvenient
Watching a movie/ TV	Laughter or escape can be very relaxing	Stressful commercials, other people, subject change to stressful	Inexpensive, relatively easy
Hobbies	Cooking, painting, gardening, or whatever makes you feel relaxed	Getting too caught up in perfectionism	You should make this inexpensive and easy!
Spending time with a pet	Studies show petting an animal reduces blood pressure	A disagreeable animal	Pets are a time and financial commitment

Life Stages

Preadolescence

Before the age of 10, learning a new sport is pretty easy. Young girls can compete with boys and juggle many activities—the more activities, the better. This will prevent burnout in a sport and also allow for muscle, bone, and posture development that is well balanced. In particular, girls are encouraged to participate in sports or recreation that requires upper arm strength such as climbing and swimming. Activities that challenge balance, such as dance, skating, or court sports are also recommended. Mixing these activities will allow muscles to develop equally and make participation in all types of sports later in life easier and more enjoyable.

Adolescence

During adolescence, there are some challenges. There is a lot of peer pressure to be thin; this is when most girls try dieting. Adolescence is actually the worst time to diet, as young women are still growing and need nutrition to supply their developing body. Girls must be especially careful to eat a diet rich in calcium, at least 1,200 mg a day. This is the time bones are gaining their greatest strength for the rest of your life.

Balancing school, sports, and social life can be difficult. There can be peer pressure to try drugs, tobacco, and alcohol. Stress levels can be high. If you are feeling overwhelmed with your schedule, consider dropping an activity. If your friends are not supportive of your busy schedule, find new ones. It should be easy with all you are involved in. Try to maintain your baseline health as much as possible by eating three well-balanced meals a day with snacks, taking a multivitamin, and drinking at least eight cups of fluid (soda does not count!). Try to get seven to eight hours of sleep and incorporate seeing your friends into your life of school and athletic activity.

As an athlete, ease into a new sport or sport season. Stay conditioned during the off season, and rest if you feel sore or tired. Maintain overall body conditioning throughout the year. Take at least one day of rest from athletics a week. These strategies will prevent overuse injuries.

Young Adult

At this time of life, you are figuring out where sports fit. If you are a college or competitive athlete, you are spending much of your day training and doing sports. You should especially make sure you are eating well and continuing with calcium and a daily multivitamin. Dieting can be tempting, but keep perspective of your healthy weight and muscular athletic physique. You should be getting your period every month. If you are not, you might be over-training or not eating enough. Discuss this with your doctor.

Adult

Regular exercise is your greatest benefit. It keeps you physically and mentally healthy, controls your weight, makes your skin glow, and energizes you. It also strengthens you and allows you to participate in all activities without problems. Nutrition, as in all stages of life, is important. Weight is often a concern. Remember, the best way to be at your optimum weight is to avoid junk foods and sugary foods and eat well-balanced meals. Take a multivitamin and calcium supplement daily.

If you are a competitive or elite athlete, make sure you allow your body to rest at least one day a week. See a doctor if you have any pain or weakness that limits you for more than a few days. You should be getting your period every month. See your gynecologist every year and do your monthly breast self-exams.

Mature Adult

Maintaining bone strength, preserving cardiovascular health with aerobic activity, and maintaining flexibility and posture are important exercise-related goals for health at this stage of life. You want to avoid the hunched posture so common to older women, as this decreases your lung and breathing capacity, decreases height, reduces overhead shoulder motion, and causes shoulder, neck, back, and rib pain. To prevent these complications, you should be doing upper body strength training with an emphasis on upper back and shoulder muscles and stretches.

As you go through menopause, your symptoms of night sweats, hot flashes, irritability, and moodiness will be reduced by regular exercise. If you are taking hormone replacement, make sure you are on the lowest dose, and do not take them for more than five years. Alternative treatments for your menopause symptoms include black cohosh and soy products. (Do not take either of these if you have estrogen-dependent cancers.) Medications to treat mood are also very effective to help with menopausal symptoms.

Incontinence can be troublesome. There are strategies to decrease this problem, including Kegel exercises, medications, insertable devices, and surgery. Other body changes that can be a problem for active older women include a decrease in sweat gland function, which can be noticed by having less tolerance to exercise in hot temperature. Also, as you age, your maximum heart rate goes down, although this should not affect your activity level.

Age-Related Changes That Improve with Exercise	
Arthritis and stiff joints	Decreased flexibility
Incontinence	Decreased strength
Slower reflexes	Slower metabolism
Decreased balance	Decreased vision

Arthritis is one of the most frequent complaints of aging without known causes other than genetic predisposition, trauma, and wear and tear. Arthritis can decrease your balance, leading to muscle weakness and increased risk of falls. This becomes worse with joint and soft tissue stiffness that occurs as collagen becomes firmer and less stretchy. Conditioning exercises and stretches can prevent most of these changes from interfering with your lifestyle and activity level. Other tips to prevent arthritis from worsening include wearing well-cushioned shoes, having injuries evaluated and treated early to prevent weakness and loss of motion, and avoiding pushing through severe pain in the joints. If arthritis affects your hands, larger, more comfortable grips and vibration absorbing sports equipment can be very helpful.

Balance is an essential component of fitness, as good balance decreases falls and injuries such as sprained ankles. Balance becomes impaired over time due to muscle and joint stiffness and weakness, slower reflexes and nerve firing, and core weakness. Fortunately, balance can be improved with practice. Correcting vision trouble, making it easier to see little bumps in the road, can prevent accidents and injuries. Having good balance can help you right yourself in unstable situations and prevent falls. Therefore, you should work on your balance daily. Walking heel to toe and standing on one leg with your eyes closed are simple exercises that improve balance.

Ways to Improve Age-Related Problems That Affect Balance

PROBLEM	IMPROVEMENT
Stiffness of joints and muscles	Stretch daily
Weakness of muscles and bones	Strength train
Slower reflexes	Train reflexes with ball sports
Weakness of your core	Exercise and stretch on a stability ball
Vision problems	Have your vision evaluated and corrected
Nerve slowness	Nurture them with a B complex vitamin

Exercise is the best way to maintain your health and fitness throughout all stages of life. Learning a new sport or athletic activity challenges your body in new ways to increase its strength, nerve functioning, balance, and endurance. Regular daily activity keeps the heart and muscles strong. Sleep is improved, and metabolism is maintained to accommodate to a healthy appetite and prevent weight gain. Posture is maintained to prevent height loss, and bones are protected from osteoporosis. Be aware of your osteoporosis risk, know your bone density, and take your calcium.

Maintaining a healthy, athletic attitude allows for graceful transitions through more challenging activities. Regular exercise manages the stress that can occur later in life and keeps you in top form to prevent injuries and maintain strong immunity. Being socially involved in teams or sports stimulates your mind and elevates mood. These activities are the most effective ways to stay young.

With regards to exercise and aging, there are no restrictions. You should do what feels good. There are many older women who run marathons, climb mountain peaks, and downhill ski aggressively. Women in their 70s have completed Ironman triathlons, and women in their 80s have completed marathons.

Your Best Type of Workout

There are so many types of exercise available to girls and women, you should be able to find an exercise program that makes you feel great and brings you joy. If you are a competitive athlete, try to expand your fitness horizon off season by doing more recreational activities. When choosing your type of exercise, consider if you have any weaknesses or past injuries and make sure the new activity does not stress that area (see chapter 16, "Sports-Specific Injuries").

If you go to a gym, it should be a conveniently located place that makes you feel energized. Comfortable temperature should be maintained, equipment and changing rooms clean, and machines have enough variety that you can find the ones that are right for you. All gyms should also have free weights and stability balls, which are essential tools for injury prevention and recovery. Exercise classes should be enjoyable, with instructors who do not pressure you to do activities you do not feel comfortable with. Staff should be helpful and friendly.

Joining a sports team can be an important decision, especially as a young girl. Sports and athletic activities can define you and should build you up mentally and physically. You should be comfortable with your teammates and especially your coach. If the team is too competitive, or not competitive enough for you, consider changing teams. Participating in sports with other motivated, hard-working athletes will not only improve your performance, but also your enjoyment.

If you feel like your workout is getting boring or easy, try something new or change the intensity. (Do not do this two days in a row to prevent injury.) A good workout should leave you tired but energized. You might be a little sore, but you should not have pain. Sometimes even a small change, such as a new playing partner, new equipment, or new coach or trainer, can renew your enthusiasm and participation in an activity. Always remember how many sports and activities there are out there; if you feel you are not a "natural," get easily frustrated, or do not enjoy it, change! Reviewing your exercise and fitness goals each month will keep you on track.

Exercising properly with a program including strength training, aerobic conditioning, and flexibility is the best way to stay fit and healthy. You should know your risk of injuries and diseases and how to decrease them. Make sure you are going for regular check-ups and tests as recommended. Manage stress, and enjoy your workouts. Reevaluate your training goals periodically to make sure you are doing what is best for your health. Maximizing health and preventing illness and injury are paramount to happiness, health, and well-being.

Self-Empowerment

Self-empowerment is a feeling of being in control. This is a very important element of personal happiness and life fulfillment. In these modern times, women have no limits and are able to enjoy the freedom to be able to be self-empowered in any way they like. As a physically active female, you have established yourself as a strong, confident person. You feel no different from anyone else and know that you can perform under any circumstance. You have chosen a life of strength and activity, and your ability to multi-task, harness creativity, communicate, nurture effective social interactions, and use finesse over power make you amazingly efficient.

Sometimes there is a delicate balance of power over one's self—the need for maintaining healthy functioning must be preserved, as self-empowerment should not be confused with self-discipline. Discipline in moderate amounts is good; too much discipline can lead to extreme behaviors such as eating disorders and overuse injuries. The optimum healthy, active life is one that is challenging, exciting, and respectful of your body. Battling constant illness or injury is not beneficial to you.

The best recommendation is to remain physically and mentally fit to feel strong, confident, and happy with yourself. This way, you can get through anything. Being physically fit leads to being mentally fit. Having a strong body leads to a strong mind. Being healthy leads to being happy and allows you to help others to be strong, fit, healthy, and happy as well. These positive features result in a wonderful life. And remember, rest is a vital part of successful activity. Do not feel guilty if you are resting, if you did not work out as hard as you expected, or if you did not perform as you hoped. Focus on the positive successes—your incredible fitness, agility, flexibility, speed, strength. Use and flaunt these qualities. Share them with others. Inspire girls younger and women older. Embrace yourself; embrace your health; embrace your life!

RESOURCES

Chapter One

GENERAL HEALTH INFORMATION
Center for Health Information, OSU Medical, 614-293-3707,
www.WebMD.com
National Institute of Diabetes and Digestive and Kidney Diseases, www.niddk.nih.gov
American Association Complete Guide to Women's Health, Ramona I. Slupik, M.D.,
   Random House, 1996.

QUITTING SMOKING
American Lung Association, 1-800-LUNG-USA
www.quitnet.com
greatstartquitline, 866-66-START (quit-smoking hot line).
American Cancer Society, 1-800-ACS-2345, for state quitlines.

Chapter Two

Mind/Body Medical Institute, www.mindbody.harvard.edu
Peak Fitness for Women, Paula Newby Fraser, John M. Mora. Human Kinetics, 1995.
The Female Stress Survival Guide, Georgia Witkin, Newmarket Press, 2000.

Chapter Three

BOOKS ON NUTRITION
Nutrition and the Female Athlete, Jamie S. Ruud. CRC Press, 1996.
The American Dietetic Association Guide to Women's Nutrition for Healthy Living,
   Susan Finn, Janet Tougas. Perigee, 1997.
Strong Women Eat Well, Miriam E. Nelson. Perigee, 2001.
The Glucose Revolution, Jennie Brand-Miller, et al. Marlowe & Co., 2000.
Nancy Clark's Sports Nutrition Guidebook, Nancy Clark, Human Kinetics, 1996.

EVALUATING VITAMINS AND SUPPLEMENTS
www.fda.gov
www.ConsumerLab.com

HELPFUL WEBSITES ON NUTRITION
American Dietetic Association, 800-366-1655, www.eatright.org
National Institute of Health, www.nih.gov
U.S. Dept of Agriculture Food and Nutrition Information, www.usda.gov/cnpp
U.S. Government Department of Food Safety, www.Foodsafety.gov
Center for Food Safety and Applied Nutrition, www.cfsan.fda.gov (click on "Women's
   Health")
Environmental Protection Agency, epa.gov (water purity)
Center For Food Safety and Applied Nutrition, 1-888-SAFEFOOD

Chapter Four

HELP WITH EATING DISORDERS

Anorexia and Bulimia Treatment Center, 800-841-1515.

Harvard Eating Disorders Center, 617-236-7766, www.hedc.org

National Eating Disorders Association, 800-931-2237, www.nationaleatingdisorders.org

National Association of Anorexia Nervosa and Associated Disorders, 847-831-3438, www.anad.org

GENERAL DIET INFORMATION

National Institute of Health weight control information network, 877-946-4627, www.niddk.nih.gov,(click on weight control).

Diet Reviews and Information, www.chasefreedom.com

WEB-BASED HELP WITH DIETS

www.dietwatch.com

www.nutrio.com

www.Ivillage.com, diet and fitness page

www.cyberdiet.com

www.tops.org

BOOKS

The Athletic Woman's Survival Guide, Carol Otis, Human Kinetics, 2000.

The Bodywise Woman, Judy Mahle Lutter and Lynn Jaffee, Human Kinetics, 2000.

101 Ways to Help Your Daughter Love Her Body, Lane Richardson, Elaine Rehp, Harper Collins, 2001.

Eating Well for Optimum Health, Andrew Weil, Random House, 2000.

Teenage Fitness: Get Fit, Look Good and Feel Great, Kathy Kaehler, Harper Collins, 2001.

Chapter Five

BOOKS

Strong Women Stay Young, Miriam Nelson, Bantam Books, 2000.

Osteoporosis: How to Make Your Bones Last a Lifetime, Wanda Lyon and Cynthia Sulton

RESOURCES

National Osteoporosis Foundation, 202-223-2226, www.nof.org

National Bone Health Campaign, www.cdc.gov/powerfulbones

Powerful Bones, Powerful Girls: National Bone Health Campaign. Targeted for girls 9 to 12 and their parents.

Chapters Six Through Twelve

EQUIPMENT

888-556-7464, www.performbetter.com.

   Hand weights, stability balls, exercise mats, rock ankle boards, ankle weights, stretch cords.

OPTP: 888-819-012, 1 www.OPTP.com.

   Stability balls, exercise mats, rock ankle boards, stretch bands, glacier ice packs.

BRACES/SPLINTS/BACK SUPPORTS

1-800-803-2352, www.supportsusa.com

1-888-498-8587, www.painreliever.com

CHAPTER 6

Recommended book: *Treat Your Own Neck*, Robin McKenzie.

Tempur Pedic Brand (recommended) and other neck pillows available at:

877-COMFORT, www.healthyback.com

866-203-5023, www.cheaprelief.com

CHAPTER 9

The Balance Ball Workout, www.gaiam.com

Stretch strap: 888-819-0212, OPTP.com

Supportive ergonomic pillows, painreliever.com, 888-498-8587, www.OPTP.com, 888-819-0121.

Book: *The Core Program*, Peggy Brill, Bantam, 2001.

CHAPTER 10

SI belt: 888-819-0121, www.OPTP.com

Pelvic Pain and Low Back Pain, A Handbook for Self-Care and Treatment, Janet Hulme,

1-800-549-8371, www.phoenixpub.com

CHAPTER 11

Balance board, also called "rock board" or "wobble board:"

888-556-7464, www.performbetter.com

888-819-0121, www.OPTP.com

Cryocuff available at:

877-633-9464, www.buyaircast.com

1-800-390-1114, www.jointhealing.com

CHAPTER 12

Sports ankle braces, supportive inserts, heel cushions

800-803-2352, www.supportsUSA.com

888-498-8587, www.painreliever.com

CHAPTER THIRTEEN

American Physical Therapy Association Section on Women's Health: physical therapists trained in women's health issues and incontinence: 1-800-999-2782 x3230, www.womenshealthapta.org

Aquajogger, for in water training while recovering from injury: www.Performbetter.com

Sports bras in all sizes:

773-385-9557, www.x-chrom.com

972-475-8110, www.biggerbras.com

CHAPTER FOURTEEN

BOOKS ON SPORTS NUTRITION FOR WOMEN

Women's Sports Medicine and Rehabilitation, Nadya Swedan ("Sports Nutrition" chapter) ProEd Inc, 2001.

Women's Sports Nutrition, Edmund Burke, Keats Publishing, 1996.

Nutrition and the Female Athlete, Jamie S. Ruud, CRC Press, 1996.

WEBSITES

The Glycemic Institute, www.glycemic.com

Memorial Sloan Kettering Herb and Supplement Information: www.nskcc.org/aboutherbs

www.sportsmedicine.about.com (click on hydration and sports nutrition).
What you need to know about sports medicine and peak performance: www.ppon-line.co.uk (click on nutrition).

CHAPTER FIFTEEN
NUTRITION IN PREGNANCY
Center for Food Safety and Applied Nutrition, 888-SAFEFOOD
cfsan.fda.gov

SUPPORTIVE BRACES
Mommy and Me Brace, Maternity SI lock brace, 888-819-0121, www.OPTP.com
Prenatal Cradle, 1-800-383-3068, www.aboutbabiesinc.com
Mom-EZ full support brace, 435-752-9794, www.maternitystop.com
1-800-DRUGSTORE, www.drugstore.com

MATERNITY PILLOWS
Comfortchannel.com, 800-303-7574
Maternitystop.com, 435-752-9794

BOOKS
Essential Exercises for the Childbearing Years, Elizabeth Noble, New Life Images, 1995.
Exercising Through Your Pregnancy, James Clapp, M.D., Addicus Pub, 2002.
Expecting Fitness, Biritta Gallo, Renaissance Books, 1999.
Pilates Pregnancy, Mary Winsor, Perseus Publishing, 2001.
The Pregnancy Exercise Book, Judy DiFiori, Harper Information, 2000.
Pregnancy Fitness, *Fitness* magazine, Crown Publishing Group, 1999.
Yoga for Pregnancy, Francoise Barbita Friedman, Cassell PLC, 2003.
Yoga Mom, Buddha Baby, Jyothi Larson, Bantam Doubleday Dell, 2002.

WEBSITES
National Women's Health Information Center, www.4women.gov/pregnancy
www.ivillage.com
www.babycenter.com

HOT LINE FOR OB QUESTIONS
1-888-MODIMES

CHAPTER SIXTEEN
BOOKS OF INTEREST:
Boxing: The Complete Guide to Training and Fitness, Danna Scott, Perigee, 2000.
Complete Conditioning for the Female Athlete: A Guide for Coaches and Athletes, O'Connor, Fasting, Dahm, Wells. Wish Publishing, 2001.
Golf Is a Woman's Game, Jane Horn, Adams Media, 1997.
Five-Star Girls' Basketball Drills, edited by Stephanie V. Gaitley. Wish Publishing, 2000.
Women Ski, C. Carbone. World Leisure Corporation, 1996.

CHAPTER SEVENTEEN
The Change Before the Change, Laura Corio, M.D. Bantam, 2000.
The Wisdom of Menopause, Christiane Northrup. Bantam Doubleday Dell, 2001.

Index

Page numbers in *italic* indicate illustrations; those in **bold** indicate tables.

ABOUT THE AUTHOR

Nadya Gabriele Swedan, M.D. is a physiatrist and specialist in recovery from and prevention of injuries. In private practice with Manhattan Orthopedics and Sports Medicine, she is known for her expertise in women's health, pain syndromes, and athletic injuries. She is also the fitness doctor on the diet and fitness channel of ivillage.com and an advisor for the Women's Sports Foundation.

A graduate of Brown University, University of Cincinnati College of Medicine, and Northwestern University's Rehabilitation Institute of Chicago, Dr. Swedan lectures in both the academic and public arena on issues specific to women's fitness health, pain, and injury recovery and prevention. She has been quoted in numerous magazines including *Elle, Prevention, Fitness,* and *Self* and has appeared on nationally syndicated television. Her first book, *Women's Sports Medicine and Rehabilitation,* is a resource for doctors, therapists, and fitness professionals.

Her athletic history began in fourth grade, when she was an active member of a state-ranked AAU swim team, competed in state meets in junior high and high school, and also played on the varsity tennis team. College athletics was on the nationally ranked Brown women's varsity crew team. In medical school, she escaped competition and joined the fitness world as an aerobics instructor. Currently, she trains for and competes in local triathlons in the summer season; enjoys recreational golf, tennis, and downhill skiing with family and friends; and also keeps fit with step aerobics, yoga, and power walking through Manhattan. She is married to her athletic partner, Robert McIntyre, the best skier she knows. At time of publication, they eagerly await the birth of their first athlete!